HANDBOOK OF PSYCHOTHERAPY IN CANCER CARE

WATSON
KISSANE

HANDBOOK OF PSYCHOTHERAPY IN CANCER CARE

Maggie Watson
Consultant Clinical Psychologist, Psychological Medicine
The Royal Marsden NHS Foundation Trust, Sutton, Surrey
Honorary Senior Lecturer, Institute of Cancer Research
Honorary Professor, Research Department of Clinical
Educational and Health Psychology, University College London
London, UK

David W. Kissane
Jimmie C. Holland Chair, Attending Psychiatrist and Chairman
Department of Psychiatry and Behavioral Sciences
Memorial Sloan-Kettering Cancer Center, Professor of Psychiatry
Weill Medical College of Cornell University
New York, NY, USA

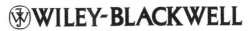

WILEY-BLACKWELL
A John Wiley & Sons, Ltd., Publication

Library of Congress Cataloguing-in-Publication Data

Kissane, David W. (David William)
  Handbook of psychotherapy in cancer care / David Kissane and Maggie Watson.
    p. ; cm.
  Includes bibliographical references.
  ISBN 978-0-470-66003-4 (pbk.) – ISBN 978-0-470-97516-9 (ePDF) – ISBN 978-0-470-97517-6 (Wiley Online Library) –
ISBN 978-1-119-99051-2 (ePub)
  1. Cancer–Psychological aspects. 2. Cancer–Treatment. 3. Psychotherapy. I. Watson, M. II. Title.
  [DNLM: 1. Neoplasms–psychology. 2. Psychotherapy–methods. QZ 200]
  RC271.P79K53 2011
  362.196′994–dc22

                                                                                    2011008396

A catalogue record for this book is available from the British Library.

This book is published in the following electronic formats:
ePDF: 978-0-470-97516-9; Wiley Online Library: 978-0-470-97517-6; ePub: 978-1-119-99051-2.

Set in 9.5/11.5pt Times by Laserwords Private Limited, Chennai, India.

First impression 2011

Contents

Section B: Group Models of Therapy   105

List of Contributors

Allison Applebaum
Research Fellow
Department of Psychiatry and Behavioral Sciences
Memorial Sloan-Kettering Cancer Center
1275 York Avenue
New York, NY 10021, USA

Lea Baider
Professor, Psycho-Oncology
Sharett Institute of Oncology
Hadassah University Hospital
Jerusalem 91120, Israel

Lodovico Balducci
Senior Member, Program Leader
Senior Adult Oncology Program
H. Lee Moffitt Cancer Center and Research Institute
12902 Magnolia Drive, Tampa, FL 33612, USA

Abraham S. Bartell
Assistant Attending Child Psychiatrist
Department of Psychiatry and Behavioral Sciences
and Department of Pediatrics
Memorial Sloan-Kettering Cancer Center
Assistant Professor of Psychiatry and Pediatrics
Weill Medical College of Cornell University
1275 York Avenue, New York, NY 10021, USA

Bo Snedker Boman
Consultant Clinical Psychologist
Department of Oncology and Hematology
Roskilde Hospital
7, Koegevej
DK4000 Roskilde, Denmark

William Breitbart
Attending Psychiatrist, Chief, Psychiatry Service, and
Vice-Chairman
Department of Psychiatry and Behavioral Sciences
Memorial Sloan-Kettering Cancer Center
Professor of Clinical Psychiatry
Weill Medical College of Cornell University
1275 York Avenue
New York, NY 10021, USA

Jack E. Burkhalter
Assistant Attending Psychologist
Department of Psychiatry and Behavioral Sciences
Memorial Sloan-Kettering Cancer Center
1275 York Avenue
New York, NY 10021, USA

Harvey Max Chochinov
Canada Research Chair in Palliative Care
Director Manitoba Palliative Care Research Unit
Cancer Care Manitoba
Distinguished Professor, Department of Psychiatry
University of Manitoba
3017 - 675 McDermot Avenue
Winnipeg, Manitoba, R3E 0V9, Canada

Catherine C. Classen
Associate Professor
Department of Psychiatry
Women's College Hospital
University of Toronto
76 Grenville St., 9th floor
Toronto, ON, M5S 1B2, Canada

Mary Jane Esplen
Professor, Department of Psychiatry
Faculty of Medicine
University of Toronto
Director, de Souza Institute
Head, Program of Psychosocial and Psychotherapy
Research in Cancer Genetics
University Health Network
200 Elizabeth Street, 9-EN-242a
Toronto, ON, M5G 2C4, Canada

Fawzy I. Fawzy
Professor, Department of Psychiatry and
Biobehavioral Sciences
David Geffen School of Medicine at the University of
California, UCLA Neuropsychiatric Institute
760 Westwood Plaza at University of California
Los Angeles, CA 90024-1759, USA

Nancy W. Fawzy
Assistant Clinical Professor
School of Nursing at the University of California
Los Angeles, CA 90095-001, USA

Luigi Grassi
Professor of Psychiatry, Section of Psychiatry
Department of Medical Science of Communication
and Behavior
University of Ferrara
Corso Giovecca 203, 44100 Ferrara, Italy

Jimmie C Holland
Wayne Chapman Chair of Psychiatric Oncology
Attending Psychiatrist
Department of Psychiatry and Behavioral Sciences
Memorial Sloan-Kettering Cancer Center
Professor of Clinical Psychiatry, Weill Medical
College of Cornell University
1275 York Ave, New York, NY 10021, USA

David Horne
Consultant Clinical Psychologist
Department of Medicine and Psychiatry
The University of Melbourne
Level 1 North, Main Block, Royal Melbourne
Hospital
Albert Road Clinic Ramsay Health, Melbourne
Victoria 3050, Australia

Mary K Hughes
Clinical Nurse Specialist
M.D. Anderson Cancer Center
The University of Texas
1400 Pressler St., Unit 1454
Houston, TX 77030-3722, USA

Jonathan Hunter
Associate Professor
Head, Psychiatry, Health and Disease Program
Department of Psychiatry
University of Toronto
1285-b Mount Sinai Hospital
Joseph and Wolf Lebovic Health Complex
600 University Avenue
Toronto, ON, M5G 1X5
Canada

Mikael Birkelund Jensen-Johansen
Consultant Clinical Psychologist
Psychooncology Research Unit
Department of Oncology
Aarhus University Hospital and Department
of Psychology
Aarhus University, Aarhus, Denmark

Julia Kearney
Assistant Attending Child Psychiatrist
Department of Psychiatry and Behavioral Sciences
Department of Pediatrics
Memorial Sloan-Kettering Cancer Center
1275 York Ave, New York, NY 10021, USA

Ian B. Kerr
Consultant Clinical Psychologist
Coathill Hospital, Coatbridge, ML5 4DN, UK

David W. Kissane
Jimmie C. Holland Chair, Attending Psychiatrist
and Chairman
Department of Psychiatry and Behavioral Sciences
Memorial Sloan-Kettering Cancer Center
Professor of Psychiatry, Weill Medical College of
Cornell University
1275 York Avenue, New York, NY 10021, USA

Marguerite S Lederberg
Attending Psychiatrist
Department of Psychiatry and Behavioral Sciences
Memorial Sloan-Kettering Cancer Center
Professor of Clinical Psychiatry, Weill Medical
College of Cornell University
1275 York Ave, New York, NY 10021, USA

Emma J. Lewis
Consultant Clinical Psychologist
Oncology Health Service, Queens Centre for
Oncology and Haematology
Castle Hill Hospital, Cottingham, HU16 5JQ, UK

Frances Marcus Lewis
Virginia and Prentice Bloedel Professor
University of Washington, Seattle, WA 98195, USA
Adjunct Professor, Public Health Sciences Division
Fred Hutchinson Cancer Research Center, Seattle,
WA 98109-1024, USA
University of Pennsylvania, Pennsylvania, PA 19104,
USA

Nancy A. Mackeen
Research Associate, Manitoba Palliative Care
Research Unit
University of Manitoba
St. Boniface General Hospital
8006 – 409 Tache Blvd
St. Boniface, Manitoba R2H 2A6, Canada

Sharon Manne
Professor and Chief Section of Population Science
Cancer Institute of New Jersey
195 Little Albany Street
New Brunswick, NJ 08901, USA

Robert A. Neimeyer
Professor of Psychology
Department of Psychology
University of Memphis
400 Innovation Drive, Room 202
Memphis, TN 38152-6400, USA

Jamie Ostroff
Chief and Associate Member
Behavioral Sciences Service
Department of Psychiatry and Behavioral Sciences
Memorial Sloan Kettering Cancer Center
1275 York Avenue
New York, NY 10021, USA

David K Payne
Instructor in Psychology
Department of Psychology, Wallace Campus
Wallace Community College
1141 Wallace Drive, Dothan
AL 36303-0943, USA

Carolyn Pitceathly
Consultant Clinical Psychologist
Psycho-Oncology Service, Christie Hospital
Deputy Manager and Senior Trainer
Maguire Communication Skills Training Unit
The Christie NHS Foundation Trust, Manchester,
M20 4BX, UK

Donald M. Sharp
Senior Lecturer in Behavioural Oncology, Honorary
Consultant Clinical Psychologist
Oncology Health Service, Queens Centre for
Oncology and Haematology
Castle Hill Hospital, Cottingham
University of Hull, Institute of Rehabilitation
215 Anlaby Road, Hull, HU3 2PG, UK

David Spiegel
Willson Professor and Associate Chair of Psychiatry
and Behavioral Sciences
Stanford University School of Medicine
Stanford, CA 94305-5718, USA

Iñigo Tolosa
Consultant Clinical Psychologist
Pan Birmingham Cancer Psychology Service
Cancer Centre, Queen Elizabeth Hospital
University Hospital Birmingham
Edgbaston, Birmingham B15 2WB, UK

Maggie Watson
Consultant Clinical Psychologist
Psychological Medicine
The Royal Marsden NHS Foundation Trust
Downs Road, Sutton, Surrey SM2 5PT, UK
Honorary Senior Lecturer
Institute of Cancer Research
Honorary Professor, Research Department of Clinical
Educational and Health Psychology
University College London, London, WCIE 6BT, UK

Robert Zachariae
Professor, Psychooncology Research Unit
Department of Oncology
Aarhus University Hospital and Department of
Psychology
Aarhus University, Aarhus, Denmark

Talia Zaider
Assistant Attending Psychologist
Department of Psychiatry and Behavioral Sciences
Memorial Sloan-Kettering Cancer Center
1275 York Avenue, New York, NY 10021, USA

Foreword

Most of us know very little about cancer – until it happens to us. How we deal with what is usually a shock diagnosis depends on many things, including our personality type, but most of all – as a leading patient advocate over the last 10 years – I know it depends on the quality of the support we get through a difficult time.

I had not even heard of colon cancer before my diagnosis out of the blue with advanced cancer 20 years ago. My husband and I were presenters of a peak-time BBC TV show and our son was just three years old. The hairs on the back of my neck stood up in fear when I read that, on paper, my chances of survival were 34% and I suffered from insomnia for a long time afterwards.

A medical delay in diagnosis of almost a year made the prognosis even harder to bear – the thought that my life and my family's happiness was now in the balance, perhaps because of this long delay in diagnosis.

Cancer is an emotional roller coaster – it will affect approaching half of us in our lifetime – and most of us need help to get through it. To be diagnosed when you have dependent children or parents is an even greater worry. How will we cope? Why did we get it? What are the chances of it coming back? Who can we turn to for help?

When my best friend of 34 years was diagnosed with a Stage D stomach cancer, I witnessed the worst of care (physical, psychological and emotional) in one large city hospital – and the best of care when I was able to move her to another specialist cancer hospital, through a doctor I knew who was running a clinical trial on her cancer. There she died happy because of the way she was treated – with dignity, respect, support, great care and, she felt, love. She even married in the hospital the week before she died, calling it "the happiest day of my life".

As a result we, her friends, are left with happy memories of the end of her life and with great gratitude that we were able to access such wonderful support. Sadly, not everyone can and psycho-oncology is still largely an underrecognised yet vital part of the cancer journey for patients.

I co-founded the European Cancer Patient Coalition and ran it as Chair/President for seven years, building up a network of 300 member patient groups in 41 countries. We adopted three mantras to summarise how we wanted to be treated:

- Nothing about us without us

- See us – not our disease

- Patients as partners in our care

Too often the medical profession concentrates on healing our bodies and not enough on caring for our heads. Many national cancer plans have inadequate, or even no, coverage of the importance of psycho-oncology to patients.

The **Handbook of Psychotherapy in Cancer Care** is a welcome addition to the learning which cancer patients, their families, friends and colleagues would like to see practised in our lives after a diagnosis of cancer. We hope to see the benefits in more of our lives in the years to come.

Lynn Faulds Wood
Lynn's Bowel Cancer Campaign
European Cancer Patient Coalition

Preface

This book has been developed as part of the International Psycho-Oncology Society's (IPOS) educational strategy with the aim of sharing ideas and experience of psychological therapies being developed for cancer patients, their families and carers. Each chapter introduces the reader to the background and techniques as well as the existing evidence on efficacy of a number of therapeutic approaches and some ideas on service implementation. The chapters are not intended as stand alone therapy manuals but as an introduction to each therapy.

Psycho-oncology is a young discipline that developed during the second half of the last century in response to the many psychosocial challenges that cancer brings. Its clinical focus is to foster active coping and facilitate a healthy adaptation as each patient journeys through their cancer treatment and beyond. Its integrated multi-disciplinary approach complements the biomedical model led by cancer doctors. The expertise of psychologists, psychiatrists, social workers, nurses, chaplains, general practitioners and a range of other health care providers ensures comprehensive attention to the biopsychosocial and spiritual needs of patients and their families.

Psychotherapy encompasses a range of skilful interpersonal interventions able to be applied by the psycho-oncologist to support coping by patients and families. Psychotherapy is both patient- and family-centred in its focus, insightful through its deep understanding, respectful in its application and yet as varied as the practitioners in the field. As a result, it utilises a sizeable range of models to better define what it does and how it is applied. Moreover, these are adapted not only to the needs of patients within different cultures and educational groupings, but also in response to the demands of different cancers and their treatments. Applied psychotherapy has emerged as the art of the skilled practitioner in cancer care.

In this book, the many models of psychotherapy used by psycho-oncologists across the world are reviewed and authors offer guidelines intended to optimise the delivery. We cover its application in individual, group, couple and family settings, alongside the differing issues that emerge in different cancer stages – onset and early stage, survivorship or progression, palliative care and bereavement. Some exciting new models of intervention are presented that point the way to vastly improve the care of our patients. Our authors have been drawn from the international Psycho-Oncology community, many of whom have taught regularly in the Psychosocial Academies that have accompanied IPOS World Congresses. Indeed, they have led much of the research that has adapted psychotherapeutic interventions to the oncology setting and ensured that these are truly responsive to the needs of patients, families and carers. In this book, they describe the application of each model, together with clinically illustrated strategies that help generate beneficial outcomes.

As editors, we have been honoured to work with our esteemed authors in generating this book; they are leaders in this field. We thank them deeply for the time and effort put into sharing their wisdom and skill in the chapters they have written. We are especially grateful for their collegiality and friendship, their scholarship and their commitment to IPOS and the discipline of psycho-oncology. We also thank our readers for their interest and hope this handbook will guide their thoughtful and sensitive therapy in the years ahead. Specific thanks go to Joan Marsh and Fiona Woods at Wiley-Blackwell, Sue Davolls at the Royal Marsden Hospital supporting Maggie Watson, Laurie Schulman at Memorial Sloan-Kettering Cancer Center supporting David Kissane and finally Elliott Graham and her administrative team at IPOS Headquarters. This book results from a wonderful team effort, which exemplifies the very essence of a cohesive psychosocial care team needed to deliver excellent cancer care.

Cancer affects nearly one out of every two people over their lifetime and three out of four families, serving as a leading cause of death across the world. It brings a great challenge to those so diagnosed, while its treatments can also be demanding. Just as progress is being made every day with targeted anti-cancer therapies, so also has much been accomplished with the psychological therapies described in this book.

We hope that physicians and surgeons, psychologists and psychiatrists, nurses and social workers, indeed, health care professionals from many disciplines, will learn from the varied techniques and strategies described herein. As a result, we trust that patient care will continue to improve and healing result, so that no matter how stressful the diagnosis or treatment of a cancer proves to be, any inherent suffering can be ameliorated and quality of life helped to prevail.

Maggie Watson and David W. Kissane
11 October 2010

Section A

Individual Models of Therapy

1 Supportive Psychotherapy in Cancer Care: an Essential Ingredient of All Therapy

Marguerite S. Lederberg and Jimmie C. Holland

Department of Psychiatry and Behavioral Sciences, Memorial Sloan-Kettering Cancer Center, New York, NY, USA

1.1 Introduction

Supportive psychotherapy for patients with cancer and their families is the single most important tool of the psycho-oncologist (or psychosocial oncologist). With it, patients are often sustained through the whole fragmented course of their illness. Supportive psychotherapy is both the most simple and the most complex tool we have. Therapists must be knowledgeable about cancer as a medical disorder, skilled at assessing and managing patients psychologically and comfortable with their own subjective experience in the face of complex and tragic medical situations. It also requires sound clinical judgement to recognise the patient's changing psychological needs and to match them accurately with the flexibility of our therapeutic approach.

Psycho-oncologists come from different disciplines, use different theoretical frameworks and have different cultural backgrounds, yet all converge to deliver this vital service. Clearly, there is a human interaction, a crucial piece, that is hard to fit into so many different theoretical frameworks for which technical and theoretical terms are inadequate. We should not sound apologetic but speak of supportive psychotherapy with pride, as it requires the highest level of clinical skills and taxes our own emotional capacities to the fullest. It also cannot be done without personal involvement and 'caring'. Francis Peabody in 1927 wrote in the JAMA that 'the secret to caring for the patient is CARING for the patient' [1]. This is no less true today, almost a 100 years later. Human emotions are universal and unchanging – only medical treatments change.

In this chapter, we define supportive psychotherapy in cancer care and provide the beginner with the basic principles that guide therapy with patients and their families. It may give more experienced therapists a fresh overview. Most lessons apply equally to patients with other life threatening illnesses. We do not seek to provide solutions, but rather identify techniques to manage situations that could otherwise be overwhelming.

1.2 Definition

Supportive psychotherapy is a therapeutic intervention utilised intermittently or continuously that seeks to help patients deal with distressing emotions, reinforce pre-existing strengths and promote adaptive coping with the illness. It explores the patient's self, body image and role changes within a relationship of mutual respect and trust. The range of approaches includes:

- Knowing how to clarify and discuss highly charged information, which arouses overwhelming emotions that interfere with processing, and helping to manage those emotions constructively.

- Being familiar with methods of promoting learning and problem-solving and using cognitive and behavioural techniques at any stage of disease.

- Being comfortable with a range of therapeutic activity including crisis intervention and a quiet, supportive presence for patients too weak to interact, an exploration of deep dynamic patterns operating in

Handbook of Psychotherapy in Cancer Care, First Edition. Edited by Maggie Watson and David W. Kissane.
© 2011 John Wiley & Sons, Inc. Published 2011 by John Wiley & Sons, Inc.

the patient's psyche as well as family counselling in many constellations.

• Standing ready to guide the patient and family to available resources.

• Working well with the medical caregivers and understanding the system in which they operate so as to allow the reciprocal flow of useful information. This means knowing how to discuss the coping abilities and the vulnerabilities of the patient, in ways that humanise without violating confidentiality.

• Understanding the medical information you are given, and asking if you need more help.

• Understanding your own emotional responses, especially in your early years as you learn to manage yourself for the long haul, in these demanding situations.

1.3 History and Evidence Base

Given its core requirement for flexibility, supportive psychotherapy is difficult to study in randomised controlled trials that follow strict guidelines and manuals to assure treatment fidelity. As a result, there are far more studies of cognitive behavioural therapy and other more focused therapies, because of their easier study design. However, numerous compelling studies from the last 20 years were reviewed in 2007 by a multidisciplinary committee of the Institute of Medicine (IOM), National Academies of Science and the Committee concluded that a sound evidence base exists to recommend supportive psychotherapy as a valid therapeutic intervention. This landmark IOM report, *Care for the Whole Person: Integrating Psychosocial into Routine Care*, highlights the vital quality standard of integrating the psychosocial domain into routine cancer care [2]. It recommends that all cancer patients be screened for distress/psychosocial needs, which should then be addressed in the patient's treatment plans. Those with a level of distress identified in a rapid screen which fits an algorithm for 'caseness' should be referred to a proper psychosocial resource for help. Caseness identifies the level of symptoms without providing a diagnosis, but raises a 'red flag' about unmet needs. A two-phase screening is recommended, first rapidly via one or two questions, (such as the Distress Thermometer) followed by a more in-depth appraisal as needed.

In the US, the Alliance for Quality Psychosocial Cancer Care is educating patients, families, oncology 'front line' doctors, nurses and social workers about

this mandate [3]. It is an official paradigm change wherein clinical practice guidelines and accreditation documents for training in different disciplines include psychosocial care as one of the criteria for good overall care. Supportive psychotherapy is an effective management of anxiety, depression and distress across all stages of cancer. In complex cases, it is the 'default condition', that is the home base from which the therapist guides the patient to other helpful therapies and resources.

1.4 Qualifications for Clinical Privileges to Provide Supportive Psychotherapy as a Psycho-Oncologist

Psycho-oncology is an inclusive discipline to which different professions make unique contributions. We assume appropriate psychotherapy training, which can come from many different programmes. Each therapist needs a framework to organise psychosocial data and the conclusions drawn from it. This is the structure on which new knowledge can more easily be incorporated as part of a coherent whole. We also assume basic familiarity with recognition and treatment of anxiety and depressive disorders, cognitive disorders and delirium [4].

Today, a number of different theories commonly underlie any therapist's technique. Some are psychoanalytically derived, like modern supportive-expressive psychotherapy, object relations theory, self psychology and relational approaches. They deal with self awareness, managing emotions and relationships, absorbing losses and struggling with existential issues. Cognitive and behavioural therapies, learning theories and problem solving techniques have a critical role in improving adaptive skills but can be applied across many points of the disease trajectory. Many varied approaches are detailed in the rest of the book.

1.5 Application of Supportive Therapy in Cancer Care

1.5.1 Location

This approach spans the outpatient, inpatient and home care settings; sometimes the telephone or e-mail must suffice to stay in touch. The important issue is that the patient knows you remain 'there for him'.

1.5.2 Timing

The patient's level of energy will vary, necessitating that some sessions be shortened, based on fatigue or level of illness. These are still extremely important. Even with curtailed dialogue, the session may be meaningful, particularly when the patient is very ill.

1.5.3 Frequency

Again, this varies with level of illness. As patients recuperate and feel able to address issues beyond illness, outpatient visits are reinstated with the rules akin to those conducted with physically healthy patients. But each medical setback restarts the cycle.

1.5.4 Sense of Urgency

Patients often have a strong sense of their time being limited, with a need to work out problems and family conflicts rapidly, yet realistically. Therapists must maintain an accurate sense of time within which the work can be accomplished.

1.5.5 Flexibility of Approach

Good therapists are always flexible, but psycho-oncologists need to be gymnasts as patient's concerns change repeatedly, and change seems the only certainty [5]. The fears during the diagnostic work-up are different from the pain of adapting to its result. The toll of treatments with their significant side effects may be severe. Some refuse further treatment because the drugs are 'too toxic'. Others, who were focused on 'healthy living', feel betrayed by treatment side-effects, even when the treatment is effective. Much as they hate treatment, patients experience paradoxical anxiety when it ends, as they no longer have the security that came with it. This needs to be recognised, normalised and occasionally treated.

During difficult periods of acute illness, emotional reassurance and support may be all that should be attempted. Patients may have to adapt to an unexpected recurrence that forces them to face dark realities they had kept at bay. Or they have to accept the permanent loss of a body part or functions like walking, sexuality, sight, hearing or speech. These are devastating losses with profound grief. Listening, exploring and not offering false comfort is itself a gift which not all provide. Gentle exploring may or may not follow.

Patients are very anxious about the unpredictability of cancer. They repeat, 'If only I knew what was going to happen next! How long do I have? If only someone would tell me what to expect?' Helping the patient cope with uncertainty remains a central challenge, irrespective of the medical information they

receive. Patients struggle with anger at the doctors who tell them truthfully that they don't know what will happen next. Yet they feel stricken when given a prediction about survival. When they exceed that time, they crow with satisfaction and feel triumph over the doctor's inaccuracy – he does not begrudge them that pleasure.

As illness improves, patients may explore family issues or deeply personal problems. Shifting to a more dynamic approach gives patients something meaningful besides cancer to work through and allows them to relate consciously to who they were and how they got that way. This engagement is usually welcomed. The work may be disrupted by the next medical event, but it leaves greater trust between patient and therapist, while the latter has gained a better understanding of the patient's motivation and reactions. The course of many cancers is like a roller coaster, with sudden, severe episodes interrupting tolerably stable periods. Expect the therapy to have similar characteristics.

1.5.6 The Need for the Therapist to Understand the Disease

The initial evaluation must include the diagnosis, staging, prognosis, current therapy and usual side-effects of the treatment. You need this overall view to be able to match it against the patient's awareness of the illness and its seriousness. The patient's own subjective formulation is often very different from what you know to be the reality. Obtain permission to call the primary physician, the oncologist, a prior therapist and anyone who can help you to understand the medical facts that direct the patient's current existence. It is impossible to give valid psychological support if you do not understand the medical reality.

A man, whose self-esteem had been battered all his life, was afraid to make demands by asking questions, out of fear that he might push away the doctors. He presented himself as the ideal patient. The therapist was familiar with his disease and thus able to discuss his fears in concrete and practical ways. This made him feel more accepted and helped his trust of the therapist to develop.

1.5.7 Denial

In response to severe physical illness, patients employ remarkable flexibility in their use of denial, particularly in dealing with prognosis. It functions as a 'cushion' to give them time and space within which to absorb 'bad news'. It allows the development of two levels of co-existent knowledge, one realistic, one wishful. The words of a young woman with advanced colon cancer expressed it well: '*I know I am going to die, but I can't believe I am going to die*'.

Denial ranges from a nearly psychotic reaction to mature coping skills, with all intermediate variants. Distinguishing between pathological denial and affective denial is useful: (i) pathological denial is destructive because it delays consultation, invites poor compliance and embraces risks, all in the service of avoidance and (ii) affective denial can help the patient focus on hopeful options, without interfering with optimal care. Pathological denial is distressing to all, while positive avoidance may interfere with open communication in the family, but creates an atmosphere, that is easier for all, at least temporarily. If denial gets more intense as the disease progresses, it risks depriving the patient of a powerful source of comfort. In general, denial as a coping strategy varies considerably. Inconsistency should not cause surprise, but instead, define an area of fruitful exploration.

1.5.7.1 Ambivalence and Ambiguity

Both of these are often in the service of denial. Sometimes the treating team become frustrated when patients and families have unexpected and radical shifts in their thinking about important issues and decisions. One day they discuss a difficult option; the next, they ignore it. Or they withhold their decisions and keep things unsettled. This commonly relates to prognosis but can also occur when choosing between two equally undesirable treatments or when the needed decisions are too painful to face. It can be the main reason for avoiding medical care altogether. If it does not interfere with a necessary decision, it need not be addressed. But eventually, the reality must be discussed, and many doctors are able to do so in a kind and non-confrontational way.

A single mother had an aggressive, metastatic cervical cancer. She did not allow her daughter, aged 7, to visit because it would upset them both. They had cheery conversations over the phone and she talked to her therapist about 'fighting' so as to get home to her daughter. Yet she had already arranged for her brother, a family man, to be her daughter's guardian, had made financial arrangements and had been sending the child for visits there. Fortunately, the uncle was sensitive and after talking with the psychiatrist, was able to introduce a successful visit

between mother and child. Over time, the topics that would permit a loving farewell were covered.

1.5.8 The First Visit

For many, psychiatric referral adds insult to injury. Patients say 'I don't know why my doctor sent me!' or; 'My sister dragged me here!' Often a therapeutic alliance is created despite the odds, and the patient can acknowledge grief, suffering, fears and relief as they are normalised. If no change occurs, it is best to respect patients' wishes and let them go in a way that will allow them to return when ready with minimal embarrassment. They often get referred again or come back voluntarily.

A 58-year old business man with a recent diagnosis of lung cancer was being evaluated for secondaries before deciding on surgery. He was blunt about his low opinion of therapy and grumbled about his wife's insistence. The therapist commented that he seemed like a man who was not used to being ill and pressured by other people. He agreed. The therapist kept that theme unobtrusively present and he cooperated with a brief review of his current life and a few questions about depressive symptoms, which he denied, and anxiety symptoms, which were more prominent. He remained uninterested in treatment, so the therapist took the initiative and, emphasising his strengths, commented that his anxiety was not only understandable given what he was going through, but even inevitable. Saying that there were good medications for anxiety much more severe than his, she said he did not seem to need them right now, but should feel free to return if things got more difficult. He did return.

1.5.9 'I Am OK, Just Out of Control!'

We are trained to evaluate symptomatic patients according to DSM-IV, but cancer patients may not fit these diagnostic boxes. Some acutely distressed patients are upset at the referral, because they have always been cheerful, happy, resilient and competent; in brief, 'normal'. They feel that cancer is their only ticket of admission to our office, not 'psychiatric problems'. Even if we see issues, we must acknowledge and respond to their self-description. After all, they may be right. They were 'normal'. If we focus on the disrupted self too exclusively, the patient may feel diminished and unheard. We want to build a therapeutic alliance and avoid anger or demoralisation. We emphasise the strengths of the psychological self, because there can be no reassurance about the physical self. Acknowledging life's accomplishments, both worldly and psychological, can be productive, at the right moment.

The mere suspicion of cancer, and the workup that ensues, generate a sense of loss of control which patients describe accurately as frightening and depersonalising. If the illness gets worse, patients may become depressed or demoralised as they absorb the reality of permanently losing the roles and human functions that defined them most deeply. Acknowledge their grief about losing their pre-illness self-image, because it is in their thoughts every waking moment and probably in their dreams as well. Help them remember the strengths that may still be theirs. This kind of early intervention may avoid the need for medication, because it helps patients hang on to their healthy self and gives them some continuity with 'who I was before', even as they become sicker.

An accomplished woman, always a support to others, presented in a tearful, disorganised state four months after diagnosis of stage II breast cancer. Her reaction was out of character and appalled her. 'I am a totally different person. It's terrifying!' She needed crisis intervention, medication and monitoring of her mood disorder. Only after several weeks did her strengths resurface and she began to cope in more characteristic ways. Throughout her treatment, the therapist recognised how important it was to acknowledge and honour her ability to manage again on her own.

1.5.10 All Patients Need to Tell Their Story

When you ask, it just comes tumbling out! Sometimes the story is about anger, disappointment or mismanagement; sometimes the impact of the illness is so strong that facts get lost along the way. Patients may be tired, agitated or anxious and do not remember events well. It helps if your familiarity with the disease enables you to volunteer information that allows the patient to realise you understand something about his ordeal. Unless there is a compelling reason to obtain other details, let the patient unburden. The story usually reveals interesting emotional information. Collaborative history from family members, with the patients' permission and a signed release for reports from other physicians are important. It reassures the patient that you are a member of his 'team'.

1.5.11 The Body Has a Voice; Listen to It

A patient may be suffering pain, revulsion or heartbreak at changes to the body. The therapist must be able to stay with it, without displaying discomfort or waning involvement. It is not always easy. While we are accustomed to focusing on the psychological aspects of patients' disclosures, we must also focus on the immediacy of the body, its losses, humiliations, embarrassments and exhausting routines that now dominate life. This requires varying degrees of conscious effort for different therapists. Many patients declare that the best support comes from fellow patients, who 'really know' what they are going through. The therapist cannot provide that, but must provide a helpful equivalent.

The opposite may also occur, when the body is initially silent. The diagnosis is made accidentally, and the patient never feels ill until treatment ushers in significant side effects. For such a patient, the diagnosis can bring unreality and bewilderment. He may be angry and develop a resentful attitude, or even a paranoid tinge. It is useful to normalise it by bringing it out in the open. If not, it may persist into the later phases of the disease, when the cancer is all too evident and anguish becomes high. Angst and anger will combine and be projected even more negatively, usually onto the medical caregivers, but also onto relatives in dysfunctional families.

Some patients go through treatment with minimal interference with normal life. Not all treatments are equally rigorous and not all patients are equally resilient. It is important to be aware of what your patient is going through. Some patients are proud and/or relieved to have gone through treatment without missing work. But they do feel fatigued and require rest. Others never return to work again, and it is not always obvious why from their physical state. If the outlook is not bleak, it is worth exploring why.

1.6 Boundaries in the Therapy Relationship: Therapeutic Activism

Much of what is taught about the boundaries of the therapeutic encounter with physically healthy patients must be modified when working with the medically ill [5]. Touching, usually taboo, becomes acceptable as a hug or a pat on the arm for encouragement. As a psychosocial-oncologist, you are more participatory as a fellow human being, but must always be conscious of valid therapeutic reasons for all your actions, and alert to patients who need the security of physical distance.

Hospital consultations make short work of standard guidelines. The ill patient can be positioned uncomfortably, unable to move or pull blankets higher. He may be thirsty and can't reach the glass, lost the call bell or dropped the phone. Ignoring these obvious facts limits the effectiveness of any contact. The therapist must feel comfortable helping out with small problems that respect the patient's privacy and do not replace nursing care. Pulling up blankets, altering the bed controls to make it more comfortable, moving the glass and replacing the call bell can be viewed as the opening conversation. Ignoring those needs, while interviewing, is like neglecting verbal messages. The patient's body has betrayed him, and has been assaulted by rigorous treatments. The therapist must welcome any discussion of distortions in body image or sense of self, so as to encourage verbalisation of thoughts and feelings. This may extend to questions about physical details that may be upsetting. Every mental health professional should be attentive to an ill patient. But in psycho-oncology, it is part of the therapeutic duty. Ignoring the body sends the wrong message, one the patient dreads to hear, because in his own life, it happens all too often, and painfully isolates him from the healthy world.

When a patient is weak, in pain or in a wheelchair, attention to promoting comfort should not depend on being invited. The therapist must remain actively interested in the patient's medical course throughout. She will be committed to careful surveillance of the patient's overall state, the extent of compliance with treatment and the judgement used in seeking extra care when needed.

1.7 Themes Met in Advanced Cancer

Legacy, guilt, fear of dying, spirituality, transition to palliative care and end-of-life themes are grist for the mill in supportive therapy with patients with advanced cancer.

1.7.1 Family Legacies

These can find expression through the meaning of both the cancer and the illness.

1. **The meaning of cancer**: Despite many commonalities, having cancer means something different to each individual. It is essential to understand this fully, including aspects that may be unconscious. The loss of parents, other family members or a close friend to cancer all have a bearing on how the patient experiences the illness. Difficult memories become haunting and may need to be aired and discussed. Often they are decades old and seem writ in stone. But they belong to another age and the patient must be helped to confront

the difference between themselves then and now, and the treatment between then and now. It may address unfinished business, re-awakened grief, frightening memories of illness in the family, guilt around imagined misdeeds and usually, unrelieved, lonely suffering and helplessness never shared with a supportive adult. Thus, exploring a patient's associations with cancer is quite revealing. When not volunteered, it is elicited through a detailed family history, preferably using a genogram that includes grandparents and asks about good friends as well.

2. **The meaning of illness**: Being ill is somewhat different. It can be part of the family culture, or even more, the family of origin. It may never have been explicitly stated, but has been absorbed nonetheless and has strong ethnic variations. In some families, one does not complain and is as independent as possible. Any neediness is suspect, unless its causes are blatant. For others, illness itself carries a covert message of ill-doing or retribution. Some family members are illness-phobic and want to minimise it at any cost; others are too frightened to help. In such families, severe illness can be catastrophic. Sometimes one sees a role reversal with the patient providing comfort to distraught family members. In other families, being ill is a favoured status. The patient receives a freely offered cornucopia of extra care and attention, sometimes too much, if it interferes with the level of desired independence. But it is usually welcome. Fortunately, there are many families where there is a loving and competent caregiver, fewer where support from others prevents caregiver exhaustion. An awareness of the stresses and the price paid by primary caregivers is required to enable the therapist to ease their burden.

Discussion of these issues helps the therapist understand more, and helps the patient gain insight into his formative experiences. Most find these explorations interesting and feel a sense of release after discussing them. As the disease progresses, activities drop away and old interests no longer have the same traction, at which point this new self-understanding becomes even more important as it gives life greater coherence and meaning.

1.7.2 Guilt

Guilt is a common issue. Many feel they are being punished for previous misdeeds which they identify with unjustified certainty. This is not truly guilt, but attribution as to cause. They can feel guilty about what they are doing to their family, leaving them to fend for themselves and causing grief and disruption. In turn, the families may contribute through blunt accusation about causality, or by nagging about self-care and having the 'right attitude to beat the cancer'. For other than heavy smokers, 'blaming the victim' is generally toxic and unjustified. (Not helpful to the lung cancer patient either.) Most other toxic exposures were not in the patient's control, although diet is being identified as causal for some. Human beings are well versed in the art of making themselves and others feel responsible for uncontrollable negative events.

Guilt is important in diagnosing major depression. The physically ill, depressed patient may not always display overt depression or active suicidality and the usual physical symptoms of depression are attributed to the cancer. Depressed patients are typically guilty, convinced they are not really worth saving, will not be saved and have lost agency over their life. This state of mind is accompanied by loss of interest in the things they once enjoyed, constricted affect, poor eye contact, personal neglect and imperviousness to outside input [6]. Such a patient needs referral for medication, as do patients with severe anxiety and panic attacks or confusional states [4–6].

1.7.3 Fear of Death

The thought of death barrels instantly into the mind of all newly diagnosed patients unless the tumour is so curable that the patient believes the physician's reassurances. Even then, the word 'cancer' is enough to bring fear into people's minds, sometimes overwhelming all else. For some, it is not fear of death but of dying, for which it is easier to offer some reassurance. But some patients are terrified at the prospect of being dead, which is much harder to explore. It may be related to some personal history, but often it is very primitive, and not readily available. It is not age related, since many children and adolescents face death with impressive courage, but it is a fear with deep and early roots. It is asking a lot to expect the patient to manage this amidst the insults and injuries of the disease. Discussing it repeatedly in a calm and secure setting can begin to make it a little easier. A life review with an emphasis on the underlying meanings that made it what it is, and some psychodynamic observations that highlight the unity of the narrative, can bring the patient to feeling better about what he has done and who he has been, thus capturing some of his attention. Medication for anxiety is usually beneficial,

but does not obviate the role of human conversation. The presence of a loving family or other valued friends lowers much anxiety. Relaxation techniques can bring momentary relief.

Some patients have an excellent prognosis, have already been discharged and yet are convinced they are going to die. This usually relates to the pre-morbid personality and is best treated outside a cancer centre or clinic.

1.7.4 Spirituality and Religion in Supportive Therapy

The need for cultural and religious sensitivity is well recognised. But in fatal illnesses, they play a very intense role. Patients with strong religious or spiritual beliefs will adapt to the illness and their death within these constructs. They may have a religious counsellor who will help maximise support and access to community resources. Clearly, the therapist supports the patient's prior beliefs. It is important not to impose one's own meanings and perceptions about existential issues. Obviously there is no place for proselytising.

For patients without such pre-existing resources, a number of relaxation and breathing techniques can relieve anxiety, while guided imagery can get the patient in touch with the inner self. Use conversations in which the patient describes the most meaningful, happy or peaceful moments or scenes in his life, and offer to make a tape based on that information and enriched by constructive and realistic elaboration. Patients often use them repeatedly. For people who do not locate transcendent feelings in a particular practice, moments of intense, facilitated introspection may bring them a different kind of peace.

1.7.5 Transition to Palliative Care

Ideally, the transition from curative to palliative care should be introduced early. Late transitions are psychologically more difficult, especially if the patient and/or family are shocked by the news. Therapists can alert oncologists to what patients/family are thinking about end-of-life concerns. They can help patients and families explore further, in a hypothetical mode: 'What would you do if . . . ?' Existential issues come to the fore and the therapist is well positioned to discuss them with the family, and suggest a meeting with the medical staff. This speaks yet again to the necessity of being known and trusted by the staff.

1.7.6 End-of-Life

As death becomes a fully acknowledged outcome, education is needed about what to expect, what dying may be like, and most of all, what can be done to insure comfort for the patient and support for the family. Therapists can help the patient and family process medical information that was emotionally so loaded that it was misheard, altered by wishful thinking or forgotten. It is impossible to exaggerate the family's need for explanations about what is happening, what it means and what may come next.

Honest communication is critical at this time. The therapist can help the patient address unfinished business and support better communication about dying and saying goodbye. It is moving to see a family that is open about what is happening and hence surround the patient with warmth and love until the end. A patient who has been 'protected' from the truth, or, even more ironically, knows the truth, but has received the unspoken message that he cannot talk about it, dies alone no matter how many people are in the room. Therapists should try to minimise this. If the patient is dying at home, a therapist visit will be very meaningful. Being a welcome presence at such a profound moment is a privilege. Attending a funeral or a memorial is a personal choice, depending on one's need to honour the patient's memory, support the family and assist closure for one's self. Recognising this personal involvement is important. Not infrequently, the caregiver will seek bereavement therapy since the therapist is already known and trusted.

1.7.6.1 Controversies

Unfortunately, many difficult choices may arise in the final days [7], including decisions about what treatments to have or not have, whether to start protocols, when to stop nutrition and hydration. Family members may insist on useless, inappropriate care and become threatening about it. At such times, therapists can support the staff. Some patients want to select the time of their death and want staff help in achieving it, which is illegal in most venues. Such requests must be handled sensitively with advice about legal options, such as stopping treatments, nutrition and hydration. The proxy may be in a difficult position if the family is not united and should receive therapist attention. The best stance is to remain constant in support.

The completion of advanced directives is becoming more common and greatly facilitates clarity over the patient's wishes. Therapists do well to encourage completion of these when issues likes completion of wills, estate planning and appointment of health proxies are being considered.

1.8 Families as Part of Patients' Supportive Psychotherapy

1.8.1 What Is a Family?

For our purposes, a family is the collection of individuals recognised by the patient as an important part of their life and who are themselves very attached and emotionally impacted. We are not here to define it for them.

1.8.2 Healthy Families

Many patients show remarkable fortitude, courage and generosity while their families are loyal, loving and stay the course. They are realistic, show initiative in organising care, look after each other, discuss painful truths openly, take care of unfinished business and cherish their time together. But there are different profiles of strength and vulnerability in all families. Family members often cope differently and use different strategies that conflict with each other. Therapists must evaluate these differences and develop a plan to manage them that troubles the patient as little as possible.

1.8.3 Patients without Social Support

For patients who have no family or loyal friends, the course is infinitely more difficult. The therapist often becomes a crucial resource and must take on a heavier burden of fidelity than with more embedded patients. Finding support groups, calling in religious and community sources if appropriate and identifying community volunteers, becomes very important.

1.8.4 Patient's Need for and Reaction to Family Involvement

Dealing with the patient's family is not a choice, but a necessity. Relational concerns must be appraised and discussed. A surprisingly large number of patients request psychotherapy, not for their cancer, but for family or relationship concerns. Some of their issues are completely unrelated to the cancer, others were precipitated by it, but are not integrally related to it. Even patients, who initially focus on the disease, will sometimes in the first or second session move into a pre-existing personal problem. As the disease progresses, it eventually displaces these private concerns, yet even stage III or IV patients will still focus on the personal problem.

A 76-year old school principal came for therapy during chemotherapy for locally invasive colon cancer. But she only wanted to discuss her profound guilt about the way she neglected her other children when her eldest daughter had died of Ewing's sarcoma at age 6, almost 45 years ago. She quickly bore a 'replacement child' and believed he must have been damaged too. She felt responsible for all their problems but had no other symptoms of depression. We reviewed the customs around handling childhood cancer at the time, as well as aspects of her childhood and adolescence that made her over-responsible and guilt-prone. One day, she announced that she could see her children were doing well and did not bear grievances and she terminated therapy.

A patient may initially be too stunned with his own fear and grief, and too consumed by his illness to process what is going on in the family, especially if there is a 'conspiracy of silence' meant to spare him. But quickly enough, the family attitudes intrude and generate varied feelings in the patient, ranging from gratitude, guilt and worry, to disappointment, resentment at lack of engagement or a deep yearning for signs of love, understanding and reassurance. These powerful feelings need to be explored.

A 58-year old man had stage IV renal cell cancer and depression, which responded fairly well to medication, but he continued to be unhappy and disaffected because he felt uncared for by his wife and teenage children. When his cancer took a turn for the worse, his family changed suddenly, with all of them showing affection, engagement and grief. He then became much more active and energetic, explored experimental options and went to another hospital for another protocol, while remaining in touch with the therapist.

1.8.5 The Family's Need for Involvement

1. **Emotional stressors**: Cancer is a family crisis. With a more serious diagnosis, family members react strongly. Some are grief stricken and jump to the worst conclusion; others are reassuring, present and supportive. They cry a lot, explore other treatments and often get contradictory advice. Finding out about a bad prognosis at the computer is a lonely way to learn about it. Guide the family to select a trusted person to do the online searches, if they are inevitable.

Losing one member to cancer and another to caregiving requires extensive reorganisation and cooperation from the remaining family members to fill the void and keep going. Many times, it cannot be done. There are many small, isolated families for whom the demands are overwhelming and the social safety net inadequate. It is crucial to search for outside support of any kind for them.

2. **Primary caregiver**: Usually one person takes on, by choice or by adjudication, the role of primary caregiver. They are at risk for anxiety, depression, neglect of their own health and a permanent downward mobility, yet moments of transcendence can give them joy and meaning. Many patients are very difficult, in which case the caregiver needs more support. Caring for the primary caregiver, or referring her for her own treatment, should always be on the therapist's radar [8].

3. **Environmental stressors**: In countries lacking socialised medicine, the financial stresses are severe and inevitable. Families can easily spend all their savings. Many bankruptcies are not due to profligate spending, but to medical expenses assumed out of devotion. This might be an issue to explore with the proxy or caregiver. There are many secondary losses, such as the loss of the patient's income, the caregiver's loss of work or shift to lower pay so as to accommodate more time off. Adolescents may stop college for financial reasons, but also because they are being parentified. Young children are shunted aside 'for their protection' and develop guilt-ridden fantasies to explain their exile. The therapist should address parenting issues early. Families always welcome reliable advice about how to manage children in dire situations and discussions of other issues will usually follow [9].

The family rallies during the acute periods, but attention wanes during remissions or lengthy, stable treatments. Devotion fatigue and variably controlled resentments may be expressed. If mild or episodic, they can be managed, but they can easily disrupt the fragile equilibrium. The therapist can discuss the siblings' simultaneous jealousy and guilt about the patient, help the parents understand and re-integrate the farmed-out children, work with a couple that is drifting apart and help them develop better communication, encourage the adolescent's continued education and support the family in seeking and accepting outside help. Highly stressed family become isolated and withdrawn and may neglect local resources. Most of these events become known to the patient who may be very anxious about them.

1.8.6 Family Bereavement

The death of a loved one can be a profound loss but also a major trauma. Therapists have a responsibility to try to minimise traumatic outcomes from the circumstances of the death. Some terminal events such as acute bleeds or unhelpful customs like giving the proxy full responsibility for 'pulling the plug' despite complicated relationships in the family that lead to significant distress, anger or guilt, cannot be erased. Sometimes one of the health care team is unthinkingly brusque and offends the family that has little tolerance at this time. In fact, family members are easily oversensitive to any behaviour they construe, or misconstrue, as heartless and uncaring. The worst of all is when they feel the patient's suffering has not been well treated. On the other hand, a sensitive physician, nurse or therapist will be long remembered with deep gratitude. Either way, these actions are deeply imprinted in the family's memory bank, whether accurately interpreted or not.

> *A patient's widow, who had had a good experience with the staff, and had good relationships with her children and friends in her community, came eight years later to speak to a group of oncology fellows about her experience with the death of her husband. Her first words were: 'It is still in my mind as if it happened yesterday. It was his decision to disconnect the respirator. It was his decision alone. He did it'.*

The last days of any patient's life deserve the utmost attention, support and respect. This effort will bring comfort to the survivors instead of painful memories that rankle for the rest of their days, especially because they often embrace unjustified or unconscious guilty feelings for having 'failed' to prevent them.

The therapist can be helpful at defusing the impact of the events, but more importantly, should be available for bereavement therapy after the death. It is important to send a letter to the family, which confirms for them your understanding and concern for the patient and family. A phone call is good but does not carry the weight of a letter that families will cherish long after.

1.8.7 Working with Patient and Family: It's about Communication!

Families that communicate well manage better after the death. Communication is an essential factor in family adaptation, even when members differ with regards to other variables. The therapist must be attuned to family members' coping and strengths, be ready to refer those in need and give special support to the caregiver and proxy, both in formal sessions or more casual meetings. The therapist needs to identify unspoken painful issues that have a bearing on the present and gently bring them out into the open. These can involve reactions to the illness and things too difficult to talk about, especially dying. But it can also be an inability to plan for the future, unresolved conflicts and an avoidance of sharing real feelings and grief. When a family fails to communicate openly, the patient will die more alone and family members will feel more isolated from one another. There will have been no goodbyes, no asking for forgiveness, no shared planning and no shared memories. For families with cohesiveness and an ability to manage conflict, opening communications may not be too difficult; indeed it is very powerful in its ability to promote changes. See Chapter 14 on Family therapy for further discussion.

1.9 Therapist Issues

Working almost exclusively with cancer patients is not easy. Many professionals cannot imagine doing it, and as a result, psycho-oncologists are a highly self-selected group. This does not diminish the need to monitor ourselves. Keep in mind the limits of what we can do and keep a good perspective on what we can't do along with a healthy sense of humour. Among ourselves, 'gallows humour' certainly has a place in helping us cope, but nowhere else. Awareness of our counter-transference reactions is necessary given the exposure to wrenching human tragedies and death, the latter always hovering in the thoughts of both patient and therapist. This makes self-examination all the more important.

1.9.1 When the Therapist Is a Cancer Survivor

A number of cancer survivors wish to help patients going through the same ordeals they faced. They must have developed a stable adaption to their disease, and be immune to being hijacked by bursts of emotional memory. They must have the discipline to stay focused on the patient's story despite their own dramatic experience. In truth, they do have special knowledge, but, as with other boundary crossings, they must only share what they clearly know will benefit the patient.

1.9.2 Role of Medications

Psychotropic medications can and must complement supportive therapy when patients need treatment of depression, anxiety or confusion. Refer these patients promptly [10].

1.10 Service Development Issues

Both identifying services and both building and sustaining skills are key issues.

1.10.1 Use of Referrals

Most cities today have cancer support groups, including telephone and online ones. Chat rooms and bulletin boards provide unsupervised support from others sharing the same experience. They bring both excellent and unhelpful support. Large advocacy groups such as Gilda's Club, Wellness Community and Cancer Care have online and 'buddy' systems which are reliable. They also offer a large variety of other helpful on-site activities. The American Psychosocial Oncology Society has a helpline to assist patients in finding a counsellor with knowledge of cancer (1-866-APOS-4-HELP). Some well-developed, focused group approaches are described in other chapters.

Supportive therapy supports patients, it does not bind them. Realistic improvement is celebrated, safe exploration is encouraged and interruptions are appropriate. We cannot 'fix' all our patients' problems. Referral for complementary therapies, like art, music, meditation and yoga is helpful for patients who find 'talk' therapy difficult. There are limits to what our interventions can do and times when referral to someone else is the best option. The patients usually experience it as taking care of them.

1.10.2 The Psycho-Oncologist

Last but not least, we all need to review our life, especially our losses and must try to understand our motivation for doing this work. Many of us, not all, come because of personal losses or ordeals. They need not disqualify us, but we must be aware of them and how they might affect us. It is usually a satisfying awareness that solidifies our motivation and helps us understand ourselves. We need to recognise when a patient is touching us more deeply than others and put ourselves on alert about over-involvement or over-identification that will warp our judgement. We must also think about patients whom we dislike or who make us angry. This is the usual counter transference work, except it is in a context which is skewed by illness, suffering, injustice and death. This is not a trivial difference. The same examination is appropriate for caregivers and family members [11].

We must learn to be involved enough to be authentic with patients, but not so involved that we let them invade our personal life more than rarely. Whenever it happens, we must pay attention and talk to a colleague, a mentor or a professional until it abates. We must give young therapists a lot of support because we have been there. If working in isolation, seek out peers, even if only by email, get on professional list-serves. Stay connected to them, do peer supervision if it is feasible, attend meetings and enjoy socialising as much as learning. Join a national psycho-oncology organisation or become part of the International Psycho-Oncology Society (IPOS) (www.ipos-society.org).

Recommended Reading & Resources

American Psychosocial Oncology Society (2006) in *Quick Reference for Oncology Clinicians: The Psychiatric and Psychological Dimensions of Cancer Symptom Management* (eds J.C. Holland, D.B. Greenberg and M.K. Hughes), IPOS Press, Charlottesville, VA.
A small basic handbook with handy tables, written for non-psychiatric physicians, but useful for everyone.
Holland, J.C., Breitbart, W.S., Jacobsen, P.B. *et al.* (2010) *Psycho-Oncology*, 2nd edn, Oxford University Press, New York.
A new edition of an exhaustive text, with clearly laid out sections and chapters that cover many topics.
Kissane, D.W. and Bloch, S. (2002) *Family Focused Grief Therapy*, Open University Press, Buckingham, PA.
A clear and detailed book which explains and manualises a powerful method of family therapy around the death of the patient. But it also teaches a great deal about family therapy at any time.
Rauch, P.K. and Muriel, A.C. (2005) *Raising an Emotionally Healthy Child When a Parent is Sick*, McGraw-Hill, New York.
The welfare of children in families of cancer patients is rarely optimally sustained without input from therapists or other knowledgeable health professionals. It can seem counter-intuitive and deserves some attention.
Sourkes, B.M. (1982) *The Deepening Shade: Psychological Aspects of Life-Threatening Illness*, University of Pittsburgh Press, Pittsburgh, PA.
A short and elegant classic that discusses both therapy and the needs of the therapist. As good now as when it first came out.
Wise, M.G. and Rundell, J.R. (eds) (2005) *Clinical Manual of Psychosomatic Medicine: A Guide to Consultation-Liaison Psychiatry*, American Psychiatric Publishing, Inc., Washington, DC.

A short, well organised and readable manual that covers other diseases as well as cancer. Will be useful to therapists with a less specialised practice.

References

1. Peabody F.W. (1927) The care of the patient. *Journal of the American Medical Association*, **88**, 872–882.
2. Institute of Medicine (IOM), Committee on Psychosocial Services to Cancer Patients/Families in a Community Setting, Board on Health Care Services (2008) in *Cancer Care for the Whole Patient: Meeting Psychosocial Health Needs* (eds N.E. Adler and A.E.K. Page), The National Academies Press, Washington, DC.
3. Alliance for Quality Psychosocial Care http://www.cfah.org/activities/alliance/cfm, Access, 2010.
4. Holland, J.C., Greenberg, D.B. and Hughes, M.K. (2006) *Quick Reference for Oncology Clinicians: The Psychiatric and Psychological Dimensions of Cancer Symptom Management*, IPOS Press.
5. Lederberg, M.S. (2010) Negotiating the interface of psycho-oncology and ethics, in *Psycho-Oncology*, 2nd edn (eds Holland, J.C., Breitbart, W.S., Jacobsen, P.B. *et al.*), Oxford University Press, Oxford, NY, pp. 625–629.
6. Miller, K. and Massie, M.J. (2010) Depressive disorders, in *Psycho-oncology*, 2nd edn (eds Holland, J.C., Breitbart, W.S., Jacobsen, P.B. *et al.*), Oxford University Press, Oxford, NY, pp. 311–318.
7. Lederberg, M.S. (2009) End of life and palliative care, in *Comprehensive Textbook of Psychiatry* (eds B.N. Sadock and V.A. Sadock), 9th edn, Lippincott Williams & Wilkins, Philadelphia, pp. 2353–2378.
8. Northhouse, L.L. and McCorkle, R. (2010) Spouse caregivers of cancer patients, in *Psycho-Oncology* (eds Holland, J.C., Breitbart, W.S., Jacobsen, P.B. *et al.*) 2nd edn, Oxford University Press, Oxford, NY, pp. 516–521.
9. Moore, C.W. and Rauch, P.K. (2010) Addressing the needs of children when a parent has cancer, in *Psycho-oncology*, 2nd edn (eds J. Holland *et al.*), Oxford University Press, Oxford, NY, pp. 527–531.
10. Holland, J.C., Breitbart, W.S., Jacobsen, P.B. *et al.* (2010) Psycho-Oncology, 2nd edn, Oxford University Press, New York.
11. Sourkes B.M. (1982) *The Deepening Shade: Psychological Aspects of Life-Threatening Illness*, University of Pittsburgh Press, Pittsburgh.

2 Cognitive-Behavioural Therapies in Cancer Care

David Horne[1,2] and Maggie Watson[3,4,5]

[1]Department of Medicine and Psychiatry, The University of Melbourne, Royal Melbourne Hospital, Victoria, Australia
[2]Albert Road Clinic, Ramsay Health, Melbourne
[3]The Royal Marsden NHS Foundation Trust, Sutton, Surrey, UK
[4]Institute of Cancer Research, UK
[5]Research Department of Clinical, Health and Educational Psychology, University College London, UK

2.1 Background

Cognitive Therapy (CT) and Cognitive-Behaviour Therapy (CBT) are both terms used to describe a variety of similar psychological therapies. The essential aim is to understand how a person's cognitive distortions, and subsequent irrational thinking, adversely affect their ability to cope optimally with stressful life events and then to help them to both identify their own distorted beliefs and Negative Automatic Thoughts (NATs), and to challenge these in the light of evidence from actual behaviours of both themselves and others; often leading to an improvement in mood and a reduction of depressive symptoms. Beck's work is probably the most well known as clearly showing how distortion of beliefs and thinking can lead to depression [1]. Other pioneers of CT during the 1960s and 1970s include Ellis [2], Mahoney [3] and Meichenbaum [4] who all demonstrated that what we believe (even unconsciously) influences our emotions, which in turn affects our behaviour. Today, CT and CBT research provides substantial evidence demonstrating effectiveness in the treatment of many anxiety disorders and depression, for example Clark and Fairburn [5]. Evidence for the effectiveness of CT in treating depression is now so strong that it is comparable to antidepressant medication for at least mild to moderate depression and the American Psychiatric Association Practice Guidelines [6] indicated that among psychotherapy methods, CBT and interpersonal psychotherapy were the most efficacious for treatment of major depression.

More recently, the UK National Institute for Health and Clinical Excellence [7] review of Depression in Adults with Chronic Health Problems recommended the use of group CBT, individual CBT and Computer-delivered CBT. The review concluded that: (Section 7.5) '. . . the most substantial evidence base (for moderate to severe depression) is for CBT'. CBT is the treatment of choice for depression in patients with chronic health problems given the weight of evidence on efficacy. While there is limited evidence for the effectiveness of combined antidepressant treatment and CBT in depressed patients, the National Institute of Health and Clinical Excellence (NICE) review concluded that there was uncertainty about benefit in the medium-term and the potential for interactions with medications prescribed for physical health problems 'is a concern'.

Cognitive and emotional processing theories attempt to provide some scientific basis for the links between emotions, cognitions and behaviour, through theory, hypothesis testing and empirical research, for example, Wells [8]. The development of Behaviour Therapy (BT) in the late 1950s and throughout the subsequent two decades was initially focused on treating anxiety but soon, also, focused upon depression [9–11] and can be seen as an important antecedent to the later cognitive therapies. BT showed that, in some instances, focusing upon avoidant behaviours and distressful arousal, associated with learned (conditioned) fears, could lead to effective and quite brief treatments; such as, systematically exposing a person to a hierarchy of their feared stimuli (even in imagination), whilst simultaneously lowering their anxiety arousal using a form of relaxation. This became known as Systematic Desensitisation. In some instances, simple exposure whilst preventing avoidance (called 'flooding therapy' or 'implosive therapy') produced experimental extinction of fearful reactions to perceived harmful stimuli and a decrease of inappropriate avoidance or protective behaviours. These approaches had notable success particularly for the treatment of phobic anxiety and some obsessive compulsive behaviours [12].

This earlier antecedent of CT and CBT is important to bear in mind whilst working with cancer patients because phobic anxiety and obsessive thoughts and behaviours can be serious problems for a significant percentage of patients who may, for example, have acquired 'irrational' fears (i.e. exaggerated appraisals of threat associated with certain stimuli, such as needles, blood, medical settings, and so on) due to prior learned associations of pain or threat, perhaps as a result of clumsy medical experiences in childhood (conditioning) or by early modelling or social learning, for example from a parent with a phobia of blood, needles, and so on. Such fears may result in avoidance of anything that reminds the person (even unconsciously) of them and may lead to preventive action to ensure they never encounter any cues or triggers that serve as reminders. This can produce excessive rumination (worry about what might happen) or the carrying out of ritualistic (compulsive) behaviours as a form of protecting themselves from ever encountering any threat. The use of behavioural interventions, such as Systematic Desensitisation for cancer patients with medical phobias, may be crucial to the acceptance of an important cancer treatment [13]. In some instances such psychological intervention, prior to undergoing medical or surgical treatments, may actually contribute to saving a person's life because, without it, they would have avoided having what may eventually be life saving, or at least life prolonging, treatment, such as chemotherapy or radiotherapy. Certain treatments for cancer, such as chemotherapy with its associated nausea, may in themselves provide an aversive conditioning experience for a patient so that a reminder or the mere mention, or thought, of chemotherapy, even when no active treatment is taking place, can cause the patient to experience nausea and even overt vomiting [13–16].

CBT takes into account complex interactions between thoughts, feelings and behaviours, and allows the therapist to provide the cancer patient with a dynamic formulation of the problems they are experiencing. It also provides a brief structured approach to psychological treatment that relies on the collection and feedback of clinically relevant data about all three processes in order to determine where to focus an intervention most effectively at any point in time (e.g. more cognitive or behavioural), and to change this focus according to the feedback data obtained. CBT has a major contribution to make to any overall improvement to the emotional, psychological and social wellbeing of cancer patients because of its well established effectiveness in the treatment of depression, anxiety disorders and Post Traumatic Stress Disorder (PTSD) and Post Traumatic Stress Syndrome (PSS). In recent years there have been concerted attempts to introduce CBT as an effective part of enhancing the psychological care of cancer patients.

2.1.1 Target Groups

CBT is particularly useful for patients with early stage cancers but has also been used with some success in advanced and terminally ill patients. It is less appropriate in patients with organic mental syndromes such as psychosis, schizo-affective disorders or delirium. For patients showing clear evidence of severe clinical depression (e.g. as detected by using the American Psychiatric Association Diagnostic and Statistical Manual-IV [17] or similar diagnostic criteria) it may be important that anti-depressant therapy is considered initially. The patient can then be reviewed after an appropriate interval for any therapeutic benefits of anti-depressant therapy. However, for clinically depressed patients it is not always necessary to wait for any benefits of anti-depressants if the patient expresses a desire to work on problems themselves. Also, many cancer patients diagnosed with clinical depression may be reluctant to take anti-depressants for a variety of reasons including concerns about interactions with drug regimens for their cancer treatment and an associated desire to minimise taking further medications. In this situation it is worth working with the patient to use the CBT model and hold anti-depressant therapy as the second line treatment option. CBT is also effective for patients with chronic psychological symptoms and entrenched problems.

With cancer patients CBT is often adapted to allow a focus on problem-solving where issues to be resolved are targeted and worked on using techniques that impact on thinking and the degree/intensity of negative ruminations. More psychologically-minded patients (i.e. those who feel comfortable with ideas such as self-reflection, examination of their thinking; those more likely to show a tendency to be introspective, able to step back and reflect upon problems and why they are affected; more inclined to be analytic thinkers) seem to do better with cognitive techniques. Behavioural techniques are usually straightforward to grasp and seem to apply more generally across the patient spectrum. Specific problems can be targeted using CBT.

2.1.2 Procedural and Treatment Related Anxiety

Early intervention using some form of CBT, such as Systematic Desensitisation, modelling and cognitive restructuring, can effectively reduce levels of anticipatory anxiety associated with medical and surgical treatments and, also, lead to reductions in post-treatment distress, including pain. Despite few reports of this approach being used systematically for cancer patients, evidence from other patient groups shows CBT to be consistently valuable for ameliorating procedural anxiety [18–20].

2.1.3 Post-Traumatic Stress Disorder

Related to high levels of anxiety adversely affecting patients' ability to cope with treatment is PTSD [21, 22]. CBT has proven to be one of the most effective therapies for this severe emotional disorder (see: Resick, Monson and Gutner [23], for a contemporary review). So, it is important to detect its presence in cancer patients as research shows it may be quite common [24]. If left untreated a significant number of cancer patients may experience unnecessary long term distress.

2.1.4 Fatigue Management

Post-treatment fatigue is another problem some cancer patients experience that can be helped by CBT. Most commonly fatigue is reported as a result of chemotherapy or radiotherapy. Beyond chemotherapy-induced anaemia, medical research remains unclear about the pathophysiology of fatigue, but many patients do complain of it. Patients participating in a psycho-educational post Bone Marrow Transplant adjustment group, run by one of the authors (DH), agreed that the tiredness they experienced was like no other kind of tiredness they had felt in all their previous life; describing it as being like an absolute dead loss of energy or total exhaustion (see Cure Leukaemia, 2008). The use of CBT can help patients develop less catastrophic thinking about this new phenomenon, aided by sharing the experience with the group and gaining some reasonably factual information. An important component of managing the effects of fatigue is learning to monitor and moderate their behaviour in an explicit manner, so they can pace their activities and use rest/relaxation techniques to prevent the feeling of total exhaustion occurring so frequently. Exercise programmes have indicated clear benefits and where elements of CBT are used to manage resistance to continuation of exercise, such as the experience of fatigue, a more sustained effect is obtained [25].

2.1.5 Survivorship Issues

Readjustment or transition concerns are important after having experienced the emotional trauma of cancer and its treatments and research in this important area is beginning to develop [26]. In understanding the nature of stressful situations that cancer patients have to learn to manage, it is useful to differentiate between Major Life Events and Daily Hassles. Major Life Events in cancer concern the diagnosis process, the treatment of the disease itself and establishing a new 'normal' life after regular treatment has finished. The consequences of these events can be profound and the basis of extreme levels of anxiety and, sometimes, of depression or demoralisation [27]. Psychological therapy can help with these readjustment and coping issues, and CBT certainly has a role to play; particularly in helping a person to re-orient themselves in their self-appraisals and use of more adaptive coping strategies. However, perhaps surprisingly, Daily Hassles can also be a source of major distress [28] because they require constant attention and problem solving. An example of this is frequent, often externally determined, attendance at follow-up outpatient appointments which can serve as a cue, trigger or simply a reminder, that one is still a cancer patient; even when the disease is in remission. Such hassles also demand ongoing energy to overcome what might normally be seen as minor frustrations, such as finding a car park space at the hospital. This might not appear to be a major problem but when energy is low, and dependence on others is high, these routine tasks can become very stressful. So, by ascertaining the presence of NATs and less than optimal coping behaviours, using CBT may be effective in helping the patient develop both more effective styles of thinking and coping behaviours; thus reducing levels of distress. The psychological and emotional impact of cancer, therefore, remains an issue across the whole transition period from primary therapy to follow-up with consequent late or long-term effects in survivors.

2.1.6 Pain Management

Pain is an area of health care that receives much attention from both a pharmacological and psychological perspective. Cancer is no exception. There is wealth of evidence that CBT has an important contribution to pain management, particularly for chronic (duration of more than six months) pain, but also, as mentioned above, in acute pain, such as that associated with invasive procedures [29]. The CBT approach to management of chronic pain in cancer patients is not remarkably different from that used with other chronic pain conditions. However, the interpretation of pain as sinister (i.e. could be a sign of disease progression) is an idiosyncratic factor in the management of cancer pain that needs to be addressed, where it is evident.

2.1.7 Sexuality and Intimacy

One area of patient need, that is currently under assessed is the effect of cancer on intimate relationships and sexual behaviours. In a way this seems surprising since there has been much research and psychotherapeutic development in this important area of human experience since the 1960s (e.g. Masters and Johnston [30]). The use of CBT has also been shown to be effective in treating sexual dysfunction in many settings, through identifying and allaying anxieties and helping change unhelpful assumptions about sex and communication in relationships. New developments are occurring in the cancer field [D. Brandenburg, personal communication, 31]. See also Chapter by Hughes.

2.1.8 Paediatrics

The use of psychological therapies with children with cancer is an important topic. See also the chapter by Bartell and Kearney. CBT can have a useful role, if adapted appropriately; for example in managing phobic anxiety and preparation for invasive procedures [19].

2.2 Processes and Techniques

At the beginning of CBT, as with any psychotherapy, there is a clear need to ensure ample opportunity for simple *ventilation of emotions* before moving on to a more structured psychological approach. This ventilation allows the building of trust and rapport but also provides both therapist and patient with the opportunity to establish an initial process of analysis of relationships between feelings or emotions, thoughts or beliefs, and the consequences for actual behaviour; an essential exercise in reaching a clear formulation of patient needs and issues. At this early point, patients usually benefit from the process of being able to 'tell their story'. It is important, at this stage, to establish that the patient feels the need to change something about how they cope. Part of good clinical care ideally includes *an initial structured assessment* of the patient's psychological status to determine if there are any emotional or personal issues (e.g. beliefs) that could interfere with the person's ability to manage their illness and associated treatments. A good formulation will guide therapy decisions effectively.

Some understanding of the background to the presenting problems, previous coping preferences, social and contextual factors and other life stressors, need to be established at this early point through an assessment interview.

To then move forward into the therapy requires an understanding of some of the basic principles. What follows is a description of some of the more useful therapy techniques that can be used across the treatment stages.

While techniques can be divided into *cognitive* and *behavioural* it is worth keeping in mind that these are *interlinked* and influence each other. However, on occasions it may be useful to decide, together with the patient, which techniques might best be focused on the presenting problem. A simple decision tree sometimes helps (see Figure 2.1).

CBT is essentially a *collaborative therapy* which requires the therapist to be constantly aware of the patient's agenda and the need to work with this agenda to avoid therapeutic resistance. Rogerian attributes such as positive regard and warmth [32] help in the development of this collaborative relationship between patient and therapist.

Use of *Socratic questioning* is a central technique. This involves engaging the patient in a dialogue where the therapist uses questioning to encourage patients' ideas, for example by asking the patient '*How would you...? What would happen if...? Can you tell*

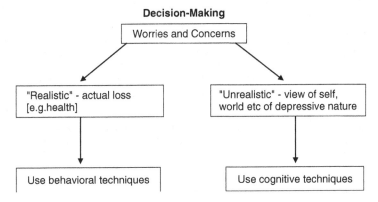

Figure 2.1 *Decision tree therapist can use to decide where to focus therapy.*

me about . . . ?' This provides a process of guided discovery.

The use of *summaries* is a helpful technique. It serves a number of purposes. For instance, the therapist can, at points throughout the session, summarise to patients what they have understood so far and check whether there have been any misunderstandings. It also tells the patient that the therapist has listened and tried to understand the issues/problems the patient is facing. A summary can be used towards the end of the session to help bring it to a conclusion and to clarify what goals have been agreed upon and what planning there will be by the patient between now and the next session. Patients can also be asked to summarise what has emerged from the session. This can be useful as it clarifies to the therapist what the patient interprets as the most important elements of the conversation in the session.

Introduce patients to the idea of *homework* early in therapy, that is the need to implement change in everyday life rather than seeing most change resulting from the therapeutic process within the actual session such as used in more psycho-analytic approaches. The term *'homework'* does not have to be used and, for some patients it has negative connotations. An alternative term might be, *'Mutually Agreed Between-Session Assignments'* (MABSAs). The main point is that patients grasp the idea, early on in therapy, that positive change requires their willingness to work on problems in their everyday life and that benefits derive from this work, that is, you get out what you put in.

What is important is that the patient learns new and better coping skills via actual practice in their day-to-day environment and keeps some explicit record of what they have done and how effective their new efforts have been. In this way, progress is largely through integrating the agreed elements of CBT into daily routines; the sessions with the therapist provide opportunities to reflect, review and change agreed upon aims and the more didactic elements of therapy are used in these review sessions to guide the patient towards effective techniques for change.

2.2.1 Cognitive Techniques

A significant part of CBT is the *self-monitoring of thoughts* using a diary (see Figure 2.2) of feelings and behaviour and carrying out *behavioural experiments* [33] to see what actually works between therapy sessions. It is quite usual for the therapist to provide some patient education which includes talking through how thoughts affect mood. The use of illustrative examples from the patient's own thinking patterns is helpful in explaining the cognitive elements of therapy. This process introduces patients to the skills model of coping. Include descriptions of identifying *NATs and thinking errors;* list classic thinking errors, for example all/nothing thinking, selective attention, should/oughts, negative predictions, and so on.

A leaflet describing thinking errors can help at this point (see Table 2.1). Introduce the patient to *cognitive re-structuring;* think of using *'hot'* cognitions in sessions, that is, when the patient describes an emotion or shows signs of distress, ask them gently to talk through what they are thinking that causes them to feel this way. You can illustrate quickly how the thoughts are linked with the emotions. Describe the use of *thought diaries for monitoring NATs*, that is, thoughts are recorded and emotions described in a diary. The diary can be used to link coping techniques to changes in thoughts and mood and can be reviewed with patients in the sessions.

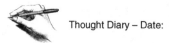

Thought Diary – Date:

Situation	Thoughts	Feelings	Behaviour
Where were you? What were you doing? Who was with you?	What were you thinking/saying to yourself?	Describe your emotions and rate the strength of these feelings from 0 to 10	What did you do? How did you respond to the problem?
Watching TV programme about cancer	*"What if the cancer comes back?"* *"I am not coping as well as those people – I am useless"*	*Anxious – 9/10* *Sad - 6/10*	*Went to bed to escape, unable to get to sleep*

Figure 2.2 *Diary for negative automatic thoughts.*

Table 2.1	Thinking errors applied to cancer patients	
Type	**Definition**	**Cancer examples**
Black or white	Viewing situations, people or self as entirely bad or entirely good – nothing in between.	'My family never understands my needs. They never get it!'
Exaggerating	Making self-critical or other-critical statements that include terms like *never, nothing, everything* or *always*.	'I always get the worst possible side-effects from chemo.'
Filtering	Ignoring the positive things that occur to and around self but focusing on and accentuating the negative.	'I'm sure that Tamoxifen will give me clots travelling to my lungs.'
Discounting	Rejecting positive experiences as not being important or meaningful.	'My oncologist was reassuring, but he's just trying to lift my morale.'
Catastrophising	Blowing expected consequences out of proportion in a negative direction.	'Although they say my prognosis is good, I'm sure that I'll die from this cancer.'
Judging	Being critical of self or others with a heavy emphasis on the use of *should have, ought to, must, have to* and *should not have*.	'My doctor should not keep me waiting for my appointment. He ought to know I keep to precise time.'
Mind reading	Making negative assumptions regarding other people's thoughts and motives.	'That worried look on that nurse's face must mean I'm in trouble with this cancer.'
Forecasting	Predicting events will turn out badly.	'This cancer is destined to return. I'm doomed.'
Feelings are facts	Because you feel a certain way, reality is seen as fitting that feeling.	'I am very sad about getting these chemo side-effects and so this illness is certain to turn out badly for me.'
Labelling	Calling self or others a bad name when displeased with a behaviour.	'I'm such a fool when I forget to ask my doctor the questions I have written out in my pocket.'
Self-blaming	Holding self responsible for an outcome that was not completely under control.	'Getting cancer is my fault as I've let too much stress affect my life.'

Table adapted from 'Negative Thoughts Trigger Negative Feelings' worksheet in Adult Psychotherapy Homework Planner. Jongsma, A.E (Eds.), 2004 to apply to cancer patients.

The therapist also needs to consider the role of 'meta-cognitions' (i.e. overarching themes in thinking) and the importance of core beliefs (see case presentations for details) which may be difficult to change; sometimes these *core beliefs* have to be worked with rather than changed.

2.2.2 Behavioural Techniques

Behavioural techniques often give rapid symptom relief and can be used by most patients without the need to be highly introspective or reflective. Techniques include; *activity scheduling* and *distraction* with use of a diary sheet.

2.2.2.1 Activity scheduling with use of diary sheet

Initially, the patient can be asked about whether they feel able to complete a diary for a one or two week period which lists the things they are doing and their associated mood. This can be used by therapists both as a baseline for amount of activity and for understanding the patient's current mood and the results used as patient feedback in the therapy session. In this way the therapist can see quickly and easily how under-occupied the patient might be (if this is the case) and, also, how mood differs depending on what the patient is doing.

When patients are diagnosed with cancer, normal daily activities can be disrupted. Activity is a process of negotiating with the patient what normal routines are possible to put back into their life (see case presentation for examples).

2.2.2.2 Distraction

Distraction is a useful mood limiting technique that most patients can use. It is helpful to talk with patients about their experiences. Methods that can be used here include asking patients to notice any variability in mood and whether this is linked to distracting activities (i.e. behaviour). The patient can be introduced to the idea of *'thought stopping'*, that is techniques and actions that limit difficult and uncomfortable thoughts. While this focuses on cognitive processes the techniques are often behavioural as they involve the patient in changing something about what they do and/or their routines in order to have the effect of stopping the uncomfortable thoughts.

2.3 Case Examples

2.3.1 Case A

A 41-year-old married woman, presented four weeks post diagnosis of breast cancer. She had had a unilateral mastectomy but the operation was complicated. Chemotherapy was being advocated but she was finding this prospect very upsetting.

She had a complex history, including a reversal of a tubal ligation when re-marrying after an unhappy first marriage. This led to a successful pregnancy and birth of an 'adorable daughter' (now five years old), but she had a subsequent traumatic miscarriage at 12 weeks into a later pregnancy, with much blood loss, blood transfusions and a five-day inpatient hospital stay.

A key critical event was her mother saying, 'It is all your fault for trying for another baby. You should have been content with x'.

The NATs to this were:

> *It is all my fault.*

> *I am convinced totally I have caught something from the transfusion.*

These were associated with a feeling of *'being guilty about everything'*.

The treatment plan comprised:

1. Being asked to write a brief autobiography to obtain some perspective on her life/her family of origin and her mother.

2. Explaining the Lazarus and Folkman [34] coping model (Primary and Secondary appraisals to threat stimuli) to her (psycho-education). The use of the coping strategies was discussed such as: Planned Problem Solving, Emotion Focused Coping and Meaningfulness Coping.

3. Then introducing her to the nature of CBT, including the types of cognitive distortions or 'thinking errors' (NATs) that are common (see Supporting materials on page 22).

4. Encouraging her to identify and map out her NATs and produce more constructive and useful thoughts and behaviours (Planful Problem Solving).

5. Training in relaxation techniques, including the use of autogenic imagery [35, 36]. See also Chapter 5.

By session 3 (six weeks post diagnosis), she was coping well with chemotherapy and acknowledging this to herself. However, she had become focused upon how unhappy her childhood was, mainly because her mother was always threatening to walk out on her children because of her own unhappy relationship with her husband.

She also admitted that working on her NATs was hard work. But she persevered with the agreed MABSA of self-monitoring and counteracting her

NATs and using relaxation to decrease her anxious arousal levels.

At session 4 (10 weeks post diagnosis), she reported she was coping reasonably well and she, her husband and five-year-old daughter were going to have a three-day beach holiday. She no longer believed or 'felt' the cancer was her fault and was no longer angry with her mother. She reported she was more able to see life from her mother's perspective, which made her threats of leaving more understandable. She also said she was able to give herself permission to be upset without feeling guilty and she continued to use her new skills, learned from CBT, to manage life better on a daily basis. Four sessions of CBT, albeit spread over 10 weeks, was all that was required to change breast cancer and its treatment from a major threat to something to be managed whilst working on enjoying life with her husband and 'adorable daughter' to the maximum.

2.3.2 Case B

Mrs. A had given up her main social activity, which was golfing, due to her mastectomy and worries that she would not be able to limit her upset when talking with friends at her golf club.

Two elements were targeted for therapy:

1. A behavioural experiment: [33] where she was asked if she could test the idea that going into the golf club to meet friends for coffee always leads to her emotions becoming out of control. This also involved having a strategy for how to deal with being upset, that is, going to the ladies room to take some moments to recover her composure and explaining to friends, in advance, that if she didn't feel up to it she would not stay. In this way she did not need to explain herself at the time when she was more emotionally fragile. She was also encouraged to make repeated attempts, if possible using a graded approach, that is, initially using 10 minute visits, gradually increasing in length, as a way of normalising the situation.

2. Goal-setting: Exploring how would she be able to join her friends on the golf course without playing herself? The patient was asked to consider how this might work in a brain storming session with the therapist. A plan emerged of setting modest targets in order to avoid any failure experiences that would reinforce her feelings of helplessness and lack of engagement in usual activities.

At this goal-planning session, she was able to consider phoning a friend in advance and asking about

doing some walking round the course with them for about half-an-hour. She was also considering meeting them outside the club house towards the end of their game and joining them at that point.

She was encouraged to use *flexible planning* and asked to consider having a Plan B, so that if Plan A proved to be too difficult, there was another option. In this way she was encouraged to *review her goals* and test out what she could realistically cope with.

The idea that this could allow her a sense of success and progress was emphasised. The notion that helplessness and low mood was linked to failure to control aspects of normal life was discussed in the session.

The aim of the behavioural experiment in enhancing her sense of control was discussed. The solutions were not suggested by the therapist; rather *the patient was encouraged in the session to explore how she might tackle the problem*.

Solutions offered by the therapist may not be helpful for three reasons:

1. The patient is more likely to find barriers to change when plans are not linked to self-generated ideas.

2. It disempowers the patient whose sense of control is more likely to be enhanced if they have generated their own ideas.

3. Finally, the patient is more likely to generate ideas that are part of their normal life.

At the next session she described telephoning her friend to ask about joining them for some of the nine holes of the golf round. The friend actively encouraged her to join them at the beginning to see how she managed with the proviso she could leave early if it was too much. She described how together, she and the friend came up with a plan whereby the friend would help the patient achieve the round of golf by doing the drives, leaving the patient to do the easier swings. In this way she was able to do nine holes without being too limited by her breast surgery. She described how she then entered the club house at the end of the game of golf and only realised later that she had not been upset at all and had felt quite normal.

Possible setbacks were discussed in therapy sessions so she could anticipate and build upon success experiences and maintain her sense of control over normal activities of life.

Further goal-setting was planned including a discussion of behavioural techniques that she might use. Towards the end of therapy the discussion was focused on whether the patient now felt able to use the methods she had acquired through therapy and apply these independently to any future issues. Once the patient was able to express confidence in her coping abilities, she was discharged with the proviso that, should she encounter difficulties, it would be possible to return for further consolidation sessions.

2.4 Evidence on Efficacy

Greer *et al.* [37] showed that CBT adapted as an individualised therapy for cancer patients (Adjuvant Psychological Therapy) could significantly reduce anxiety and helplessness compared to a no treatment control group. This was one of the earliest large randomised controlled trials evaluating CBT with screened cancer patients. Subsequent studies have focused on evaluation of application to the group context [38, 39], application to specific cancer problems such as insomnia [40] and efficacy linked to delivery by type of professional [41]. Overviews have generally concluded that there is sufficient efficacy with cancer patients [42–44] but further evidence with large samples using RCTs is still indicated. There is very little evidence on cost effectiveness as yet in the cancer context, although Simpson *et al.* [45] were able to demonstrate modest cost-offsets of CBT groups for breast cancer patients. An advantage of CBT, demonstrated clearly by a number of studies, is its utility to bring positive benefits over a relatively short number of sessions [37, 46]. The gold standard for psychotherapy research is based on the randomised controlled trial and outcome studies based on RCTs will continue to provide the type of evidence that service commissioners seek.

2.5 Service Development

The provision of effective interventions raises questions about who is able to deliver what type of counselling, support or actual psychological therapy. In some countries, national guidelines are being developed on the level of formal psychosocial skills required of all health care professionals working in cancer care (e.g. NICE, UK [47]). Once such standards of care are established, there arise major implications for the training of both the psycho-social professionals working in cancer care, including psychologists, psychiatrists, social workers, and so on, and, also, those professions with little formal training in psychological aspects of care. Thus, different levels of skills need to be clearly defined and appropriate training and supervision provided, as with the four tier system advocated in the UK [47]; a stepped model of care ranging from general psychological support at level 1 through to specialist psychological and psychiatric interventions at level 4.

In the UK the programme to facilitate Improved Access to Psychological Therapies (IAPT) involves providing a workforce of therapists, who have a somewhat lower level of training than clinical psychologists and psychiatrists, who can be skilled up to offer brief therapies based on efficacious methods such as CBT. This pragmatic approach is likely to become more favoured as intervention programmes for cancer patients and their families are developed and made more accessible.

2.5.1 Key Issues

2.5.1.1 Training and Supervision

Methods of therapist training and supervision need to be established. For CBT, it may be possible to use an established therapist rating scale [48] to evaluate success in training. The use of audio-taped sessions for peer supervision is a technique to be encouraged. Many organisations will require patient consent to the use of audio recordings for therapist training purposes. Observational sessions can be used so that trainee therapists can be observed by more experienced CBT therapists and vice versa. Sharing of therapy notes in peer supervision sessions is straightforward. However, issues about patient confidentiality need to be clarified within the organisational structure when deciding upon which supervision methods are most appropriate. External supervision can be of benefit where therapists feel it important to discuss emotions and thoughts about patients which might be inappropriate to discuss with colleagues. Therapists may require time to discuss their own emotions and coping strategies (reflective practice and self-care).

2.5.1.2 Recruitment of Patients

Policies on how to reach patients with high levels of need are not limited to therapy services using CBT but are common to many services. Evidence suggests that identifying patients with high needs is complex for the staff that routinely provides cancer treatments. Service providers need to consider methods of screening for distress and psychological problems and to provide guidelines to front-line cancer staff. The provision of good information directly to patients is important. Self-referral to services should be something that is made as easy as possible for patients who want access to support. Issues about screening and distress recognition are outside the scope of this chapter but have been well described elsewhere [49–52].

2.5.1.3 Development of Outcome Assessment

It is important to ascertain how to use measures that capture the core elements of CBT [53], alongside more conventional measures of distress (e.g. Hospital Anxiety and Depression Scale [54]; Distress Thermometer [50]). All service providers need to have available evidence on efficacy of outcomes. This can be achieved through audit or research. Individual patient (i.e. N = 1) outcomes can also be used, especially if systematic measures are used from the first contact with the patient, such as the Distress Thermometer.

2.5.1.4 Who Will Deliver the Therapy?

This raises issues about use of CBT by non-mental health professionals. However, there is a need for skill-sharing with nurses, allied health professions (e.g. social workers, occupational therapists) and doctors to have some understanding of the model and techniques so that they can use these in a limited, but effective way within their regular clinical practice. In the UK this is being achieved through the IAPT programme driven by the need to provide accessible and cost effective psychological treatments for those who may benefit.

2.6 Summary

We have presented a brief account of the theoretical and research bases of CBT and its relevance to contemporary adjunctive psychological therapies for patients experiencing cancer and the associated medical treatments. It was demonstrated that early developments in BT have implications for the use of behavioural interventions in cancer, including treating aspects of anxiety (e.g. medical phobias), but also, in helping rehabilitation of patients to achieve the most normal level of lifestyle possible following treatment of cancer.

Cognitive therapies, with their early focus on depression, highlighted the importance of understanding the interactions between unhelpful, automatic thoughts and assumptions people may have about themselves because of the negative consequences of these on their mood state, which, in turn, strongly affects their coping behaviours. Powerful, negative thoughts and feelings are naturally common in people with cancer but can lead to significant levels of psychiatric disorder [24]. There is some evidence that cancer clinicians are better at detecting anxiety than depression, but are not particularly good at either. However, unrecognised and, therefore, untreated anxiety and depression, can significantly negatively impact a cancer patient's ability to cope with the disease and its distressful physical treatments.

CBT provides a flexible but structured approach to psychological therapy for cancer patients. It allows the treatment emphasis to shift between cognitive or behavioural modalities according to patient need, as determined by feedback obtained from between therapy monitored activities, including completing rating scales of thoughts and feelings in association with an activity diary. CBT has been shown to have a strong evidence-base to the extent of being as effective, and sometimes even more effective, as psychotropic medication. This is especially true for depression.

Specific target groups of cancer patients were identified where CBT is of particular use, including: procedural and treatment-related anxiety, fatigue management, both acute and chronic pain, sexuality and intimacy and, last but not least, longer term survivorship issues. A brief guide to the processes and techniques of CBT was provided, along with a couple of case examples that illustrated both behavioural and cognitive interventions. Finally, some comments were offered about how to implement service delivery of psychological support to cancer patients.

2.7 Supporting Materials

Supporting materials have generally been developed from mainstream CBT and adapted for use with cancer patients. These include: (i) diaries for NATs used to guide patients towards awareness of how thinking impacts mood and allows for the recording of coping techniques (Figure 2.2). (ii) lists describing thinking errors (Table 2.1).

Other more specific materials (can be obtained direct from the authors) include:

- DVD Stem Cell Transplant: A Users' Guide. E-mail: cureleukaemia@mac.com;

- Pamphlet – Managing Nausea and Anxiety associated with chemotherapy. E-mail: cancer.psycholgy@uhb.mhs.uk;

- CBT-based patient guide (Watson M. and White C. *'Coping with Cancer: A Patient Guide©'*. E-mail: maggie.watson@rmh.nhs.uk.

References

1. Beck, A.T. (1976) *Cognitive Therapy and the Emotional Disorders*, International Universities Press, New York.
2. Ellis, A. (1962) *Reason and Emotion in Psychotherapy*, Lyle Stuart, New York.

3. Mahoney, M. (1974) *Cognition and Behaviour Modification*, Ballinger, Cambridge.

4. Meichenbaum, D. (1977) *Cognitive Behavior Modification: An Integrative Approach*, Plenum Press, New York.

5. Clark, D.M. and Fairburn, C.G. (eds) (1997) *The Science and Practice of Cognitive Behaviour Therapy*, Oxford University Press, Oxford.

6. American Psychiatric Association (2000) *Diagnostic and Statistical Manual of Mental Disorders, Text Revision (DSM-IV-TR)*, 4th edn, American Psychiatric Association, Arlington, VA.

7. (2009) Depression in Adults with a Chronic Physical Health Problem: Treatment and Management. National Clinical Practice Guideline Number 91. National Collaborating Centre for Mental Health commissioned by the National Institute for Health and Clinical Excellence.

8. Wells, A. (2000) *Emotional Disorders and Metacognition. Innovative Cognitive Therapy*, John Wiley & Sons, Ltd, Chichester.

9. Lewinsohn, P.M. (1974) A behavioural approach to depression, in *The Psychology of Depression: Contemporary Theory and Research* (eds R.J. Friedman and M.M. Katz), Winston, Washington, DC, pp. 157–185.

10. Rachman, S.J. (1997) The evolution of cognitive behaviour therapy, in *The Science and Practice of Cognitive Behaviour Therapy* (eds D.M. Clark and C.G. Fairburn), Oxford University Press, Oxford, pp. 3–26.

11. Wolpe, J. (1958) *Psychotherapy by Reciprocal Inhibition*, Stanford University Press, Stanford.

12. Rachman, S.R. and Hodgson, R.J. (1980) *Obsessions and Compulsions*, Prentice-Hall.

13. Horne, D.J.de L., McCormack, H.M., Collins, J.P., Forbes, J.F. & Russell, I.S. (1986) Psychological treatment of phobic anxiety associated with adjuvant chemotherapy. *The Medical Journal of Australia*, **145**, 346–348.

14. Horne, D.J.de L. and Coombes, E.A. (2007) Vomiting and nausea, in *Cambridge Handbook of Psychology, Health and Medicine*, 2nd edn (eds S. Ayers, A. Baum, C. McManus *et al.*), Cambridge University Press, Cambridge, pp. 929–931.

15. Morrow, G.R. and Dobkin, P.L. (1988) Anticipatory nausea and vomiting in cancer patients undergoing chemotherapy treatment: prevalence, etiology and behavioral interventions. *Clinical Psychology Review*, **8**, 517–556.

16. Watson, M. (1993) Anticipatory nausea and vomiting: broadening the scope of psychological treatments. *Support Care Cancer*, **1**, 171–177.

17. American Psychiatric Association (1994) *Diagnostic and Statistical Manual of Mental Disorders (DSM-IV)*, 4th edn, American Psychiatric Association, Washington, DC.

18. Horne, D.J.de L., Vatmanidis, P. and Careri, A. (1994a) Preparing patients for invasive medical and surgical procedures 1: adding behavioural and cognitive interventions. *Behavioural Medicine*, **20**, 5–13.

19. Horne, D.J.de L., Vatmanidis, P. and Careri, A. (1994b) Preparing patients for invasive medical and surgical procedures 2: using psychological interventions with adults and children. *Behavioural Medicine*, **20**, 15–21.

20. Johnston, M. and Vogele, C. (1993) Benefits of psychological preparation for surgery: a meta-analysis. *Annals of Behavioural Medicine*, **15** (4), 245–256.

21. Brewin, C.R., Watson, M., McCarthy, S. *et al.* (1998) Memory processes and the course of anxiety and depression in cancer patients. *Psychological Medicine*, **28**, 219–224.

22. Kangas, M., Henry, J. and Bryant, R. (2002) Posttraumatic stress disorder following cancer: a conceptual and empirical review. *Clinical Psychology Review*, **22**, 499–524.

23. Resick, P.A., Monson, C.M. and Gutner, C. (2007) Psychosocial treatments for PTSD, in *Handbook of PTSD: Science and Practice* (eds M.J. Friedman, T.M. Deane and P.A. Resick), The Guilford Press, New York, pp. 331–358.

24. Smith, M.Y., Redd, W.H., Peyser, C. and Vogl, D. (1999) Post traumatic stress disorder in cancer: a review. *Psycho-Oncology*, **8** (6), 521–537.

25. Courneya, K.S. (2009) Physical activity in cancer survivors: a field in motion. *Psycho-Oncology*, **18**, 337–342 (Editorial special issue physical activity in cancer survivors).

26. Brennan, J. (2001) Adjustment to cancer – coping or personal transition. *Psycho-Oncology*, **10**, 1–18.

27. Kissane, D.W., Wein, S., Love, A. *et al.* (2004) The demoralization scale: a report on its development and preliminary validation. *Journal of Palliative Care*, **20**, 269–276.

28. Ho, S. (1999) Development of a stress and coping model of bone marrow transplantation procedures. Unpublished Ph.D. thesis. University of Melbourne, Victoria, Australia.

29. Morley, S. (2007) Pain management, in *Cambridge Handbook of Psychology, Health and Medicine*, 2nd edn (eds S. Ayers, A. Baum, C. McManus *et al.*), Cambridge University Press, Cambridge, pp. 370–374.

30. Masters, W.H. and Johnson, V.E. (1966) *Human Sexual Response*, Little Brown, Boston.

31. Hersch, J., Juraskova, I., Price, M. and Mullan, B. (2009) Psychosocial interventions and quality of life in gynaecological cancer patients: a systematic review. *Psycho-Oncology*, **18**, 795–810.

32. Rogers, C.R. (1951) *Client-centred Therapy*, Houghton-Mifflin, Boston.

33. Bennett-Levy, J., Butler, G., Fennell, M. *et al.* (2004) *Oxford Guide to Behavioural Experiments in Cognitive Therapy*, Oxford University Press, Oxford.

34. Lazarus, R.S. and Folkman, S. (1984) *Stress, Appraisal and Coping*, Springer, New York.

35. Horne, D.J.de L., Taylor M. and Varigos, G. (1999) The effects of relaxation with and without imagery in reducing anxiety and itchy skin in patients with eczema. *Behavioural and Cognitive Psychotherapy*, **27**, 143–151.

36. Walker, L.G., Walker, M.B., Ogston, K. *et al.* (1999) Psychological, clinical and pathological effects of relaxation training and guided imagery during primary chemotherapy. *British Journal of Cancer*, **80**, 262–268.

37. Greer, S., Moorey, S., Baruch, J.D.R. *et al.* (1992) Adjuvant psychological therapy for patients with cancer: a prospective randomized trial. *British Medical Journal*, **304**, 675–680.

38. Edelman, S., Bell, D.R. and Kidman, A.D. (1999) A group cognitive behaviour therapy programme with metastatic breast cancer patients. *Psycho-Oncology*, **8**, 295–305.

39. Watson, M., Fenlon, D. and McVey, G. (1996) A support group for breast cancer patients: development of a cognitive-behavioural approach. *Behavioural and Cognitive Psychotherapy*, **24**, 73–81.

40. Savard, J., Simard, S., Ivers, H. and Morin, C.M. (2005) Randomized study on the efficacy of cognitive-behavioural therapy for insomnia secondary to breast cancer, part I: Sleep and psychological effects. *Journal of Clinical Oncology*, **23**, 6083–6096.

41. Moorey, S., Hotopf, M., Monroe, B. *et al.* (2007) Can home care nurses apply CBT methods in their home visits with terminally ill patients? A randomized controlled trial. *Psycho-Oncology*, **16**, S1–S287, 19A.

42. Newell, S.A., Sanson-Fisher, R.W. and Savolainen, N.J. (2002) Systematic review of psychological therapies for cancer patients: overview and recommendations for future research. *Journal National Cancer Institute*, **94**, 558–584.

43. Rehse, B. and Pukrop, R. (2003) Effects of psychosocial interventions on quality of life in adult cancer patients: meta analysis of 37 published controlled outcome studies. *Patient Education and Counselling*, **50**, 179–186.

44. Tatrow, K. and Montgomery, G.H. (2006) cognitive behavioural therapy techniques for distress and pain in breast cancer patients: a meta-analysis. *Journal of Behavioral Medicine*, **29** (1), 17–27.

45. Simpson, J.S.A., Carlson, L.E. and Trew, M.E. (2001) Effect of group therapy for breast cancer on healthcare utilization. *Cancer Practice*, **9** (1), 19–26.

46. White, C.A. (2001) *Cognitive Behaviour Therapy for Chronic Medical Problems: A Guide to Assessment and Treatment in Practice*, John Wiley & Sons, Ltd, Chichester.

47. National Institute of Clinical Excellence (2004) Guidance on Cancer Services. Improving Supportive and Palliative Care for Adults with Cancer. www.nice.org.uk/csgsp. Access year 2004.

48. Blackburn, I-M., James, I.A., Milne, D.L. and Reichelt, F.K. (2001) The Revised Cognitive Therapy Scale (CTS-R): psychometric properties. *Behavioural and Cognitive Psychotherapy*, **29**, 431–446.

49. Zabora, J., Brintzenhofeszoc, K., Curbow, B. *et al.* (2001) The prevalence of distress by cancer site. *Psycho-Oncology*, **10**, 19–28.

50. Jacobsen, P.B. and Ransom, S. (2007) Implementation of NCCN distress management guidelines by member institutions. *Journal of the National Comprehensive Cancer Network*, **5**, 99–103.

51. Mitchell, A.J., Kaar, S., Coggan, C. and Herdman, J. (2008) Acceptability of common screening methods used to detect distress and related mood disorders – preferences of cancer specialists and non-specialists. *Psycho-Oncology*, **17**, 226–236.

52. Mitchell, A.J., Baker-Glenn, E.A., Granger, L. and Symonds, P. (2010) Can the distress thermometer be improved by additional mood domains? Part I. Initial validation of the Emotion Thermometers tool. *Psycho-Oncology*, **19**, 125–133.

53. Moorey, S., Frampton, M. and Greer, S. (2003) The cancer coping questionnaire: a self-rating scale for measuring the impact of adjuvant psychological therapy on coping behavior. *Psycho-Oncology*, **12**, 331–344.

54. Zigmond, A.S. and Snaith, R.P. (1983) The hospital anxiety and depression scale. *Acta Psychiatrica Scandanavica*, **67**, 361–370.

3 Cognitive Analytic Therapy in Psycho-Oncology

Carolyn Pitceathly,[1] Iñigo Tolosa,[2] Ian B. Kerr[3] and Luigi Grassi[4]

[1]Psycho-Oncology Service, Christie Hospital, Maguire Communication Skills Training Unit, Christie Hospital Manchester, UK
[2]Pan Birmingham Cancer Psychology Service, Cancer Centre, Queen Elizabeth Hospital, University Hospital Birmingham, Edgbaston, Birmingham, UK
[3]Coathill Hospital, Coatbridge, Scotland, UK
[4]Department of Medical Science of Communication and Behavior, University of Ferrara and Unit of Clinical and Emergency Psychiatry, Integrated Department of Mental Health and Drug Abuse, Local Health Agency, Ferrara, Italy

3.1 Introduction

Cognitive analytic therapy (CAT) is a recently developed integrative model of psychotherapy with a major focus on relational aspects of development and psychological distress [1–3]. It is especially helpful with psychologically distressed, complex or 'hard to help' patients. CAT can also be a consultancy tool to assist stressed staff teams and services as well as patients. We consider, in this chapter, the use of CAT in different domains of psycho-oncology.

Broadly, our therapeutic approaches help patients to deal and cope with the acute distress and anxiety associated with serious and life-threatening illnesses such as cancer, and address a patient's habitual self management and coping patterns, which may otherwise compromise their coping. Models of psychotherapy need to be flexible and pragmatic, with a focus that may need to vary from the practical and behavioural to the more philosophical or existential. CAT does exactly that.

Help is sometimes needed when well-intentioned counselling and advice from staff may paradoxically provoke 'difficulty' or 'resistance'. This distresses and isolates patients, causes frustration and 'burns out' staff attempting to help, and ultimately leads to poor outcomes for medical treatment. Therapy must also address socio-cultural factors, meaningful social support and/or rehabilitation for patients with cancer.

3.2 Theoretical Background of CAT

CAT utilises an integrative model of psychological development, which stresses the social and relational formation of the self, with its potential 'psychopathology'. It was initially formulated by Anthony Ryle across several decades and further extended both theoretically and clinically by a range of other workers, most notably Mikael Leiman in Finland [1–4].

Although initially seeking to integrate psychoanalytic object relations theory with cognitive therapy, including Kelly's personal construct theory [5–7], it has been further transformed by three contributions. First, Lev Vygotsky's activity theory incorporated the role of cultural mediation and internalisation to guide the construction of the self, scaffolded with the support of an adult/other [3, 8–10]. Second, Mikail Bakhtin's notions of a dialogical self [9, 11, 12] are incorporated, where a person's thoughts are understood as an internal conversation. Third, developments from infant psychology are seminal and stress the need for active, playful, collaboration and 'companionship' [13–15].

Some key definitions will help therapists understand the CAT model:

1. *Reciprocal Roles* (RRs) are the early internalised, formative, relational experiences that develop with key figures and form a repertoire of relational styles that the person enters into throughout life.

Handbook of Psychotherapy in Cancer Care, First Edition. Edited by Maggie Watson and David W. Kissane.
© 2011 John Wiley & Sons, Inc. Published 2011 by John Wiley & Sons, Inc.

2. *Reciprocal Role Procedures* (RRPs) are the habitual coping or 'responsive' behavioural patterns that are an effort to avoid or manage the often unbearable feelings associated with experienced role positions, for example, humiliated; abused; abandoned [16].

3. *Reformulation* is a process of summarising the formative RRs and the negative or unhelpful consequences of particular RRPs as behavioural responses. It understands the source of the pattern in early experience and its relationship to the patient's recurrent intrapersonal and interpersonal difficulties. The reformulation provides a 'route map' that describes how problems occur and so, potentially, how they might be avoided.

Examples of common RRs that might describe a child's early relationships with parent or other key caregivers range from '*properly cared for (child)-properly caring for (caregiver)*' through to the other extreme of '*neglecting and abusing (caregiver)–neglected and abused (child)*'.

In its relational focus, CAT stresses the importance of 'internalisation' within a developing 'individual' of surrounding social structures and conditions, and of interpersonal experience. The outcome of this process is an 'individual' who is socially formed and constituted by these developmental interpersonal experiences and cultural values, and whose very sense of subjective self, relations with others, behaviour and values are socially-determined and relative, and for the most part unconscious. This viewpoint is further supported empirically by observational and experimental studies [15, 17].

An important corollary of the process of internalisation is that although it is an individual who experiences and presents with distress and disability, there is no such thing as individual 'psychopathology', but only 'socio-psychopathology' [18] (see Box 3.1).

3.3 CAT Concepts and Cancer

CAT concepts inform the understanding of behaviours seen with medical illness through the association between interpersonal processes in childhood and adult illness behaviour [19]. Early relationship patterns formed between a child and his or her primary caregiver are strongly re-activated by stressful situations, such as physical and/or life-threatening illness, with the purpose of maintaining close bonds with trusted others to assist coping with the illness-related dangers and fear of loss [20–22].

Box 3.1 Key Concepts of the CAT Model of Development and Psychopathology

- Predicated on a fundamentally relational and social concept of self. This implies that individual psychopathology cannot be considered apart from the socio-cultural context from which it arose and within which it is currently located.

- Early socially-meaningful experience is internalised as a repertoire of RRs influenced by individual genetic and temperamental variation.

- A RR is a complex of implicit relational memory, which includes affect and perception, and is characterised by both child-derived and parent/culture-derived poles; a role may be associated with a clear inner 'voice' or internalised conversation.

- Enactment of a RR always anticipates or attempts to elicit a reciprocal reaction from an historic or current other.

- RRs and their recurrent procedural enactments determine both subsequent interpersonal interactions and also internal dialogue and self-management.

- All mental activity, whether conscious or unconscious, is rooted in and highly determined by our repertoire of RRs.

- Human psychopathology is rooted in and highly determined by a repertoire of maladaptive or unhealthy RRs.

Cancer presents patients with multiple challenges, losses and threats. Surgical treatments may be disfiguring, chemical treatments potentially toxic and radiation therapy causes late effects. After pursuing curative treatments, many patients must manage uncertainty about the future, that is, will the cancer return? The impact of the illness and treatment may challenge patients in several domains of their lives (physical, social, emotional, psychological, spiritual), sometimes permanently. Key reciprocal relationships with cancer as the object are commonly experienced as *controlling, attacking, threatening, unpredictable – trapped, threatened, helpless*. Threats to mortality and leaving loved ones are commonly experienced as *abandoning – abandoned, isolated, alone*. Experiencing themselves in such controlled, trapped or threatened positions, patients might feel intense emotions of distress, anger, fear and guilt. For those with early experiences of neglect, abuse or trauma, including death or divorce, re-emergence of these patterns brings a powerful resonance. This re-activation of memories and intense emotional responses can be alarming and overwhelming. Emotions that had been 'boxed away' for years suddenly appear.

Each person has an established style of coping that aims to move away from any position of feeling threatened or being abandoned to lessen the intensity of otherwise unbearable emotions. Sometimes these ways of managing are effective. For example, to gain control, a patient can seek to become better informed about the illness and its treatment and may invest considerable trust and confidence in the medical team caring for them. They might think, 'I can't do anything about this illness, but it helps to know I have the best care I could have'. However, patients with prior traumatic relationships (neglectful, abandoning, attacking or abusing) may feel intensely threatened, fearful and lack confidence in achieving support and care from family, friends and health professionals. Their potential RRPs may be to withdraw and avoid treatment and hospital appointments or to be inconsistent or ambivalent about treatment plans. Staff generally experience these patients as 'difficult' because of the emotionality, disengagement or challenging interpersonal behaviours.

The usefulness of these concepts with a focus on early, internalised RRs is in keeping with recent data stressing the importance of a comprehensive understanding of the role of early relationship styles in cancer patients [23, 24]. Adverse childhood experiences can damage the ability to form supportive relationships as adults, and specifically, with clinical staff when dealing with cancer treatments [25]. Furthermore, the dysfunctional strategies patients use to cope with their cancer and their relationship with the supporting system follow RRPs [26–30]. In turn, problems interacting with staff are related to greater cancer-related traumatic stress, reduced emotional self-efficacy, less satisfaction with informational support from family, friends and spouse, and a tendency to perceive those sources of support as more aversive [31].

3.4 Process of Application of CAT in Cancer Care

CAT has been typically employed for the most part as an individual therapy offered on a time-limited basis. This time limit and the process of 'ending well' are seen as of fundamental importance (see Box 3.2). In oncology, the 'ending' of therapy may resonate with the finitude of life that patients fear. Recognising these parallels and achieving a 'good enough' ending in therapy could be a key modelling of what might be possible with family and friends if the cancer were advanced. In early stage settings, the process might facilitate consideration of what is important in life.

Box 3.2 Key Therapeutic Strategies in the Application of CAT

- Pro-active and collaborative ('doing with') style, stressing active participation of the patient.
- Non judgmental description of and insight into origins and consequences of relationship patterns (RRs) and associated dialogic voices. With more complex trauma, aim at description of various possible dissociated self states.
- Therapy offers a new way of relating with a benign, thoughtful other, which may be internalised as a new pattern of relating, and enable the exploration of new perceptions of self. This is conceived of in terms of recognition and revision of maladaptive patterns of relating.
- Therapy seeks to mutually construct written and diagrammatic tools to illustrate these relational patterns by the end of the initial phase of therapy. These serve as 'route maps' for therapy and also as narrative and validating 'testimonies' of personal strengths.
- Therapy subsequently focuses on revision of maladaptive relational patterns with their associated perceptions, affects and voices as they are evident in internal self-dialogue and self-management, through enactments in the outside world, and also as manifest in the therapy relationship ('transference' and 'counter transference').
- A range of other techniques may facilitate this, including challenging inner self dialogue, behavioural experiments, mindfulness exercises, 'empty chair' work or active processing of traumatic memories.
- Focus from the beginning on a time limited therapy, so that 'ending well' is seen as an important part of therapy (experience of new RRs), as a means of addressing issues around loss, and of avoiding protracted and collusive relationships.
- Social rehabilitation is seen as an important, although often neglected, dimension of therapy.

A typical initial contract would be of the order of 16 sessions on a weekly basis, although this schedule is flexible depending on needs and setting. A very brief CAT intervention leading to reformulation (i.e. a joint understanding and appreciation of the interpersonal origins and nature of relevant coping strategies (RRPs) and their consequences) has been used as preparation for (i) time limited group therapy [3]; (ii) as an assessment prior to recommending appropriate psychological intervention; and (iii) to provide a dynamic understanding of cancer patients in crisis.

Very brief CAT intervention (one to four sessions) that offers a reformulation of a patient's current problems and identifies the relevant RRs and RRPs can provide insights that help patients in crisis to take control and identify effective coping behaviours. An example follows:

Michael was diagnosed with leukaemia and, after admission to hospital, was refusing to eat. The nurses were concerned about his volatility and lack of motivation to do anything but sleep. They were concerned that he might be depressed but also recognised that his wife was very distressed by his irritability. He was able to identify that the diagnosis had turned his world upside down. Having been an active and enthusiastic sportsman and father, he was experiencing enforced inactivity, was unable to leave his room and had no certainty yet about his treatment plan. His young children were unable to visit. The RRs re-enacted by his illness and hospitalisation were understood as powerful attacking, controlling, confining – trapped, powerless, isolated, injured. He could see the similarity to how he responded in childhood to an overly-controlling father. He recognised that he was angry that others, including his wife, were able to leave the hospital and go on with their lives. His behaviour was aimed at re-gaining a sense of power and autonomy by refusing to eat food he would not normally choose, and rejecting family offers to bring in DVDs that he would normally enjoy because any adaptation to his situation felt like submission to the dominant, powerful other. However, these strategies also emphasised his isolation and sense of separation, and contributed to a feeling of guilt that he was so 'snappy'. The CAT reformulation of his behavioural pattern prompted him to introduce photographs and music into his room and he negotiated with staff to achieve some modification to his meals.

An increasing use of CAT has been as a common language to guide team-based care provision [3]. The use of shared contextual reformulation, either implicitly or explicitly by treating teams, has value in a variety of settings, including intensive chemotherapy, transplant and extended day hospital services. This application involves broader consultancy work, without necessarily including direct, individual therapeutic work.

Michael's experience shows the benefit of sharing such a psychodynamic formulation with staff. He agreed to ward staff being told about his difficulties with issues of control. This enabled nursing staff to respond to his behavioural patterns by providing slightly 'special' meals. More importantly, they were able to anticipate when other ward routines might present difficulties for him and modify their approach (e.g. giving him advance warning of medical procedures so that he could plan his own routines round them). So, what might have been

their critical, rejecting – criticised, rejected RRPs for Michael became valuing, respectful – valued, respected. While not a complex example, this was an effective intervention.

The therapeutic style of the therapist is proactive and collaborative, consistent with more recent findings on the nature of normal human growth and development emerging from infant psychology and also with emerging evidence about the features of successful therapies. This is particularly important in oncology where an active therapeutic alliance that is clear and coherent is extremely important to avoid reinforcing the unhelpful *expert, powerful, controlling – needy, dependent, controlled* RRP, that is often an automatic feature of patients' RRs with cancer and cancer professionals.

CAT focuses on the internalised social and relational origins of a patient's difficulties and problems (in terms of their repertoire of RRs and RRPs) and offers a means of addressing these both in general, but also as they may be enacted within the therapeutic relationship. Thus a major focus in therapy is work on what is traditionally called 'transference' and 'counter transference' (with its obvious overlap with attachment repertoire) although these are conceived of and described rather more specifically in terms of named RR enactments. The use of summary 'reformulation' letters and diagrams, or 'route maps', aid the subsequent course of therapy. In the language of Vygotsky, these letters and diagrams act as psychological tools. By making problematic RRs and RRPs explicit, there is a clear context for conversations between patient and therapist about how they are enacted in *'self to other'* and also *'self to self'* relationships.

Therapy in CAT focuses initially therefore on making sense of the formative interpersonal and social experiences to understand the RRs and related coping patterns (RRPs) emanating from them and, importantly, their consequences. The latter usually reinforce initial formative experiences in 'vicious cycles'. Many of these procedures and self states may be identified from the 'psychotherapy file' (PF), which offers a list of these based on earlier process research by Ryle and which can be completed by the patient at the beginning of therapy.

Therapy encourages patients to recognise RRPs and to try things differently in the context of a more benign and facilitating relationship. This will also ideally be internalised as an important aspect of therapy. However, this latter experience is rarely in itself enough and may actually also constitute colluding with, for example, a *'needy victim-sympathetic carer'* RR to the neglect of other more 'difficult' RR enactments. Such collusion may perpetuate or exacerbate unwittingly the difficulties with which a patient may present.

A further aim in work with extreme damage to the self is the clear depiction of various self states which a patient may experience, what provokes their switches and the consequences of coping procedures (RRPs) emanating from them. This offers a coherent overview of often confusing and distressing subjective states, which can be containing for the patient and also, through its collaborative construction, strengthens the therapeutic alliance.

Although comprehensive mapping of relational patterns is normally only attempted after several sessions, with very disturbed or distressed patients, it is often helpful to attempt a rudimentary version as quickly as possible – perhaps in the first meeting. For patient and therapist, identifying a key relational pattern can provide clarification, acknowledgement and recognition of a patient's confusing, traumatic and otherwise lonely experience.

The written narrative reformulation and the diagram (or map) in CAT are conceived of as helpful psychological tools. They provide (i) powerful summaries; (ii) imply the need to articulate 'exits' from problem patterns and (iii) support patients' attempt to try things differently. There is good evidence for the usefulness of such written tools [1, 3]. Later phases of therapy offer an opportunity to process and 'work through' often painful formative experience and possibly major losses, if appropriate. These aims may include simply not repeating familiar coping RRPs but also perhaps noting and challenging a critical inner voice.

Practical or 'behavioural' work in CAT is always undertaken in the context of a shared reformulation. This explicit and collaborative approach seeks to avoid the risk of colluding with underlying RRs (e.g. *'done to-doing to'*, *'not listened to – not listening'* and *'expected to perform-expecting to perform'*) with which patients may present. Collusion may strengthen and reinforce those RRs and result in 'resistance' to therapeutic work. For example, a patient may be reluctant to begin chemotherapy because of fears about toxic substances entering their body. If the therapist 'recommends' that the patient try one cycle of treatment to test out this hypothesis, this might reinforce *pressuring – pressured, trapped*; *overlooking – overlooked, unsupported* RRs and result in withdrawal from therapy and more emphatic reluctance to consider treatment. The therapist who listens carefully to the patient's explanation of the relevant RR (e.g. *attacking, intruding – attacked, vulnerable,*

intruded upon) maintains a *respectfully listening, clarifying – valued and listened to* RR with the patient. This, hopefully, allows for a shared exploration of the consequences of this course of action and provides an opportunity to discuss possible behavioural strategies that might help with decision-making or the feared symptoms (e.g. observational visits to the chemotherapy suite; relaxation/hypnotherapy interventions to manage anxiety; further discussion with medical staff or other patients).

Other complementary approaches can be used within a CAT framework such as dream work, creative therapies or 'empty chair' work attempting to access and process 'difficult' memories. Somatosensory approaches [32], CBT style desensitisation or approaches centred on traumatic experiences, such as Eye Movement Desensitisation Reprocessing (EMDR) can be 'nested' within a traditional CAT therapy [3]. As an integrative framework, CAT can therefore be helpful for cancer patients in enabling the use of all possible tools to help in coping with difficult situations, such as post ICU stays, traumatic isolation after bone marrow transplantation, and so on (see Box 3.3).

Box 3.3 Key Processes and Techniques Used in CAT for Cancer Patients

- Listen to the patient's story and hear about current problems. Some patients identify immediately that 'the problem' started before the cancer.
- Identify key problematic relationships and make patterns explicit.
- Take a history from earliest memories to the present day to identify the origins of any less adaptive relationships or traumatic experiences.
- Link early RRs and RRPs with current relational patterns.
- Identify that the aim of coping styles is to manage feelings associated with traumatic relationships (e.g. the fear and shame associated with feeling abused, attacked, rejected, abandoned).
- Identify that these coping styles reinforce the difficult nature of experiences and feelings they aim to avoid.
- Ask patients to monitor experiences and predicaments, recognise what emotions are generated and identify interpersonal and behavioural response styles (RRPs).
- Therapist and patient identify RR patterns and RRPs that occur in therapy.
- CAT is a collaborative therapy. Any insights gained are mutually understood and shared between therapist and patient.

3.5 Supporting Materials

3.5.1 Psychotherapy File

The 'PF' offers a repertoire of examples of problematic patterns of interpersonal behaviour. For example: Low Self esteem *I feel worthless and that I can't get what I want because I will be punished, rejected or abandoned → I feel that all is hopeless → Then I give up trying to do anything → This confirms that everything is hopeless and I am worthless*. Patients identify those that seem relevant to them. How the file is completed gives additional insights into patients' difficulties and patterns. For example, patients who suppress strong feelings in relation to others may acknowledge part of the pattern but cross out emotional words such as anger. Some patients may write long explanations on the file to clarify cycles they have identified as relevant. This might be an indication that the patient has an *'overlooking – overlooked'* RRP and so is not confident that they will be understood.

3.5.2 The Letter

After about four sessions, the therapist writes a reformulation letter to the patient, summarising the understandings that have been reached about key RRs and their roots in the patient's early life, including problematic response styles that have been identified and how these are continuing to affect the patient's life and relationships. The letter predicts how these might affect the process and experience of therapy. Particularly important in the letter is the acknowledgement of the traumatic early experiences, alongside evident strengths and abilities that the patient has. The letter often has a major impact, particularly for patients who feel overlooked, uncared for and not valued. The letter honours their experience and describes their life experiences chronologically, so they become a narrative, that is heard, often for the first time, at the reading of the letter. Patients are often shocked at the therapist's understanding, even though many of these ideas and experiences have been shared in the sessions. Patients with complex problems often have little experience of someone else wanting to deeply understand their thoughts and feelings.

Reading the letter may be a poignant experience for patient and therapist because it may be the first time patients have reflected on and felt sadness and hurt for the abused or neglected child in their 'story'. Sometimes patients refuse to take the letter because it is too painful or too intimate to risk others seeing it. As with all enactments in therapy, the response informs the therapy.

Making RRs and RRPs explicit and predicting that there will be enactments of these between therapist and patient during therapy provides a clear and valuable reference point for when those enactments occur and, hopefully, allows those enactments to be recognised and understood by both patient and therapist.

3.5.3 The Diagram

Therapist and patient often begin to map out RRs and problematic RRPs in diagrammatic form from the first session, but once the reformulation letter is read and given to the patient, the diagram forms one of the major tools of therapy. Difficult experiences that the patient brings to therapy are discussed and understood in the light of the reciprocal relationships on the diagram. For instance, Stephen (see case example below) and his therapist were able to monitor how he reacted to experiences of feeling ignored or overlooked by tracking them round the diagram. This also allows patient and therapist to acknowledge 'exits', that is, occasions when the patient finds a way to 'step out' of a habitual pattern and achieve a more positive outcome.

Seeing the RRs on a diagram may be the first step to acknowledging that whilst a patient may experience being at the victim end of a *bullying – bullied, humiliated* relationship, he or she can sometimes take the bullying position to avoid feeling humiliated. Similarly, we 'internalise' our RRs from childhood and patients will speak to themselves in a harsh way (e.g. 'I'm just so stupid'). Often the work of therapy is focused on acknowledging with patients that they consistently fail to respond to themselves with respect and care.

Patients who feel unrecognised and unacknowledged often respond positively to the summary letter. Patients who feel disorganised and chaotic and who may be fearful of the lack of structure or the 'mystique' in therapy, often find the diagram very 'containing'. It describes clearly, can balance strengths with vulnerabilities and it provides potential for change. Patients who are fearful of being 'found out' can struggle to hear their difficulties clearly described and may need help developing a 'kindest and wisest' position from which they can accept their shortcomings as human and manageable, instead of destructive flaws of character.

3.5.4 Goodbye Letter

Towards the end of therapy, usually session 15 or 16 within 16 sessions of therapy, both therapist and patient write each other a letter reflecting on the changes that have taken place during therapy, naming the experiences and acknowledging when there were difficulties. Goals achieved are identified and those that are still left to be targeted in future work are acknowledged. The letter is an explicit acknowledgement that a 16-session therapy can only be 'partial', but it also gathers the positives and validates them clearly. Patients' letters often identify similar outcomes, but can be more powerful than therapists. Sometimes patients do not write the letter, perhaps because it makes the ending too 'real' or because there is a powerfully problematic RR, for example, *controlling – controlled*, and the patient is reluctant to 'conform'.

3.5.5 Monitoring

Monitoring week by week is central to the work of therapy. Patients may monitor their own response styles using *monitoring sheets* or they may keep *diaries* of events and problem situations encountered to be explored in therapy. The act of monitoring brings perspective and alerts patients to how quickly they become aware of 'going into' a problematic RRP. After a few sessions of monitoring, patients begin to find effective ways of responding differently. These achievements are also part of the monitoring process and may be included on the diagram as 'exits' from problematic patterns. Sometimes patient and therapist may think together about potential exits, but often these occur spontaneously and it always seems more effective when patients find a solution that works for them. For instance, a patient struggled with periods of depression and the 'exit' she valued most was that, given her history, she felt she had good reason to be depressed sometimes and decided to just 'accept it'. As a result, episodes of depression became less severe because she avoided becoming depressed about being depressed!

3.6 A Brief Overview of Evidence on Efficacy

As a generic form of psychotherapy with a proactive, collaborative style and with its roots in cognitive and dynamic therapies, CAT would clearly be expected to be an effective intervention. The more pertinent question – as for all current forms of therapy – will be to determine what aspects of which approach is most effective and user-friendly for what sorts of patient or problems. CAT conforms to recognised general criteria for effective therapies and, in particular, for those more 'severe and complex' and 'difficult' personality

type disorders [33, 34]. An increasingly 'formal' evidence base, both naturalistic and controlled, has been accruing over recent years, despite its relative youth as a model.

Personality disorders have been the object of several research and clinical trials [35, 36], with data showing the efficacy and the fast improvement when CAT has been added to specific interventions in comparison with treatment as usual and manualised good clinical care [37, 38]. Other psychiatric disorders, such as anorexia, emotional problems secondary to sexual abuse, self-harm behaviours and psychosis have been also been reported to respond to CAT in its classical form or adapted to specific target populations [39–42]. Some studies in cancer settings are in progress, with the aim of demonstrating the feasibility and effects of CAT and adapted CAT strategies on cancer patients in different clinical situations.

3.7 Target Groups of Patients for Whom CAT Is Appropriate

On the basis of what we have described, CAT may be useful in several oncology settings:

1. Cancer patients affected by the most common emotional disorders, such as depressive disorders (e.g. major depression, minor depression), anxiety disorders (e.g. phobia, posttraumatic stress disorder).

2. Cancer patients with personality disorders.

3. Cancer patients with problems in their relationships with staff and/or maladaptive coping (e.g. abnormal illness behaviour, non-compliance, poor self care).

4. Family members experiencing dysfunctional relational patterns during different phases of the disease, in palliative care and bereavement, when complicated grief might occur.

3.8 Case Example

This case example describes a presentation, not uncommon in oncology, where a patient's experience of early interpersonal RRs is mirrored by the reciprocal relationship with his illness. The CAT reformulation of the patient's difficulties in the form of RRs and RRPs was achieved with a collaborative therapeutic style, while Stephen's receipt of a therapy letter provided a powerful *'attentive – attended to and acknowledged'* RR. The containment achieved by a diagrammatic representation of his difficulties contributed to the identification of effective 'exits' from longstanding problem patterns of behaviour.

3.8.1 Referral

Stephen, aged 50, had requested a referral for psychological help from his General Practitioner because of his uncontrollable anger. He was married with two children at university. He had been diagnosed with colon cancer one year earlier. His treatment had involved bowel resection and six cycles of chemotherapy and, at referral, his cancer was in remission. He had been employed in the building trade, but other chronic health problems had prevented him working for 10 years and had affected both his strength and energy levels in day to day activities.

3.8.2 Previous Psychological Intervention

Before referral to the Psycho-Oncology Service, Stephen had received counselling, attended an anger management course and completed a course of CBT. He judged there to be no change in his feelings or behaviour as a result of these interventions. He was diagnosed with a depressive disorder but could not tolerate anti-depressants because of his other health problems.

3.8.3 Presenting Problems

Stephen was concerned that he was very irritable and he often provoked conflict with both acquaintances and strangers, if he experienced them as discourteous or rude. He had never been violent towards others, but on a recent occasion had lost his temper at home and smashed up the kitchen because guests rang to cancel at the last minute. He felt tense and anxious about becoming verbally aggressive in social situations, and so avoided them whenever possible.

3.8.4 Family History

Stephen was the youngest of three children and perceived himself to be quite different to his siblings. As a child, he was bright and wanted an explanation for everything, including parental decisions. In response, his parents seemed irritated and critical of him. He was regularly excluded from family activities and sent to his bedroom. He did not understand why and, in his rage at being confined and excluded, he would deface the furniture. In contrast, he felt that his achievements, especially at school were neither noticed nor valued.

These themes of inexplicable, unpredictable criticism and attack continued into adulthood, both in personal relationships and in relation to his health. He was

diagnosed with a serious and disabling illness before his cancer diagnosis, which left him unable to work, enjoy hobbies or provide support to his family. He felt angry and diminished as a husband, a breadwinner and as a man.

Two key RRs were evident in early relationships with his parents, in current adult relationships, in relation to his illnesses and to the medical and psychological care he had received:

1. Overlooking, excluding – excluded, isolated, unrecognised, worthless.

2. Unpredictable, critical, attacking – vulnerable, attacked, defenceless.

These RRs also characterised his internal dialogue with himself. He was ashamed and critical of himself when he lost his temper and when he avoided social situations because of his anxiety.

3.8.5 Reformulation

During the early sessions of therapy, Stephen and the therapist developed an understanding of his difficulties and their roots in early experience. Most importantly, they identified how his ways of managing interpersonal situations brought him back to the positions he was trying to avoid, either feeling excluded or feeling attacked and criticised but rarely, if ever, achieving what he aimed for – to feel valued and cared for. The reformulation was summarised in a letter and Stephen and the therapist began to plot the key RRs and RRPs on a diagram together (see Figure 3.1).

Stephen's RRPs:

1. Feeling worthless and wanting to avoid feelings of being overlooked and not valued:

    Either I avoid social situations altogether and feel even more isolated and excluded, or

    I enter into them feeling anxious, tense and agitated. As a result, when I feel slighted in any way, I lose my temper. I am then criticised by others and feel misunderstood and unfairly blamed.

2. "Wanting to avoid rejection, I conceal my feelings of hurt and distress when I feel I have been overlooked or treated badly. This leaves me feeling resentful of others and critical of myself for being weak. The feelings I suppress build up and I eventually 'explode' in response to a perceived offense. I recognise that my temper is out of proportion to the situation and feel ashamed."

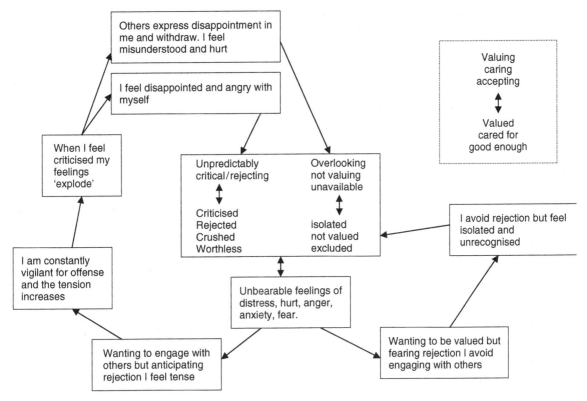

Figure 3.1 *Stephen's diagram shows how two key problematic reciprocal role procedures (RRPs) return to the problematic reciprocal role relationships (RRs) and fail to achieve the hoped for relationship.*

3.8.6 Recognition and Monitoring

Stephen began to monitor his feelings and behaviour in interpersonal situations. He realised that his behaviour towards others was either defensive or challenging. He gave no opportunity for others to be helpful or demonstrate positive regard, and so his worst expectations were regularly realised.

3.8.7 Exits from RRPs

As Stephen monitored and reported his interpersonal experiences during therapy, he became more relaxed and his speech became less pressured. This gave more opportunity for the therapist to acknowledge his experience. He risked a few social engagements and realised that friends and family valued the caring, considerate person he could often be. In spite of this, he still struggled with feelings of resentment if he felt overlooked or his opinion was challenged. He considered ways of managing those feelings and tried to show himself some care and respect when he felt excluded. So, when his wife was busy with friends,

he did something that he could enjoy alone such as a trip to a museum. He found that by providing 'self to self' acknowledgement and care, he could be the instrument of 'bringing down' feelings of anger and hurt. He accepted that he might always be sensitive to being 'overlooked'. This established a realistically valuing/accepting/caring RR with himself that was reflected in his relationship with others.

At the end of therapy, Stephen reflected on his experience in his 'goodbye' letter. He had felt heard and understood, but also had a 'description' of his problematic patterns and their roots in his early experience that was uncritical. In response to feeling recognised and accepted, he became less critical of himself and less blaming of others. There was no expectation for him to be different and so he was able to identify his own exits from the problem patterns. As the therapy was not pressuring, he was able to take time and he found that the slowing down in his speech and thoughts gave him more space to reflect and find solutions. He identified that he was also less worried about his health and the impact of his illnesses on his life.

The time limit on therapy was a challenge but he felt he could manage the feelings of loss and abandonment because he had the letters and diagram to look back on and a review session planned for three months time.

3.9 What Can CAT Offer in a Cancer Setting?

For patients:

1. A sense of being heard.

2. An explanation and validation for powerful feelings.

3. Understanding of the reciprocal relationship between their illness and other traumatic events that impact upon their sense of control.

4. Potential for change/new ways of managing.

For staff:

1. Understanding of behaviours that seem difficult or unhelpful.

2. Potential to respond in a way that will be helpful to the patients and themselves.

3.10 Service Development: Integrating CAT into Psycho-Oncology Services

CAT is widely applicable in a variety of clinical settings, and across a range of disorders and difficulties, such as depression, anxiety, personal and relationship problems, as well as more complex personality type disorders. Within the National Health Service in the UK, CAT services have been extensively developed and follow-up data show that patients treated with CAT have broadly comparable outcomes to those achieved by other well-established psychotherapy services, such as person-centred and CBT services [43].

On this basis, CAT can be readily implemented in psycho-oncology, both being valued for its flexibility and respected for its framework [44]. CAT can be modified in terms of agreed goals (e.g. focusing on specific RRPs in cancer patients), the timing (e.g. different number of sessions according to the disease stage or context, such as long-survivors of cancer vs. palliative care patients) or modality (e.g. individual vs. group, individual vs. family). Furthermore, CAT can be employed as a common language for multidisciplinary teams to understand and thus guide difficult clinical situations, as already shown in mental health settings [45, 46].

3.11 Conclusion

To summarise, CAT can offer an effective and supportive psychotherapy approach in a challenging context, both in terms of interpersonal and existential issues, and also practical coping mechanisms to better deal with illness and its treatment. It can offer a relational and systemic understanding of behaviours which may otherwise seem incomprehensible or 'difficult', and so can be helpful both to patients and staff.

Acknowledgements

The authors are indebted to Anthony Ryle and to numerous other CAT practitioners who have contributed to the development of the model and to its clinical applications. The University of Ferrara, the Fondazione Cassa di Risparmio di Ferrara and the World Psychiatric Association – Section on Psycho-Oncology and Palliative Care are also acknowledged. Carolyn Pitceathly and Iñigo Tolosa wish to thank all the patients whose therapies have informed their understanding of and enthusiasm for the application of CAT in cancer care.

References

1. Ryle, A. (1990) *Cognitive-Analytic Therapy: Active Participation in Change: A New Integration in Brief Psychotherapy*, John Wiley & Sons, Ltd, London.
2. Ryle, A. (1995) *Cognitive-Analytic Therapy: Developments in Theory and Practice*, John Wiley & Sons, Ltd, London.
3. Ryle, A. and Kerr, I.B. (2002) *Introduction to Cognitive-Analytic Therapy: Principles and Practice*, John Wiley & Sons, Ltd, London.
4. Ryle, A. (1982) *Psychotherapy: A Cognitive Integration of Theory and Practice*, Academic Press, London.
5. Ryle, A. and Lipshitz, S. (1974) Towards an informed countertransference: the possible contribution of repertory grid techniques. *British Journal of Medical Psychology*, **47**, 219–225.
6. Ryle, A. (1978) A common language for the psychotherapies? *British Journal of Psychiatry*, **132**, 585–594.
7. Ryle, A. (1985) Cognitive theory, object relations and the self. *British Journal of Medical Psychology*, **58**, 1–7.
8. Ryle, A. (1991) Object relations theory and activity theory: a proposed link by way of the procedural sequence model. *British Journal of Medical Psychology*, **64**, 307–316.
9. Leiman, M. (1992) The concept of sign in the work of Vygotsky, Winnicott and Bakhtin: further integration of object relations theory and activity theory. *British Journal of Medical Psychology*, **65**, 209–221.
10. Leiman, M. (1994) Projective identification as early joint action sequences: a Vygotskian addendum to the procedural sequence object relations model. *British Journal of Medical Psychology*, **67**, 97–106.

11. Leiman, M. (1997) Procedures as dialogical sequences: a revised version of the fundamental concept in cognitive analytic therapy. *British Journal of Medical Psychology*, **70**, 193–207.

12. Holquist, M. (2002) *Dialogism*, 2nd edn, Routledge, New York.

13. Stern, D.N. (2000) *The Interpersonal World of the Infant; A View from Psychoanalysis and Developmental Psychology*, 2nd edn, Basic Books, New York.

14. Trevarthen, C. and Aitken, K.J. (2001) Infant intersubjectivity: research, theory, and clinical applications. *Journal of Child Psychology and Psychiatry*, **42**, 3–48.

15. Reddy, V. (2008) *How Infants Know Minds*, Harvard University Press, Cambridge, MA.

16. Leiman, M. (2004) Dialogical sequence analysis, in *The Dialogical Self in Psychotherapy* (eds H. Hermans and G. Dimaggio), Brunner-Routledge, Hove, pp. 255–269.

17. Cox, B.D. and Lightfoot, C. (1997) *Sociogenetic Perspectives on Internalization*, Lawrence Erlbaum, Mahawah, NJ.

18. Kerr, I.B. (2009) Addressing the socially-constituted self through a common language for mental health and social services: a cognitive-analytic perspective, in *Confluences of Identity, Knowledge and Practice: Building Interprofessional Social Capital*, ESRC Seminar 4 Proceedings, Research Paper, 20, (eds J. Forbes and C. Watson), University of Aberdeen, Aberdeen, pp. 21–38.

19. Salmon, P. and Calderbank, S. (1996) The relationship of childhood physical and sexual abuse to adult illness behavior. *Journal of Psychosomatic Research*, **40**, 329–336.

20. Hunter, J.J. and Maunder, R.G. (2001) Using attachment theory to understand illness behavior. *General Hospital Psychiatry*, **23**, 177–182.

21. Maunder, R.G. and Hunter, J.J. (2001) Attachment and psychosomatic medicine: developmental contributions to stress and disease. *Psychosomatic Medicine*, **63**, 556–567.

22. Maunder, R.G. and Hunter, J.J. (2009) Assessing patterns of adult attachment in medical patients. *General Hospital Psychiatry*, **31**, 123–130.

23. Tacón, A.M. (2002) Attachment and cancer: a conceptual integration. *Integrative Cancer Therapy*, **1**, 371–381.

24. Tan, A., Zimmermann, C. and Rodin, G. (2005) Interpersonal processes in palliative care: an attachment perspective on the patient-clinician relationship. *Palliative Medicine*, **19**, 143–150.

25. Salmon, P., Holcombe, C., Clark, L. *et al.* (2007) Relationships with clinical staff after a diagnosis of breast cancer are associated with patients' experience of care and abuse in childhood. *Journal of Psychosomatic Research*, **63**, 255–262.

26. Grassi, L. and Molinari, S. (1987) Family affective climate during the childhood of adult cancer patients. *Journal of Psychosocial Oncology*, **4**, 53.62.

27. Schmidt, S., Nachtigall, C., Wuethrich-Martone, O. *et al.* (2002) Attachment and coping with chronic disease. *Journal of Psychosomatic Research*, **53**, 763–773.

28. Hunter, M.J., Davis, P.J. and Tunstall, J.R. (2006) The influence of attachment and emotional support in end-stage cancer. *Psychooncology*, **15**, 431–444.

29. Salmon, P., Hill, J., Krespi, R. *et al.* (2006) The role of child abuse and age in vulnerability to emotional problems after surgery for breast cancer. *European Journal of Cancer*, **42**, 2517–2523.

30. Kim, Y., Carver, C.S., Deci, E.L. *et al.* (2008) Adult attachment and psychological well-being in cancer caregivers: the mediational role of spouses' motives for caregiving. *Health Psychology*, **27** (2, Suppl.), S144–S154.

31. Han, W.T., Collie, K., Koopman, C. *et al.* (2005) Breast cancer and problems with medical interactions: relationships with traumatic stress, emotional self-efficacy, and social support. *Psychooncology*, **14**, 318–330.

32. Ogden, P., Minton, K. and Pain, C. (2006) *Trauma and the Body: A Sensorimotor Approach to Psychotherapy*, WW Norton.

33. Bateman, A.W., Ryle, A., Fonagy, P. *et al.* (2007) Psychotherapy for borderline personality disorder: mentalization based therapy and cognitive analytic therapy compared. *International Review of Psychiatry*, **19**, 51–62.

34. National Institute for Clinical Effectiveness (NICE) (2009) Borderline Personality Disorder: Treatment and Management, National Clinical Practice Guideline No 78, London.

35. Ryle, A. (1997) *Cognitive-Analytic Therapy and Borderline Personality Disorder. The Model and the Method*, John Wiley & Sons, Ltd, London.

36. Ryle, A. (2004) The contribution of cognitive analytic therapy to the treatment of borderline personality disorder. *Journal of Personality Disorders*, **18**, 3–35.

37. Chanen, A.M., Jackson, H.J., McCutcheon, L.K. *et al.* (2008) Early intervention for adolescents with borderline personality disorder using cognitive analytic therapy: randomised controlled trial. *British Journal of Psychiatry*, **193**, 477–484.

38. Chanen, A.M., Jackson, H.J., McCutcheon, L.K. *et al.* (2009) Early intervention for adolescents with borderline personality disorder: quasi-experimental comparison with treatment as usual. *Australian and New Zealand Journal of Psychiatry*, **43**, 397–408.

39. Sheard, T., Evans, J., Cash, D. *et al.* (2000) A CAT-derived one to three session intervention for repeated deliberate self-harm: a description of the model and initial experience of trainee psychiatrists in using it. *British Journal of Medical Psychology*, **73**, 179–196.

40. Clarke, S. and Llewelyn, S. (1994) Personal constructs of survivors of childhood sexual abuse receiving cognitive analytic therapy. *British Journal of Medical Psychology*, **67**, 273–289.

41. Dare, C., Eisler, I., Russell, G. *et al.* (2001) Psychological therapies for adults with anorexia nervosa: randomised controlled trial of out-patient treatments. *British Journal of Psychiatry*, **178**, 216–221.

42. Kerr, I.B., Birkett, P.B. and Chanen, A. (2003) Clinical and service implications of a cognitive analytic therapy model of psychosis. *Australian and New Zealand Journal of Psychiatry*, **37**, 515–523.

43. Marriott, M. and Kellett, S. (2009) Evaluating a cognitive analytic therapy service; practice-based outcomes and comparisons with person-centred and cognitive-behavioural therapies. *Psychology and Psychotherapy*, **82**, 57–72.

44. Strada E.A. and Sources B.M. (2010) Principles of psychotherapy, in (eds J.C. Holland, W. Breitbart, P.B. Jacobsen

et al.), *Psycho-Oncology*, 2nd edn, Oxford University Press, pp. 397–401.

45. Kerr, I.B., Dent-Brown, K. and Parry, G.D. (2007) Psychotherapy and mental health teams. *International Review of Psychiatry*, **19**, 63–80.

46. Thompson, A.R., Donnison, J., Warnock-Parkes, E. *et al.* (2008) Multidisciplinary community mental health team staff' s experience of a 'skills level' training course in cognitive analytic therapy. *International Journal of Mental Health Nursing*, **17**, 131–137.

4 Mindfulness Interventions for Cancer Patients

David K. Payne

Department of Psychology, Wallace Community College, Dothan, Alabama, USA

4.1 Introduction

The use of mindfulness as both a phenomenon and as the underpinning of psychotherapeutic interventions has grown dramatically in the Western world over the past 20 years. Due in part to the growing impact of Buddhist thought in our increasingly small global village, the concepts of Buddhism in general and mindfulness specifically have entered into the Western vernacular and experience. From this cultural introduction have flowed a variety of approaches designed to enhance quality of life.

Given the importance of the concept of mindfulness in Mindfulness-Based Stress Reduction (MBSR) and other mindfulness-based approaches, a brief exploration of this concept and a review of selected definitions is warranted. Jon Kabat-Zinn, developer of MBSR, describes mindfulness as 'paying attention in a particular way: on purpose, in the present moment and nonjudgementally' [1, p. 4]. An expanded view of mindfulness describes two components: (i) the self-regulating attention of immediate experience thereby allowing for greater awareness of mental events in the present moment; and (ii) adopting a curiosity, openness and acceptance towards one's experiences in this moment [2]. A broader and more nuanced view of mindfulness, again espoused by Kabat-Zinn, recognises that the words 'heart' and 'mind' are the same in many Asian languages and thus, to be mindful is also to be heartful, to use the heart as well as the mind as a guide to living [3].

A final point relates to a core value inherent in mindfulness-based interventions that set them apart from other psychosocial interventions. Rather than a firm distinction existing between the patient and the therapist or provider, these interventions, consonant with Buddhist belief, conceptualise people as being more alike than different. From this stance flow two observations. One, since both therapist and patient experience much of the same pain and trauma associated with life, they are more alike than different, and thus, on a more level 'playing field', rather than the power differential that typically exists in most psychotherapeutic relationships. The second observation recognises that in teaching and practicing the skills associated with mindfulness, both patient and therapist may reap benefits.

4.2 Mindfulness-Based Stress Reduction

Jon Kabat-Zinn originally developed MBSR out of his interest in mindfulness, meditation and related disciplines. He developed the Stress Reduction Clinic in the medical school at the University of Massachusetts in Worcester, where since 1979, some 18 000 individuals have completed the MBSR programme. A number of variations on MBSR have been developed, the most notable being Mindfulness-Based Cognitive Therapy (MBCT), which combines elements of MBSR with cognitive therapy to treat individuals with recurrent depression. For further information about the development of these programmes see Kabat-Zinn [4] and Segal *et al.* [5].

Although a number of variations exist, in its original form, MBSR is an eight session, manualised, group intervention that meets optimally for between 2 and 2.5 hours weekly with an 'all day of mindfulness' following the sixth session. Large numbers of patients, often ranging up to 30 or more, can participate in this

Handbook of Psychotherapy in Cancer Care, First Edition. Edited by Maggie Watson and David W. Kissane.

intervention because group interaction in this model does not necessarily constitute the essential curative element; individuals can benefit from a MBSR intervention even though they speak very little, if at all, during the course of the group session. The group serves as a vehicle in which patients participate in initial experiences with mindfulness, receive information about mindfulness and most importantly learn and practice the skills that promote the integration of mindfulness into their daily lives. In this aspect, this intervention can be useful for patients who want to learn self-regulatory skills, but do not necessarily find the ventilation of affect in a group setting to be beneficial. Group content covers an introduction to mindfulness, trouble shoots problems with the practice and offers opportunities to engage in these practices in the group session; continued home practice is essential to receiving optimal benefit from the intervention.

4.2.1 The Role of the Therapist in Mindfulness-Based Interventions

What therapist attitudes facilitate the use of mindfulness-based interventions? The mastery of psychotherapy usually requires the acquisition of knowledge related to the mechanics of the intervention, coupled with experience in delivering the intervention; personal use of the intervention is not usually considered to be necessary. The attitude in mindfulness-based interventions differs from this usual approach. In order for the teaching and discussion of these skills to be authentic, the leader needs to be personally familiar with the use of these skills. The therapist's experience with these skills lends credibility in teaching the skills. The obvious benefit for psycho-oncologists who incorporate these mindfulness skills into their daily lives is a reduction in the unrecognised or untreated psychological distress intrinsic to this field. Some therapists worry that personal discussion of these experiences may lead to breaching therapeutic boundaries. This need not occur as the knowledge and practice of these skills, given their focus on the here and now, do not necessarily lead to self-disclosure or other distortions in the therapeutic frame.

During the MBSR or therapy session, the therapist introduces these skills, helps to integrate them into daily functioning, reinforces the importance of home practice and trouble shoots with participants any of their difficulties in continuing with these skills. Although the therapist or group leader may be enthusiastic about these skills, not uncommonly participants report that the skill is 'boring', or that they can't find

time to practice the skill. For most patients, continued practice leads to positive benefit, so in the initial stages, the goal involves keeping the patient engaged in practicing the skills. Not unlike the challenge found in teaching any mind-body skill, leaders need to be persuasive in encouraging continuation of these mindfulness practices.

4.2.2 Target Populations

Originally conceptualised as an intervention to address stress related problems in general medical patients or patients with psychosomatic concerns, MBSR has expanded to successfully address the concerns of individuals with a wide range of psychological, physical and social problems. A variety of modifications of MBSR exist that address the problems of discrete populations or utilise specific techniques (e.g. MBCT as discussed for individuals with recurrent depression, or MBAT, Mindfulness-Based Art Therapy). The only requirement for participation in mindfulness approaches in psychotherapy or MBSR, aside from patient willingness, is a cognitively intact patient. Thus, this approach has usefulness for patients with all types and stages of cancer.

4.3 Content and Processes of Mindfulness-Based Interventions

The eight sessions of MBSR provide the opportunity for patients to learn and practice a variety of mindfulness skills that they will hopefully acquire and integrate into their everyday lives. The MBSR group format serves as a holding environment permitting patients to gain enough experience in the practice of the skills so they can continue following completion of the group. The eight sessions cover themes that explicate the concepts of mindfulness and provide a number of mindfulness-based skills that participants practice during the intervention and continue with following the completion of the programme.

A model developed by Shapiro and Carlson [6] encompasses the goals common to most mindfulness interventions and provides a helpful way to view the specific impact of any of the mindfulness practices taught. These objectives include: intention, attention and attitude. *Intention* involves understanding why the patient chooses to engage in mindfulness skills. Initially, the goal may be stress reduction but frequently, as the patient continues with these practices, they find that their intention moves from self-regulation to self-exploration. As they move to this phase, the patient's intention may evolve to clarify personal values, whether these values are wholesome and whether they will lead to healthy development in the individual. Not uncommonly as individuals continue with their practice of mindfulness skills, healthy physical and mental habits or behaviours are reinforced, whereas participants become more conscious of unhealthy habits or responses and may choose to change or delete these from their behavioural or emotional repertoires.

The second objective, *attention*, involves the moment by moment observation of one's internal (physical and psychological) and external experience. In this process, one cultivates a non-reactive, sustained and concentrative attention. A non-reactive attention involves seeing the events of one's mind or external world as they actually are rather than through the filters of cognitive distortion, (e.g. choosing to observe and view the contents of the mind as possibly transient perceptions rather than hard facts). Being willing to sustain an in-depth look at the phenomena of both inner and external world characterises a sustained and concentrative approach to attention.

Attitude involves the 'how' of the practice of mindfulness. It involves approaching not only oneself, but the world and the future with a sense of compassion, acceptance and curiosity. Rather than noticing with a sense of anxiety and disappointment that one is again fearful of a recurrence of cancer, choosing instead to adopt an attitude of compassion, acceptance and nonjudging about oneself and this awareness. Another aspect of a mindful attitude includes having a beginner's mind or seeing experiences through 'fresh eyes' rather than saying, 'I know all about this.' Other helpful and mindful attitudes include patience, trust, nonattachment (letting go of a predetermined view of the outcome of any event and being willing to let the process unfold) and loving-kindness (cultivating a sense of love and benevolence towards oneself and the world).

The mindfulness skills discussed below can be used to cultivate these attitudes and achieve these goals. An interesting aspect of this process is that with continued practice, patients may notice their intentions, attention and attitude changing. The positive benefit derived from these changes in focus underscores the importance in the early stages of practice, when interest can flag, of encouraging participants to continue. Although each of these skills has positive benefits in increasing well-being and relaxation, they also serve as a method that assists individuals in becoming more mindful.

Although MBSR developed as a group intervention, the skills taught and reinforced in MBSR can be taught in individual mindfulness-based psychotherapy with equally positive effect. Following the introduction of the skill, it is helpful to give the participant a CD, mp3 or audiotape for home practice. CDs are available from the Center for Mindfulness (http://umassmed.edu/cfm) for a nominal fee. Although not discussed in training on MBSR, the positive transferential advantage of therapists making their own recordings to be given to their patients is worthy of consideration.

The mindfulness practices involved in MBSR include: sitting meditation, body scan, yoga and the informal practice of mindfulness. Although MBCT will not be covered, it introduces a brief practice called the 'Breathing Break', which will be included. The yoga practices covered in both MBSR and MBCT are non-demanding forms of hatha yoga. In both *Full Catastrophe Living* and *The Mindful Way Through Depression*, the MBSR/MBCT yoga sequences are described in greater detail [4, pp 106–113]. Receiving training in this particular practice or at the least having experience with yoga is essential prior to using this with patients; this will not be covered in this chapter.

Daily practice is most beneficial in the acquisition of these skills. Understanding that patients frequently struggle with positive and negative reactions to using these skills, it is often helpful to suggest to patients in the early stages that they temporarily suspend judgement about these skills and simply set aside time to practice them. Therapists should expect a range of responses to these skills. Whereas some patients find them immediately helpful, others may struggle initially with finding time, feeling bored by the skills or other negative emotions. The non-evaluative exploration of the feelings that patients have about these self-care activities provides fruitful material for exploration in psychotherapy. Not uncommonly patients will gravitate towards one of the three core mindfulness skills (meditation, body scan, mindful yoga) and find this skill the one to which they continually return. Given that the ultimate goal of mindfulness-based psychotherapy is assisting patients in finding a mindfulness skill which will facilitate increased awareness of mindfulness in their everyday lives, any of the core skills provides a pathway that can accomplish this purpose.

4.3.1 Introduction to Mindfulness

The Raisin Exercise is an introductory experience that utilises an activity (eating) which is part of everyday experience. This exercise can be done either in a group or individually. The skills developed in this process are: (i) practicing moment by moment awareness (coming off automatic pilot) and experiencing even the most pedestrian events in as fully a way as possible; (ii) watching the tendency to judge and evaluate (good and bad) the events in life; and (iii) observing the working of the mind in a more unique way, thus cultivating the dispassionate observer within. Although this exercise is usually done with a raisin, for participants who do not like raisins, small pieces of chocolate may serve the same purpose. The following script contains suggestions for the leader, included in parentheses.

'I'm going to give you something and I'd like for you to imagine that this is something you've never seen before, maybe something you would have discovered if you'd come here from another planet. So take this in your hand, and begin to explore it, be interested in and curious about this object. How does it look? What words would you use to describe its appearance (encourage participant to speak*). Does it have texture? How does it feel in your hands? Can you squeeze it? (* Encourage tactile exploration of the raisin*). Does it have a smell? Does it create a sound (* encourage participant to squeeze it as they hold it close to their ear*)? Now, put it in your mouth, but don't bite into it. As I say that, do you notice what's happening in your mouth (* most people will say that they are salivating*)? Isn't it interesting that your mouth knows exactly what to do with this thing? Pay attention to how your tongue works with this thing in your mouth. Now, bite down just once. What do you notice? (* participants may note a burst of flavor or other experiences*) Pay attention to the experiences in your mouth. Watch the sensations that are there as they gradually change and then disappear. (* After this, ask participants to describe what this experience was like.) Have you ever paid such close attention to a raisin (or chocolate) before? Usually, we eat these things in handfuls with no attention'. (* Encourage them to describe the process, noting connections participants make between episodes of attention and lack of attention in their everyday life, e.g., the tendency in our culture to mindlessly eat large amounts of food.)*

4.3.2 Body Scan

The body scan, a foundational skill in MBSR, is usually the first formal mindfulness skill taught. Most participants find the body scan the most accessible of the mindfulness skills, in part because the focus on different parts of the body keeps the patient's experience

grounded in the current moment. Although traditionally performed while the patient is lying supine on a mat on the floor, this technique can also be done in a sitting position and, for patients who tend to fall asleep during the body scan, this may be desirable. The skills developed during the body scan involve (i) strengthening the 'muscle' of attention by working with the continual refocus of attention on the different parts of the body and (ii) awareness of how the 'chattering' of the mind influences emotions. This practice focuses on each part of the body and can be illuminating for some patients who have particular issues with certain parts of their body (e.g. women who have undergone a mastectomy may find it difficult to focus their mental attention on the site of the surgery). It is often helpful to invite the individual to focus on that part of the body, watching any emotions that arise, and then, if it becomes uncomfortable, to return to a focus on the breath until the sequence of the body scan reaches a part of the body with which they are more comfortable. This exercise can range from 20 to 45 or more minutes. As is the case with each of these exercises, the skill for the therapist involves a balance between thoughtfulness of delivery, which encourages the patient to focus, or going so slowly that the patient becomes relaxed and falls asleep. Listening to a CD of a skilled practitioner leading a body scan provides a useful model for tempo and timing.

Finding a comfortable place to sit or lie down on your back, take a moment to see that the body is reasonably comfortable, no clothing that is tight or constricting. Having the intention of 'falling awake' during the body scan rather than the tendency to fall asleep. Let your attention scan your body noting to which parts of your body your attention travels (Pause*). Now bring your focus to your left foot, more specifically to the toes of your left foot. Seeing if you can, without moving the toes, get in touch with the sensations that are there. Can you distinguish between your big toe and little toe without moving them? Is there warmth, coolness, tightness, itching, or maybe no sensation at all in your foot? Allowing all of your left foot to be center stage in your mind and continually bringing your attention back to it if it wanders. (* Pause*) Now let go of your awareness of your left foot and allowing your attention to move to your left ankle, the front of the ankle, the side, noticing whatever sensations are there, or maybe noticing that there is no sensation at all. Again, being curious about this part of your body and the sensations that are there is important. Tune into the subtlety of the sensations that may exist in this part of your body.*

Following this method, move the focus to the lower leg, thigh, right foot, calf, right thigh, hips, pelvis, abdomen, chest and back, arms and hands, shoulders, neck, face. At each of these anatomical points, focus the patient on whatever sensations exist in that part of the body, even if no sensations are apparent. Encouraging the patient to focus their breathing ('Imagine that you can breathe into your left foot.') often helps patients to keep their focus. Again, as with all of these activities, the patient needs the encouragement that 'a wandering mind' is normal and all that need be done is return the focus to the body with the next breath. In individual psychotherapy, a non-evaluative exploration of the patient's experience during the body scan can be helpful. For a more complete explanation of this technique and a more complete script see Williams [7].

4.3.3 Mindfulness Meditation

A second foundational skill in mindfulness-based interventions is the use of sitting meditation. Unlike concentrative meditation where the participant focuses on a visual or auditory stimulus (e.g. a visual object or a word), in mindfulness meditation the practitioner keeps a more open focus. The initial stage involves keeping the focus on the breath and, as participants become more skilled, they allow the attention to wander, observing where the attention goes, but using the breath as an anchor. In other words, when the attention wanders (as it most certainly will), the patient is encouraged to return to the breath. Below is a script used in teaching meditation with attention on the breath. The goals of Mindfulness Meditation include: (i) increased awareness of the body; (ii) exercising the 'muscle' of attention by continually returning to the next breath; and (iii) becoming more aware of the mental chatter that flows through the mind and having the opportunity to note, 'I am not my thoughts.' Initially this experience during a psychotherapy session should last about 10 minutes or so and should be followed with a discussion of the experience. In keeping with the nonjudgemental quality that therapists want to cultivate, the discussion should focus on curiosity and observations about the experience rather than on 'What did you like or dislike?' It will reassure participants to find that 'the wandering mind' represents a universal phenomenon rather than the reflection of some neurological aberration. Although initially therapists can suggest that participants begin with 10 minutes of home practice, over time encourage an increase to 20, 30 minutes or more.

Begin by finding a comfortable seat, one that you could maintain for a period of time. Take a moment to note any areas of discomfort and, if possible, to shift your position to make those areas more comfortable. Allow your hands to rest supported on your lap, feet comfortably on the floor, sitting with a posture of dignity. Scan your body, beginning with your feet and ankles (pause*), your calves (* pause*), thighs and hips (* pause*), abdomen and lower back (* pause*), chest and shoulders (* pause*), arms and hands (* pause*), neck and head (* pause*). Now find your breath. Being curious about where the breath seems most noticeable. Is it in your abdomen, your chest, your nose, or some other area? (* pause*). Begin to pay attention to the rise and fall of your breathing. Not forcing the breath but allowing the body to breathe itself. Be curious about the breath. Is it smooth? Even? Ragged? Is there a difference between the in-breath and the out-breath? Just allow yourself to keep this interested focus on the rise and fall of your breath (* Period of silence*). Noticing how your mind begins to chatter at you and, with gentleness and firmness, return your focus to the next breath. Each breath is a new beginning (* Period of silence*).*

When leading a meditation activity with beginners, the balance, past providing instruction and trouble shooting, rests between being too intrusive with comments or being so silent that patients get lost in their own mental chatter. Using short phrases or clauses delivered every minute or so in the early stages seems to provide the best approach (e.g. 'Always coming back', 'Each breath a new beginning', 'Where am I now?', etc.). Again, listening to a skilled meditation leader provides a useful model.

4.3.4 Informal Mindfulness

Although meditation and the body scan are considered formal practices of mindfulness meditation, the informal practice of mindfulness involves bringing conscious awareness to everyday activities. The experiment with the raisin provides an example of extending mindfulness to an ordinary daily activity. Following this activity with the raisin, patients can be given the assignment of choosing a repeated daily task and performing this task with conscious awareness. Examples include: mindfully eating a meal a day, brushing one's teeth, bathing, walking the dog or indeed any activity which is typically characterised by a lack of attention, where attention focuses on other thoughts as we are engaged in the task, rather than on the direct experience of the task. The purpose of this skill is twofold:

first, it puts into sharp relief the activity of the mind, the 'chattering of the mind', and secondly, it provides brief opportunities during the course of the day to practice the skill of mindfulness so that this becomes something not only associated with formal sitting meditation but incorporated into everyday activity.

4.3.5 Breathing Break

A modification of formal 'attention on the breath' meditation utilised in MBCT is the Breathing Space. Intended to provide a readily available tool to deal with uncomfortable situations and feelings, the Breathing Space takes about 3 minutes. Broken up into three segments that takes the patient where they are, acknowledging their current emotional or physical state, then moves them to a more specific focus on the breath and finally expands their awareness back to both body and surroundings. It serves as a technique for coming off of automatic pilot (responding mindlessly to life's events) and focusing upon the patient's current experience. The following is an adaptation of the technique found in Williams *et al.* [8].

- Step 1 (becoming aware) 'Begin by sitting or standing erect and in a position of dignity and if possible close your eyes. Ask yourself about your experience in this moment. Then bring your awareness to what is happening with you now, your thoughts, your bodily sensations, noting areas of discomfort, noticing your tendency to judge or dismiss them and, as best as you can, noting to yourself, "That's how it is with me right now." Spend about a minute with this exploration.'

- Step 2 (gathering) 'Now, gather your attention and choose to focus on the breath. Noting, with curiosity, the sensation of the breath, where do you feel the breath most? in the nose? the chest? the belly? Breath in and out and focus upon the sensation of breathing. Spend about a minute with this.'

- Step 3 (expanding) 'Now allow the attention to expand from the focus on the breath to the whole body, scanning the entirety of the body and noticing how the body is in this moment. Again observe and note without judging. Again spend about a minute on this.'

4.4 Case Example

A 53-year-old woman, Janet was diagnosed with Stage III breast cancer. After undergoing surgery,

chemotherapy and radiation, she was prescribed an aromatase inhibitor. Her understanding of the significant risk of developing metastatic disease made Janet anxious and ruminative. Seen in individual psychotherapy, her chief complaint was 'I just can't stop worrying.' With present and past symptoms of anxiety suggestive of Generalised Anxiety Disorder, she responded well to an SSRI. Cognitive-behavioural therapy focused on disputing her catastrophic thoughts, 'I can't stand not knowing what is going to happen to me' and 'I'm sure that I'm going to die a horrible death'. MBSR was suggested to provide her with a series of techniques and approaches that might help in managing her anxiety. She attended the eight session group and suspended individual psychotherapy during this period with the option of emergency sessions if needed. Her response to the group was positive as she described one of the usual epiphanies of patients in MBSR (or indeed any meditation practice) that her catastrophic ideation was simply one of a range of thoughts that would populate her consciousness, rather than facts engraved in stone. The 'not knowing about metastasis' as she called it had moved from being a foregone conclusion to just one of the possibilities of her life. She began to feel great freedom in, as she put it, 'living in the unknown'. Rather than telling herself that she faced an imminent and painful death, she found it easier to begin her day with, 'I don't know what will happen and with each breath I choose to live in this moment rather than wasting my time focusing upon a future that is quite possibly an illusion.'

Janet continued in her practice of home meditation and found the combination of sitting meditation and yoga to be especially powerful. Her surgery had left her with some degree of discomfort and a sense of betrayal in relation to her body. She joined a local yoga studio, where she found that the use of yoga with its emphasis on working with and accepting the body and its limitations in each moment provided her with an opportunity to address these issues using a discipline that also led to stress reduction. She also continued to participate in the MBSR graduates programme that met once a week for a brief discussion of the use of meditation, trouble-shooting meditation problems as well as a brief sitting period. She routinely attended the 'day of mindfulness', a part of each cycle of MBSR.

Unfortunately, Janet eventually developed metastatic disease and continued in the use of mindfulness skills as well as participation in regular psychotherapy. The psychotherapy was suffused with the mindfulness concepts that had been helpful to Janet throughout her illness. Janet's sessions often began with a period of meditation where both patient and therapist sat in silence for 5 or so minutes. Janet would often say, 'When I'm quiet, my 'wise mind', the part of me that really knows, becomes more apparent. I then have a clearer understanding of where I am in my life and what is required for this moment.' She noted that when she was in touch with that 'wise mind' her fears about the future would, if not diminish significantly, be put in perspective and therefore become more manageable. Janet continued with the use of the practices she had learned in MBSR as her disease advanced and up until the time of her death.

This case example of Janet illuminates two points about the integration of MBSR (or any mindfulness skill) and psychotherapy. As Janet practiced these skills, she noticed positive changes in her functioning. Despite the traditional view of mental health that the therapist's skills and the therapeutic relationship represent the principal source of change, the mindfulness informed therapist accepts that these practices (mindfulness, meditation, mindful yoga) may facilitate a drive for inner wholeness or equilibrium and, as they appear to be leading the patient in this direction, the role of the therapist may be to support, encourage and trouble shoot rather than direct. Secondly, Janet's personal development in meditation practice exemplifies a common pattern in meditation practitioners. Initially she came to meditation practice to seek emotional regulation and to cope more effectively with what appeared to be an unmanageable situation and the ensuing emotions. Although many practitioners remain at this level, commonly the next stage in the development of meditation practice is characterised by self-discovery and self-exploration. In this stage, patients, as they sit with their own psychological freight, come to have insights into their stereotypical and possibly maladaptive reactions to situations which may lead to options for different responses.

4.5 Efficacy of MBSR and Mindfulness Interventions

The research on the efficacy of MBSR spans a wide range of psychological and physical conditions. The psychological conditions demonstrating improvement following participation in MBSR include: generalised anxiety disorder, social anxiety, recurrent depression, eating disorders, substance abuse, bipolar disorder, with pilot work suggestive of a positive effect on Attention Deficit Hyperactivity Disorder (ADHD) and schizophrenic or psychotic disorders. Mindfulness-based interventions have also

had a positive effect on a number of psychosomatic disorders including: chronic pain, fibromyalgia, hypertension, insomnia, psoriasis and immune functioning. A meta-analysis of the unpublished and published studies examining the impact of MBSR on heterogeneous health problems demonstrates a moderate effect $(d = 0.5; p < 0.0001)$ in the amelioration of a variety of physical and psychological diagnoses [9]. Since the enumeration of the studies documenting the impact of MBSR on non-cancer patients exceeds the scope of this chapter, for a more comprehensive review of the impact of meditation in general and MBSR in non-cancer patients specifically, see Shapiro and Carlson [10]. Although not focused on cancer populations, these data need to be considered by psycho-oncologists, since cancer patients will almost certainly experience many of these problems as either co-morbid symptoms or as sequelae of cancer.

The review of literature documenting the impact of MBSR on cancer patients looks at psychological and physical symptoms. Significant support exists for the role of MBSR in the amelioration of psychological distress or mood disturbance in cancer patients. Participants in MBSR report significant improvements in mood disturbance with lower scores on measures of depression, anxiety, stress, fatigue and fear of recurrence of cancer. This includes significant increases in measures of optimism, social support, capacity to cope and quality of life. Participation in MBSR leads to a more positive adjustment to the diagnosis of cancer and an increase in internal locus of control, the sense that the patient has a greater sense of personal control over the events of their lives. Not only does MBSR demonstrate an immediate impact on mood disturbance, among other symptoms, the benefits of participation in MBSR remained present at one year follow-up. In addition to improvements in psychological outcomes, participation in MBSR has also led to significant changes in physical parameters in cancer patients. Not surprisingly given the salutary impact of meditation, cancer patients participating in MBSR reported significant improvement in sleep and a significant decrease in both heart rate and resting systolic blood pressure. More intriguingly, MBSR participants demonstrate changes in immunological functioning and a number of studies document that, following their participation in MBSR, cancer patients' immune profiles shift to ones consistent with healthier immune functioning [11]. A meta-analysis of the impact of MBSR on cancer patients provides a summary of these studies demonstrating a moderate impact $(d = 0.48)$ on the mental health symptoms of cancer patients and a small effect ($d = 0.18$) on the physical symptoms of cancer, suggesting the greater efficacy of MBSR in the amelioration of the psychological symptoms of cancer patients than the physical symptoms [12].

4.6 Service Development

Whether it is with a formal MBSR programme or the integration of mindfulness into psychotherapy, the challenge in developing mindfulness-based approaches for institutions involves finding leaders who not only embrace but practice mindfulness concepts. Rather than recruiting interested but unskilled individuals, a professional experienced in meditation would be a more efficacious choice. As mentioned before, group leaders who have no significant experience with meditation or yoga will likely be at a loss in presenting these concepts to patients in a genuine fashion, much less trouble shooting the inevitable problems that patients will have as they attempt to incorporate these techniques into their lives.

The Center for Mindfulness at the University of Massachusetts Medical School in Worcester, MA provides a comprehensive training programme for prospective MBSR leaders. Although one is not required to be certified to teach MBSR, the training programme provides a clearer understanding of how the programme is led and help in developing the leadership skills necessary for facilitating the programme. Usually this will require that the trainee attend an eight week MBSR programme, coupled with leadership training seminars, although condensed training programmes have been developed. More information about the suggested requirements to be trained as a MBSR leader and the routes for acquiring this training is available at the web site for the Center for Mindfulness (http://umassmed.edu/cfm).

In the current healthcare system in the USA, reimbursement often presents a problem in MBSR programmes. Although research supports the efficacy of MBSR and many of the variations, these programmes do not fit under the usual reimbursement guidelines for group psychotherapy, making billing and reimbursement under the current insurance driven setting in the United States problematic. The salient issue surrounds documentation of service that can be used to justify billing. Unlike group psychotherapy where, in the context of a psychotherapy group, a review of the patient's mental health status leads to documentation

of services, standard MBSR participation does not typically provide an opportunity for an in-depth session by session review of any patient's mental status.

Given these concerns, at least two approaches exist to facilitate the integration of MBSR into a standard mental health setting. The Center for Mindfulness employs a sliding scale fee structure, where prospective participants pay based upon income (see umassmed.edu/cfm for more information). Other institutions offer MBSR as a free service and obtain funding for their instructors from other means.

4.7 Summary

Mindfulness-based interventions represent an approach that both ameliorates existing psychological and psychosomatic distress as well as shoring up and improving coping responses. They represent both restorative and preventive interventions, which dovetail well with the current understanding in medicine of the role of prevention rather than an emphasis on treatment. Although there are formal group interventions (MBSR) where these skills can be effectively taught, mindfulness-based concepts and techniques can be successfully integrated into standard psychotherapy. This will be most effective when the therapist has a personal appreciation and practice of these skills.

Recommended Reading

Kabat-Zinn, J. (1990) *Full Catastrophe Living*, Random House, New York.
This seminal book describes in detail the development of the MBSR programme, the theoretical underpinnings of the intervention, and its components. Useful for both practitioners and patients, this book will serve as a resource for continuing practice.

Segal, Z.V., Williams, J.M.G. and Teasdale J.D. (2001) *Mindfulness-Based Cognitive Therapy for Depression: A New Approach to Preventing Relapse*, Guildford Press, New York.
A handbook for therapists explaining the theoretical underpinnings and execution of Mindfulness-Based Cognitive Therapy. Included are therapist transcripts, patient handouts and guidelines for carrying out this eight session intervention.

Shapiro, S. and Carlson, L. (2009) *The Art and Science of Mindfulness: Integrating Mindfulness Into Psychotherapy and the Helping Professions*, APA Press, Washington, DC.
Two researchers in the area of mindfulness-based interventions as well as practitioners and teachers of meditation and MBSR review the literature on MBSR, deconstruct the mechanisms of MBSR and mindfulness, as well as providing practical applications of mindfulness as they related to MBSR and to the broader use of mindfulness techniques in psychotherapy.

Stahl, B. and Goldstein, E. (2010) *A Mindfulness-Based Stress Reduction Workbook*, New Harbinger Publications, Oakland, CA.

A workbook that covers the skills taught in MBSR, this book would be useful for both patients who are interested in mindfulness-based approaches or as a resource guide for therapists interested in the practical integration of mindfulness into their therapy practice. An mp3 containing meditation practices is included.

References

1. Kabat-Zinn, J. (2005) *Wherever You Go, There You Are: Mindfulness Meditation in Everyday Life*, Hyperion, p. 4.
2. Bishop, S.R., Lau, M., Shapiro, S. *et al.* (2004) Mindfulness: a proposed operational definition. *Clinical Psychology: Science and Practice*, **11**, 230–241.
3. Didonna, F. (2009) *Clinical Handbook of Mindfulness*, Springer, New York.
4. Kabat-Zinn, J. (1990) *Full Catastrophe Living: Using the Wisdom of Your Body and Mind to Face Stress, Pain and Illness*, Random House, New York.
5. Segal, Z. Williams, J., Teasdale, J. *et al.* (2002) *Mindfulness-Based Cognitive Therapy for Depression: A New Approach to Preventing Relapse*, Guildford, New York.
6. Shapiro, S. and Carlson, L. (2009) *The Art and Science of Mindfulness: Integrating Mindfulness Into Psychology and the Helping Professions*, American Psychological Association, Washington, DC, pp. 8–12.
7. Williams, M. (2007) *Mindful Way through Depression: Freeing Yourself from Chronic Unhappiness*, Guilford, New York, pp. 104–106.
8. Williams, M. (2007) *Mindful Way through Depression: Freeing Yourself from Chronic Unhappiness*, Guilford, New York, p 183.
9. Grossman, P., Niemann, L., Schmitt, S. *et al.* (2004) Mindfulness-based stress reduction and health benefits. A meta-analysis. *Journal of Psychosomatic Research*, **57** (1), 35–34.
10. Shapiro, S. and Carlson, L. (2009) *The Art and Science of Mindfulness: Integrating Mindfulness Into Psychology and the Helping Professions*, American Psychological Association, Washington, DC, pp. 64–66, 76–79.
11. Shapiro, S. and Carlson, L. (2009) *The Art and Science of Mindfulness: Integrating Mindfulness Into Psychology and the Helping Professions*, American Psychological Association, Washington, DC, pp. 79–84.
12. Ledesma, D. and Kumano, H. (2009) Mindfulness-based stress reduction and cancer: a meta-analysis. *Psychooncology*, **18** (6), 571–579.

5 Relaxation and Image Based Therapy

Emma J. Lewis[1] and Donald M. Sharp[1,2,3]

[1]Oncology Health Service, Queens Centre for Oncology & Haematology, Castle Hill Hospital, Cottingham, Hull, UK
[2]Institute of Rehabilitation, University of Hull, UK
[3]Postgraduate Medical School in Association with Hull York Medical School, University of Hull, UK

5.1 Background

Herbert Benson [1] coined the phrase 'relaxation response' after taking the principles of transcendental meditation and making them more accessible to Western society. Benson and his colleagues examined the psychological and physiological components of transcendental meditation as well as the cultural, religious, philosophical and scientific underpinnings. They concluded that various forms of meditation require focusing one's attention on a repetitive word, sound, phrase or image and passively returning to this focus when distracted. These steps result in predictable physiological changes both within and outside the central nervous system promoting a sense of calm which Benson called the 'relaxation response'. Relaxation therapy consists of learning different ways in which to reduce the body's stress response in order to induce the 'relaxation response'. This is characterised by feelings of both physical and psychological relaxation. It can be viewed as a natural human response, an integrated psychobiological phenomenon which is associated with reduced heart rate, peripheral vasodilatation, diaphragmatic breathing, increased alpha activity in the brain and reduced muscle tone. One might characterise the relaxation response as the opposite of the 'fight-flight' response. The fight-flight response is one of the body's automatic and usually adaptive responses to an acute severe threat, whereas the relaxation response can be viewed as a psychobiological counterbalance to the energising fight-flight reaction; a settling of the physical and psychological arousal reactions of the fight-flight response.

One of the most commonly applied relaxation techniques is progressive muscle relaxation (or PMR) which was developed by Edmund Jacobson in the 1920s [2]. He hypothesised that because muscular tension accompanies anxiety, reducing this tension would reduce anxiety. The technique involves the tensing and relaxing of all the major muscle groups (e.g. the arms, legs, face, abdomen and chest). The patient does this in a sequential fashion with the eyes closed working through each group for approximately 30 seconds (wherein the muscles are tensed for 10 seconds and released for 20). This process should be continued with each muscle group until the patient feels that their muscles are completely relaxed. During this procedure the patient is asked to concentrate on the difference between the feeling of tension and the feeling of relaxation. Deep breathing can be used in conjunction with PMR as the process of exhaling with release of muscular tension can aid relaxation. After sustained practice the patient is able to voluntarily relax the muscles without the need for muscular tension.

Cue controlled relaxation [3, 4] combines learning to relax the muscles with a verbal suggestion. Patients can be taught to use a key phrase such as the phrase '1, 2, 3 relax' on relaxation of the muscles. This method teaches the patient to associate the words of the key phrase with the feeling of relaxation. This can be useful as once the technique is learned just saying the key phrase can induce a relaxed state. The cue becomes a trigger for the onset of the relaxation response which becomes a conditioned response to the cue. In this way the patient can develop an adaptive coping response which can be used outside the clinic and formal practice sessions. Guided imagery is a mind-body intervention that has been used for centuries to promote a sense of peace and well-being during times of stress. It is a process of incorporating cognitive techniques to assist the body to relax and in some cases maintain and promote health. As with relaxation, imagery has been found to have an effect on heart rate, blood pressure, respiratory rate, oxygen consumption, brain waves, body temperature and hormonal balances. We draw a distinction in our clinical practice between two types of imagery; guided imagery and visualisation.

5.1.1 Guided Imagery

This technique is aimed at enhancing and anchoring the relaxation response in an attempt to increase the potency and controllability of the relaxation. Imagery techniques can be particularly useful for coping with lifestyle changes and adjustments that cancer patients are often subject to as it provides an opportunity for people to focus on positive thoughts and images. The primary objective of guided imagery is to guide the patient to a state where their mind is calm and free from worry. Usually the technique begins with a general relaxation process such as progressive muscular relaxation. They are encouraged to relax, clear their mind and surround themselves in images that are peaceful and calm. To help with this the patient is asked to focus on the 'here and now' to ignore any thoughts and ideas that may be racing around through their mind. Once the patient has obtained the optimal level of relaxation they can be asked to image or imagine a 'special place'. This can be a place that the patient is familiar with, or a place they imagine to be calm and peaceful. The aim is to allow the patient to develop an image in their mind, that is associated with safety and represents an escape from present concerns. Popular 'special places' may involve, for example, a beach scene or a peaceful garden. Once the image has become vivid in the patients mind's eye they are then asked to focus on all the other senses (e.g. sights, sounds, temperature, smells) in order to allow the image to become more real for them. When patients are asked within the context of relaxation practice to imagine a particularly relaxing or 'special place', the aim is that this image of a special place becomes anchored to the relaxation

response and can therefore become another cue by which to switch into a relaxed state.

Relaxation is generally thought to be necessary for imagery to be successful as it allows the mind to be open and receptive to new information which can enhance the ability to produce an image. However, there is little empirical evidence supporting such assertions. We have conducted and are currently analysing a large scale single centre randomised controlled trial with people with colorectal cancer to investigate this issue. Patients who consent to study participation are randomised to receive a high level of support in the oncology health centre (a psychological support facility open to all people with cancer in the area – self initiated support SIS); SIS plus relaxation, SIS plus guided imagery or SIS plus relaxation and guided imagery and visualisation.

5.1.2 Visualisation

A more specific technique used to help cancer patients is visualisation wherein patients are taught to visualise their bodies own natural defences such as white cells of the immune system destroying cancer cells. The patient is asked to formulate an image that promotes health and vitality. Those patients who adopt a 'fighting spirit' use images involving a 'fight' with their cancer, for example an army who seek out cancer cells and attack them. Another form of visualisation that patients find useful is to imagine a fish swimming in the blood and lymph systems targeting any metastases, or cells of the immune system seeking out and destroying cancer cells. These are examples of phagocytic processes. For people who do not wish to employ a fighting or attacking metaphor, an alternative image of cleaning or restoration can be used. The important factor in visualisation images is that they should make sense to the individual patient and further they should be comfortable using them. Patients can be encouraged to create their own visualisation image by being shown examples of images as an aid. Examples of images from the pack that we use in our clinical practice are shown in Figures 5.1 and 5.2. Visualisation is of course a more specific and disease-related form of imagery.

5.1.3 Target Groups of Patients

Relaxation techniques are one of the most widely used psychosocial interventions in the care of people with cancer.

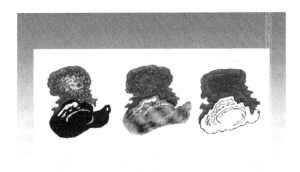

Figure 5.1 *An image of immune cells attacking cancer.* Drawn by Mr David C Chinn and reproduced with permission.

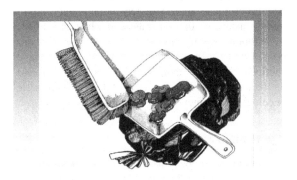

Figure 5.2 *A cleaning image.* Drawn by Mr David C Chinn and reproduced with permission.

Box 5.1 Potential Indicators and Uses for Relaxation Methods in Psycho-Oncology

- Support and promote psychological wellbeing and coping during treatment and beyond.
- Prevent the onset of psychological distress (psycho prophylaxis).
- Promote a sense of individual control and mastery during cancer treatment and over long term follow up.
- Promote the development of coping skills for treatment related side effects (nausea, pain, fatigue).
- As an intervention for procure related distress (needle phobia, scan related claustrophobia, panic anxiety related to some types of radiotherapy).
- As an adjunct to other psychological interventions (CBT plus relaxation training).

Relaxation and guided imagery techniques can be used to promote and support emotional functioning, psychological coping and general quality of life. As such they have a general application in promoting the psychological wellbeing and coping of cancer patients and may therefore play a part in preventing the development of clinically significant distress and frank psychological disorder (see Box 5.1). Given the high rates of clinically significant psychological and psychiatric disorder still demonstrated in cancer patients in recent as well as older point prevalence studies [5, 6] the potential utility of relaxation and guided imagery techniques in the arena of psycho-prophylaxis is potentially of considerable importance. However these intervention techniques also have more specific applications. Relaxation and guided imagery interventions have been shown to be useful in the control and amelioration of specific treatment related symptoms such as nausea and vomiting arising from chemotherapy and some types of radiotherapy [7–10] to promote coping and control of disease and treatment related pain, and also increasingly, fatigue [11–13] both as a current treatment related symptom and potentially as an issue of considerable relevance in the longer term in cancer survivors. Relaxation and guided imagery techniques have useful applications also in the area of procedural distress. Patients with a history of for example, needle phobia or other medical procedure related anxiety have been found to benefit from prior training in progressive muscular and cue controlled relaxation methods [13, 14]. Patients suffering from claustrophobia or with a history of current active panic disorder can find some investigative procedures such as Magnetic resonance imagery scan (MRI) scans difficult to tolerate. Patients with oral, maxillo-facial, head and neck, or some haematological cancers such as Hodgkin's Lymphoma, may receive radical radiotherapy where, to achieve the necessary treatment precision, people have to wear a close fitting mask which is fastened to the radiotherapy bench. This situation is very difficult to tolerate for people who suffer from claustrophobia or who experience anxiety or panic attacks in restricted situations from which escape is not easily achievable. Relaxation and guided imagery interventions have an important use in helping such individuals to tolerate the radiotherapy treatment and to gain an important sense of control over their treatment circumstances. The successful use of relaxation and guided imagery interventions in the amelioration and control of procedural distress can make the difference between failure to treat and the provision of vital and in some cases curative oncological treatment. Relaxation with visualisation, which involves patients imaging or visualising their bodies natural defences fighting or otherwise tackling their disease are useful for those patients who wish to engage with their treatment beyond and in addition to receiving traditional surgical medical and clinical oncological treatments. Whilst not for all patients, these techniques can give a sense of purpose, control and contribution to those patients who wish to employ them.

5.1.4 Contraindications

Whilst it is clear that relaxation techniques have great clinical utility, it should not be assumed that they can be employed in all circumstances and any consideration of their clinical use should include a discussion of a number of possible contraindications to the use of relaxation and imagery techniques. Relaxation therapy with or without imagery should be used only with caution in patients who have either a history of psychosis, or who are currently psychotic. In these individuals, any procedure which blurs the boundaries between fantasy and reality could be harmful. For these reasons we recommend that relaxation therapies should only be used by practitioners with considerable experience in mental health practice in patients who have a history and/or current presentation of psychosis.

Whilst not an absolute contra-indication, relaxation methods should be used with caution in patients with clinically significant depression. Relaxation therapy is not necessarily the treatment of choice for depression and a consequence of offering a depressed patient relaxation training might be that he or she failed to seek a more appropriate and effective treatment. Moreover, impaired concentration and low self-esteem are often symptoms of clinically significant depression: poor concentration will make learning relaxation difficult, and poor or slow progress may simply add to the individual's feelings of inadequacy.

Relaxation-induced anxiety or even panic can occur, albeit rarely, during the initial stages of learning to relax [15]. Several suggestions have been advanced for this phenomenon, the most common being that the effect may be related to a self-perceived loss of control. Depending on circumstances and individual choice, the patient may be advised to persevere or discontinue relaxation training.

For interventions which include visualisation imagery, that is imaging or imagining the body's defences fighting or dealing with the cancer there are some important considerations in deciding whether a visualisation intervention is appropriate or helpful for a patient. For patients who believe that their cancer has been cured, it is obviously inappropriate for them

to visualise their white blood cells destroying cancer cells. However, some patients still feel vulnerable about the possibility of recurrence, and for some of these patients a surveillance metaphor may be appropriate. For example, they may wish to visualise a metaphorical police force on patrol, able to deal with cancerous cells if the need were to arise. Also some patients cope well using a 'minimisation strategy' which involves a conscious attempt to keep cancer and its implication at the back of one's mind. Although not everybody can use this strategy, for those who can, it has been shown to be associated with a good quality of life and psychological coping [16]. For these patients, it may be that asking them to practice visualisation might serve as an unhelpful reminder of their history of cancer. Finally, a 'fighting spirit' coping strategy can be difficult to sustain indefinitely and it is very important to make sure that patients do not have unrealistic expectations about 'having to feel positive' as this could lead to a sense of failure and inadequacy. These cautions obviously apply for patients whose disease has recurred or shows advancement despite appropriate oncological treatment and psychological support.

5.2 Evidence on Efficacy

Relaxation and imagery are amongst the most popular complementary therapies used by patients with cancer [17, 18]. As with all interventions, there is a need to show efficacy, effectiveness and safety [19]. Studies have shown benefit in terms of psychological well-being in women with early breast cancer receiving radiotherapy [19], in colorectal cancer patients with a stoma [20], in gynaecological and breast cancer patients undergoing brachytherapy [10] and in mixed cancer patients not receiving chemotherapy [21]. However, it is not known to what extent the effects of the relaxation and guided imagery are antagonistic, additive or synergistic and to what extent they are beneficial in other cancers [22]. Luebbert et al. [23] conducted a meta analysis of randomised controlled trials employing relaxation based interventions and found considerable efficacy for the technique. Their analysis yielded effect sizes of 0.45–0.55 for the effect of relaxation methods on treatment related symptoms such as pain nausea, and also blood pressure and pulse rate. Furthermore they found effect sizes ranging from 0.44 to 0.54 for emotional adjustment variables such as general mood, tension, anxiety and depression. Interestingly, Luebbert et al. also found that relaxation techniques learned before the start of acute medical treatments had increased efficacy.

They also found that significant time input from the health care professional offering the relaxation technique was not necessary. Indeed they found that relaxation interventions requiring below 2 hours contact with the health care professional showed a greater effect on reduction of anxiety. This suggests that the input of health care professionals functions more to facilitate and support individual practice and personal efficacy of the patients. From the effect sizes yielded and the breadth of effects found for relaxation methods combined with their relative efficiency in terms of therapist input, Luebbert *et al.* concluded that relaxation training could be routinely incorporated into cancer treatment at minimal cost and with potentially considerable benefit. Roffe *et al.* [24] also concluded that guided imagery as a sole adjuvant cancer therapy may be beneficial psychologically.

For relaxation and visualisation treatments where patients visualise their bodies' natural defences tackling their disease, studies have shown efficacy in terms of improvements in psychological well-being, quality of life and mood. In addition a number of studies have shown statistically significant chasings in immune parameters as well [25–27] although others have failed to find such effect [9]. Changes in immune system parameters following psychological interventions such as relaxation and visualisation are undoubtedly interesting. However, it is not clear at present whether such changes are of sufficient magnitude or stable enough to be of direct clinical relevance. Further research is clearly warranted.

5.3 Processes and Techniques

When offering relaxation as an intervention it is always important to provide the patient with a rationale and explanation of the technique. This can help alleviate any fears of myths associated with relaxation therapy for the patient. Patients can occasionally report a 'fear of letting go' or 'being out of control' this is useful to discuss before starting the relaxation as an explanation of the techniques employed by the patient during active participation in progressive muscular relaxation and or guided imagery allow them to recognise that this is something that they are very much in control of rather than the other way round.

Relaxation is usually administered by a professional clinician and typically involves live instruction and active participation from both patient and therapist and the provision of a recording of the relaxation exercises to enable the patient to practice outside of the sessions. Often the therapy is delivered with the intention of helping the patient replicate the same relaxation response at home. As the provision of relaxation is very much a patient led endeavour the required input in terms of number of sessions required will vary between patients. This will be determined partly by individual clinical circumstances for any individual patient. In addition the need for other intervention or support techniques will have a significant effect on the number of sessions offered. As a general guide relaxation in our service is offered with two or three sessions of live practice with the therapist, and the provision of a recording of the relaxation instructions for the patients to practice with in their own time between sessions. We recommend a typical schedule of home practice of once daily although this frequency can be increased if a faster onset of effect is required for example in procedural distress where the patient is practicing relaxation prior to undergoing a forthcoming procedure such as MRI scan or radiotherapy planning. The pace of the relaxation should be delivered with the individual in mind. Most procedures include both somatic and cognitive relaxation.

Frequently in practice the patient will be asked to keep a record of their relaxation sessions and rate how successful they were at obtaining relaxation. This can be useful to review with the patient to discuss any problems with their progress. It also acts as a motivational factor and encourages the patient to practice regularly. As with the relaxation rating, a regular diary or record of the scale of relaxation obtained can also be applied to visual imagery. Patients will be asked to rate how vivid the image may be and rate this according to a Likert scale. This can help the patient identify progress in their visualisation techniques and provide instant feedback on how useful they find each session. Examples of a recording form for this propose is provided in Figure 5.3.

Regular in-vivo sessions may be held with the patient in order to hone and master the technique. Prior to beginning a relaxation session the patient should be helped to feel comfortable and at ease. Initially the patient will be taught basic progressive muscular relaxation and gradually build up to the image based relaxation. This is helpful to allow the patients to learn how to physically relax so that cue controlled relaxation becomes automatic. Once this technique is mastered the patient is able to learn the more abstract technique of cognitive relaxation. It is often easy to recognise a patient who is struggling to relax mentally but has not fully relaxed physically. This indicates that more attention should be paid to the physical relaxation techniques. Patients will also

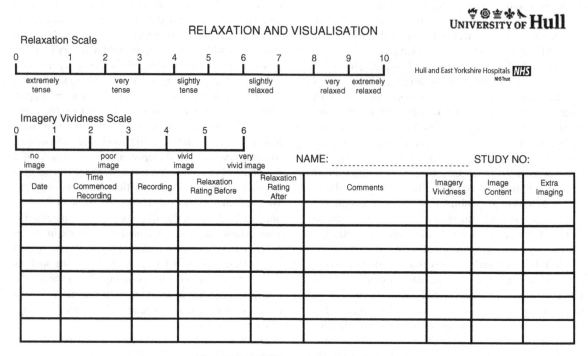

Figure 5.3 *Relaxation and visualisation diary.*

vary in the rapidity of onset of an effective relaxation response. Sessions have to be paced and structured to take account of this. For those patients who are experiencing difficulty with initial home practice, or who find it difficult to schedule time for home practice more frequent therapist led sessions may be required initially to support and facilitate practice. On the other hand some patients will master the relaxation methods quickly and with apparent ease. For these patients less frequent monitoring and consequently less frequent follow up sessions may be required. It should also be recognised that there will be a small proportion of patients who are unable to achieve adequate skill and practice with relaxation methods or, importantly, who actively choose not to use such methods. For such patients alternative interventions must be considered.

Guided imagery may be practiced as part of the relaxation practice if appropriate and if the patient wishes. Again the health professional may provide an audio recording and additional live sessions. It is usually recommended that the patient should practice learning the visualisation techniques with a trained health professional. However the use of the audio recordings should be encouraged as practice may help the patient develop a vivid image, that is relevant

to them. In addition sometimes patients may feel frustrated if they cannot obtain a clear image during the initial stages of the process. Practice in their own environment can help them gain confidence in the technique.

5.4 Case Example

Mr Smith (name altered to ensure anonymity), a man in his early 60s, was referred because of heightened anxiety and claustrophobia. He had recently been diagnosed with a stage II squamous cell cancer of the larynx and had undergone surgical biopsy. Mr Smith was then due to undergo CT planning for radical radiotherapy. CT planning involves a CT scan of fairly prolonged duration to acquire sufficient detail to permit accurate dosimetry and targeting of subsequent radiotherapy. At this stage of treatment, Mr Smith revealed that he had been claustrophobic for many years, suffering panic attacks previously in enclosed space from which he perceived escape would be difficult. Mr Smith became very anxious and panicky when it was explained that he would require a radiotherapy mask mould to be made before the commencement of his CT planning and subsequent radiotherapy treatment. This mask would be clipped to the radiotherapy bench and would prevent unwanted movement during radiotherapy planning and treatment. Mr Smith reported that he had always felt uncomfortable in enclosed spaces and often avoided using lifts for fear of experiencing panic attacks should he be trapped in an area from which escape might be difficult or socially embarrassing.

After his initial consultation with the radiotherapy team Mr Smith reported that he was unsure if he would be able to proceed with his treatment and highlighted that he was worried that he would be trapped on the radiotherapy bench with no means of escape from the room. The radiotherapy planning appointment was postponed for seven days due to Mr Smith's distress and an urgent referral made to the Oncology Health Centre for targeted psychological intervention to help Mr Smith undergo radiotherapy planning and treatment. Mr Smith was seen the same day to arrange an initial psychological assessment appointment which was arranged for the following day. A full mental state examination revealed a previous history and current presentation of panic disorder with significant avoidance of claustrophobic situations.

5.4.1 Session 1

Following mental state examination and appropriate psychosocial history taking, targeted psychological intervention was begun at this session comprising:

1. **Reframing**: Using cognitive behavioural techniques we helped Mr Smith to view the radiotherapy treatment in a more positive way. The radiotherapy mask was explained in more detail. It was explained to Mr Smith how the mask was made, how it would be fitted during planning and treatment and the role of radiotherapy staff in monitoring and supporting treatment. In particular his anxiety driven assumptions about the mask were gently challenged which helped allow Mr Smith to view the procedure as helpful rather than dangerous or life threatening.

2. **Relaxation therapy**: Mr Smith was given an explanation and rationale for the use of progressive muscular relaxation and cue controlled relaxation and encouraged to practice with an audio recording twice a day until his next radiotherapy appointment. He was particularly reassured about the role and function of relaxation in improving his psychological coping and increasing his sense of control over his emotional reaction in the radiotherapy suite.

5.4.2 Session 2

(Seven days later – or sooner to ensure that sessions co-ordinate fully with the patients other radiotherapy sessions such as CT planning.) Mr Smith had practiced the relaxation therapy as suggested and reported good initial effect, feeling calmer in general. However he continued to feel worried when he thought of attending the radiotherapy department for his forthcoming re-arranged radiotherapy CT planning appointment.

Further psychological intervention this session comprised:

1. **Relaxation therapy plus imagery**: Mr Smith was taught further relaxation this time including a guided imagery technique. This allowed Mr Smith to employ special place imagery. The purpose of the inclusion of special place guided imagery was firstly to enhance and deepen the relaxation response and secondly to generate an image whereby Mr Smith could feel more in control of his emotional reaction, safer and more able to tolerate the passing of time during the radiotherapy planning and subsequent treatment sessions.

2. **Psycho-education**: Mr Smith was given further information about the physiology of anxiety and panic and how it impacts on thoughts, feelings and behaviour. The cognitive panic model was introduced with a rationale of how techniques such as cognitive distraction can be helpful to reduce the fight or flight response and allow Mr Smith to feel more relaxed and in control.

5.4.3 Session 3

The day following this session Mr Smith attended the mask fitting which was part of his radiotherapy. He was accompanied to the room where he would undergo the mask fitting and guided through his relaxation techniques and encouraged to use his guided imagery. At the beginning of the procedure Mr Smith was asked to provide a relaxation rating on a scale of 0–5 (0 representing the most relaxed state). Mr Smith was encouraged to actively practice with progressive muscular and cue controlled relaxation and guided imagery and further ratings of his anxiety levels at different stages of the procedure. In this way Mr Smith was helped to realise that his initial levels of anxiety dissipated as the mask fitting progressed and he could feel comfortable enough to proceed with his mask manufacture and consultation with the radiotherapy team.

5.4.4 Session 4

(On the day of, and immediately prior to, radiotherapy CT planning) Mr Smith was seen immediately prior to his re-scheduled CT planning appointment at the radiotherapy department. Further discussion about the use of relaxation and visualisation techniques enabled us to provide encouragement to Mr Smith and to help him feel more confident about his ability to relax in the radiotherapy department. Prior to this appointment we had, with Mr Smith's expressed permission, discussed his case with the radiotherapy planning and treatment team so that they were fully appraised of his difficulties and therefore in a position to provide fully supportive care for Mr Smith during his planning and throughout subsequent treatment. Mr Smith was delighted to be able to complete CT planning and by employing further cognitive reframing was helped to appreciate that this was the longest duration that he would be required to wear the mask with all subsequent radiotherapy treatment sessions being of significantly shorter duration.

5.4.5 Session 5

(On the day of, and immediately prior to first radiotherapy treatment session). Mr Smith was seen immediately prior to his first radiotherapy treatment session. Progress with continued relaxation and guided imagery practice was assessed and discussed. Mr Smith volunteered that he would like to attend the radiotherapy treatment department unaccompanied as he now felt more confident to cope with treatment with the support of the radiotherapy staff. He returned to the Oncology Health Centre drop-in immediately after treatment to report that he had successfully received his first fraction of radiotherapy. As he would be returning every weekday for the next five weeks Mr Smith was pleased to understand that he could 'drop in' to the Oncology Health Centre before and after each radiotherapy treatment. Oncology Health Centre staff were aware of his psychological intervention and could thus contribute to the ongoing psychosocial support and monitoring provided by all appropriate staff to support Mr Smith throughout his treatment.

In addition to the support mentioned above, Mr Smith continued to receive some sessions with this initial psychological therapist throughout his radiotherapy sessions. Each time he was encouraged to continue rehearsing his relaxation techniques, in particular Mr Smith reported finding the cue controlled relaxation useful when he noticed his anxiety heightening before each treatment, and 'special place' guided imagery was very helpful in assisting him to distract himself from, and thus cope with, the time he spent wearing the mask during treatment. He was able to complete radiotherapy treatment without further problems or postponement.

5.5 Service Development

In an attempt to minimise distress and enhance quality of life following the diagnosis of cancer, we use relaxation, with guided imagery and visualisation interventions within the context of a comprehensive Oncology Health Service where all of the patients receive a high level of information and support. In addition, they are all screened for clinically significant distress (all our staff have been trained to identify and classify psychiatric morbidity), and a range of evidence-based interventions (psychotherapeutic and pharmacological) is available if indicated [28]. The Oncology Health Service is located in the Oncology Health Centre which is fully integrated physically, functionally, managerially and financially with the rest of the oncology services and is physically located within the Queen's Centre for Oncology and Haematology, Castle Hill Hospital, Kingston Upon Hull, UK. This close and complete integration allows the service to deliver psychological support and intervention quickly and easily and in close collaboration with colleagues in medical and clinical oncology and the chemotherapy and radiotherapy teams. The oncology in-patient wards are also located within the Queen's Centre.

This model of service organisation aims to prevent psychological problems and to enhance quality of life, to provide evidence based interventions for those who present with clinically significant psychological distress or disorder and to provide patients and their relatives with the opportunity to learn self-help techniques, such as relaxation and guided imagery. All patients with cancer and their relatives can 'drop in' to the Centre without prior arrangement or appointment. The atmosphere is informal and welcoming. Patients can also obtain information and support by telephoning the Centre. In addition, any health care professional can refer patients who are experiencing particular difficulties. The service comprises a nurse-led 'Drop-in Centre' which offers open access to all patients with a cancer diagnosis and their relatives, and a psychologist-led service to which any health care professional, in hospital or in the community, can refer patients and/or relatives for evidence-based interventions. The provision of psychosocial support within the Centre can be considered hierarchically, where basic support and the provision of instruction in self help techniques, such as relaxation and imagery, is available to all.

One of the main aims of this level of care and support is the prevention of psychological distress and disorder amongst patients and their relatives. For those who present with clinically significant distress, evidence based interventions can become increasingly complex and focussed on individual need towards the top of the suggested hierarchy. The Oncology Health Centre aims to promote a patient-centred approach by giving support, information and advice in the context of a multidisciplinary team, gain access to individually tailored information about disease, symptoms and side effects and have the opportunity to meet other patients and relatives. Staff are trained to elicit and resolve concerns quickly and effectively and offer evidence-based, self-help interventions, for example relaxation and guided imagery. The location of the Centre makes it very easy for Centre staff to liaise with medical, radiological and nursing staff and also makes it convenient and easy for patients to 'drop in' when they attend for radiotherapy, chemotherapy or follow-up appointments. The ease of access of this psychological support service has promoted a significant level of demographic equity of use in the patients attending the cancer centre [29].

5.6 Summary

Progressive muscular relaxation and cue controlled relaxation used with or without imagery techniques such as guided imagery or visualisation, are an effective and useful clinical intervention for the practitioner in psychosocial oncology. They can be deployed to improve psychological coping and general quality of life, but also have a range of specific applications in treatment related side effects and specific psychological problems such as procedure related distress. Relaxation techniques are widely used and commonly recommended and advocated. However the forgoing discussion has hopefully highlighted some of the circumstances, both clinical and individual, where relaxation techniques should be used only with caution and care. These considerations notwithstanding relaxation techniques undoubtedly provide an effective and clinically efficient means by which patients can be helped to become more skillful in the induction and use of the beneficial psychobiological state, that is the relaxation response.

References

1. Benson, H. (1975) *The Relaxation Response*, Morow, New York.
2. Jacobson, E. (1929) *Progressive Relaxation*, The University of Clinical Monographs in Medicine, University of Chicago Press, Chicago.
3. Suinn, R.M. and Richardson, F. (1971) Anxiety management training: a non-specific behaviour therapy programme for anxiety control. *Behaviour Therapy*, **2**, 498–410.
4. Russell, R.K. and Sipich, J.F. (1973) Cue -controlled relaxation in the treatment of test anxiety. *Journal of Behavioural Therapy and Experimental Psychiatry*, **4**, 47–49.
5. Hall, A., A'Hern, R. and Fallowfield, L. (1999) Are we using appropriate self-report questionnaires for detecting anxiety and depression in women with early breast cancer? *European Journal of Cancer*, **35** (1), 79–85.
6. Burgess, C., Cornelius, V., Love, S. *et al.* (2005) Depression and anxiety in women with early breast cancer: five year observational cohort study. *British Medical Journal*, **330** (7493), 702.
7. Molassiotis, A., Yung, H.P., Yam, B.M. *et al.* (2002) The effectiveness of progressive muscular relaxation training in managing chemotherapy-induced nausea and vomiting in Chinese breast cancer patients: a randomised controlled trial. *Supportive Cancer Care*, **10**, 237–246.
8. Yoo, H.J., Ahn, S.H., Kim, S.B. and Han, O.S. (2005) Efficacy of progressive muscular relaxation training and guided imagery in reducing chemotherapy side effects in patients with breast cancer and improving their quality of life. *Supportive Cancer Care*, **13**, 826–833.
9. Nunes, D.F., Rodriguez, A.L., da Silva Hoffmann, F. *et al.* (2007) Relaxation and guided imagery program in patients with breast cancer undergoing radiotherapy is not associated with neuroimmunomodulatory effects. *Journal of Psychosomatic Research*, **63**, 647–655.
10. Leon-Pizzaro, C., Gich, I., Barthe, E. *et al.* (2007) A randomized trial of the effect of training in relaxation and guided imagery techniques in improving psychological and quality of life indices foe gynaecological and breast brachytherapy patients. *Psycho-Oncology*, **16**, 971–979.
11. Fernando, F.C., Frank, T., Rabe-Menssen, C. *et al.* (2004) Effect of aerobic exercise and relaxation training on fatigue and physical performance of cancer patients after surgery. A randomised controlled trial. *Supportive Care in Cancer*, **12**, 774–779.
12. Hasse, O., Schwenk, W., Hermann, C. *et al.* (2005) Guided imagery and relaxation in conventional colorectal section: a randomized controlled partially blinded trial. *Diseases of the colon and Rectum*, **48**, 1955–1963.
13. Carlson, L.E. and Bultz, B.D. (2008) Mind-body interventions in oncology. *Current Treatment Opinions in Oncology*, **9**, 127–134.
14. Mundy, E.A., DuHamel, K.N. and Montgomery, G.H. (2003) The efficacy of behavioural interventions for cancer treatment related side effects. *Seminars in Clinical Neuropsychiatry*, **8**, 253–275.
15. Adler, C.M., Craske, M.G. and Barlow, D.H. (1987) Relaxation induced panic: when relaxing isn't peaceful. *Integrative Psychiatry*, **5**, 94–112.

16. Butow, P.N., Coates, A.S. and Dunn, S.M. (2000) Psychosocial predictors of survival: metastatic breast cancer. *Annals of Oncology*, **11**, 469–474.

17. Downer, S.M. (1994) Pursuit and practice of complementary therapies by cancer patients receiving conventional treatment. *British Medical Journal*, **309**, 86–89.

18. Maher, E.J., Young, T. and Feigel, I. (1994) Complementary therapies used by cancer patients. *British Medical Journal*, **309**, 671–672.

19. Walker, L.G. and Anderson, J. (1999) Testing complementary and alternative medicine within a research protocol. *European Journal of Cancer*, **35**, 1614–1618.

20. Cheung, Y.L., Molassiotis, A. and Chang, A.M. (2003) The effect of progressive muscle relaxation training on anxiety and quality of life after stoma surgery in colorectal cancer patients. *Psycho-Oncology*, **12**, 254–266.

21. Baider, L., Peretz, T., Hadani, P.E. and Koch, U. (2001) Psychological intervention in cancer patients: a randomized study. *General Hospital Psychiatry*, **23**, 272–277.

22. Walker, L.G., Sharp, D.M., Walker, A.A. and Walker, M.B. (2007) Relaxation, Visualisation and Hypnosis. in J Barraclough. (Ed) *Enhancing Cancer Care: Complementary, Expressive and Supportive Therapies in Oncology*. 245–256. Oxford University Press.

23. Luebbert, K., Dahme, B. and Hasenbring, M. (2001) The effectiveness of relaxation training in reducing treatment-related symptoms and improving emotional adjustment in acute non-surgical cancer treatment: a meta-analytical review. *Psycho-Oncology*, **10**, 490–502.

24. Roffe, L., Schmidt, K. and Ernst, E.A. (2005) A systematic review of guided imagery as an adjuvant cancer therapy. *Psycho-Oncology*, **14**, 607–617.

25. Walker, L.G., Walker, M.B., Heys, S.D. *et al.* (1999) The psychological, clinical and pathological effects of relaxation training and imagery during primary chemotherapy. *British Journal of Cancer*, **80**, 262–268.

26. Eremin, O., Walker, M.B., Simpson, E. *et al.* (2009) Immuno-modulatory effects of relaxation training and guided imagery in women with locally advanced breast cancer undergoing multimodality therapy: a randomised controlled trial. *Breast*, **18**, 17–25.

27. Lengacher, C.A., Bennett, M.P., Gonzalez, L. *et al.* (2008) Immune responses to guided imagery during breast cancer treatment. *Biological Research Nursing*, **9**, 205–214.

28. Walker, L.G., Walker, M.B. and Sharp, D.M. (2003) The organisation of psychosocial support within palliative care, in *Psychosocial Issues in Palliative Care* (ed. M. Lloyd-Williams), Oxford University Press, Oxford.

29. Sharp, D.M., Walker, M.B., Bateman, J.S. *et al.* (2009) Demographic characteristics of patients using a fully integrated psychosocial support service for cancer patients. *Bio Med Central: Research Notes*, **15** (2), 253.

6 Motivational Counselling in Substance Dependence

Jack E. Burkhalter

Department of Psychiatry and Behavioral Sciences, Memorial Sloan-Kettering Cancer Center, New York, NY, USA

6.1 Background

Receiving a cancer diagnosis has been framed as a 'teachable moment' when individuals may be particularly receptive to changing their lifestyle or health behaviours to reduce further threats to health [1, 2]. The harm of using tobacco, alcohol and illicit substance use, as well as physical inactivity and poor diet, may take on greater salience in the context of cancer and heightened concerns for preserving health. Despite the evidence that a cancer diagnosis can spur many patients to make health behaviour changes to reduce cancer risk [3], a substantial portion is not sufficiently motivated even by cancer to undertake lasting change [4]. In the case of substance dependence, some patients may make positive changes temporarily but then relapse after cancer treatment when the health threat recedes. Alternatively, if cancer recurs or prognosis is poor or worsens, the perceived benefits of making risk reduction changes may diminish and motivational impetus lost. Finally, individuals may have given up substance use in the past but in the context of cancer diagnosis they resume use as they try to cope. These scenarios illustrate the dynamic nature of motivation to abstain from substance use in the existential flux of cancer. Clinicians need tools to help substance-dependent cancer patients in this flux sort out their reasons for changing and maintaining the status quo, guiding them towards change in ways consistent with patient autonomy, values and goals. This chapter presents an overview of *motivational interviewing* (MI), a method with ever-widening use and extensive empirical support that counsellors can use to help patients tap motivational resources and build

momentum towards positive change. Because a full learning of MI requires considerable training and skill acquisition, this chapter is intended to introduce the reader to the method and highlight certain elements relevant to cancer care settings.

In 1991, William R. Miller and Stephen Rollnick, clinician researchers in alcoholism treatment, published their first book on MI [5], since revised [6]. Motivational interviewing is defined as 'a client-centred, directive method for enhancing intrinsic motivation to change by exploring and resolving ambivalence', [6, p. 25]. It is helpful to examine each of the components comprising the definition of MI. First, MI is a *method of communication* that applies key concepts and approaches from the client-centred, interpersonal theory of change developed by the psychologist Carl R. Rogers [7]. The authors deliberately chose the term 'interviewing' as opposed to 'therapy' or other terms, because from their perspective the term fitted with the collaborative spirit of MI and avoided an authoritarian stance of the counsellor in the relationship [6], that is 'I am the expert on how you can change.' Further, MI explicitly rejects aggressive confrontational techniques that were prominent in alcohol dependence treatment in the 1960–1980s [8, 9]. MI holds as central to its effectiveness the use of Rogers' concept of *accurate empathy*, in which the therapist skilfully helps the patient identify and clarify affective and psychological experiences in the moment to aid in self-understanding and to create a trusting and supportive environment for change. MI, however, differs from the Rogerian method in that it is openly directive, with the goal of eliciting and

---

Handbook of Psychotherapy in Cancer Care, First Edition. Edited by Maggie Watson and David W. Kissane.
© 2011 John Wiley & Sons, Inc. Published 2011 by John Wiley & Sons, Inc.

reinforcing *change talk* as it reduces patient resistance to change. *Change talk* refers to statements in which the patient recognises the need to change, or expresses intent to change or openness to the possibility of change. A second theoretical basis for MI comes from research in cognitive dissonance and self-perception theories, whereby individuals who verbally defend a position are more likely to become committed to that position, even if the defended position conflicts with current attitudes [10, 11]. Thus, facilitating patient 'change statements' is a critical step towards enabling change itself.

MI is a method that is specific about the *quality* of the motivation and which entails understanding the distinction between *intrinsic and extrinsic motivation*. Motivation can be defined along a continuum of externally versus self-determined. At one end is *extrinsic motivation* emanating from external sources (e.g. law enforcement, family), and at the other end to the most self-determined, where *intrinsic motivation* flows from deeply held values, interests and goals. Although the MI approach is most closely associated with the Stages of Change theory [12], the MI concept of motivational quality is not anchored to a specific theory. The spirit and practice of MI is highly compatible with the types of motivation specified in Self-Determination Theory [13]. This theory is concerned with 'how people internalise and integrate extrinsic motivations and come to self-regulate their behaviours in order to engage autonomously in actions in their daily life' [14, p. 5]. In this theory, only inherently enjoyable and interesting behaviours are conceived as being intrinsically motivated; thus, volitional singing or collecting stamps would meet this definition, but abstinence from substance use would not. Abstaining from substance use would always be *extrinsically motivated*, and it is in the *types* of extrinsic motivation that distinctions are crucial regarding behaviour change. It is beyond the scope of this chapter to detail these, but suffice it to say that the types range along a dimension of degree of autonomy, internalisation and integration of behaviour change with the identity, values and goals of the individual. Anchoring this continuum on one end is *externally regulated* motivation stemming from external rewards, punishments or coercion, and which yields the least stable and committed behaviour, to *integrated regulation* at the other end, in which a person identifies with the regulation and has harmonised that identification with core values, beliefs and aspirations. Because integrated regulation is fully consonant with self-determination or autonomy, it

is stable and persistent. Thus, from the perspective of empirical findings in Self-Determination Theory, MI aims to promote a more autonomous form of motivation, that is, towards an integrated regulation of extrinsic motivation, rather than draw upon intrinsic motivation *per se* [14].

This exposition on motivational theory is particularly relevant to the cancer context. Extrinsic forces for change are intensified for a substance-dependent patient due to the setting of acute medical illness and health care providers' concerns for patient safety during cancer treatment. An oncologist may insist that a patient stop smoking, drinking in excess or alter other behaviours prior to or over the course of treatment. The abrupt abstinence from substance use is more likely to convert to longer-term maintenance of abstinence if the sources of motivation for that change are congruent with important goals, such as the desire to stay healthy in service of achieving specific goals, or cherished values, such as nurturing one's spiritual life. If the patient is not aided in internalising the behaviour change and motivation stays primarily externally regulated, strong resistance may be activated and the abstinence is unlikely to persist once the external pressures subside. Providers skillful in MI can help patients internalise and integrate the extrinsic forces pushing for behaviour change by adopting an autonomy-supportive stance and guiding them in the discovery of how change resonates with their aspirations and values.

The last element of the definition of MI entails exploration of the person's conflict about changing versus maintaining a current behaviour or perspective, and facilitation to resolve the ambivalence in a manner congruent with the person's values and goals. This entails a nuanced approach to exploring with the patient the pros and cons of maintaining the status quo versus making a change. The means by which this is done will be described later. Next, the core features or *spirit* and general principles of MI are elaborated.

The *spirit* (tone and intent) of MI embraces collaboration, evocation and autonomy [6]. To foster collaboration the counsellor skillfully avoids the 'expert trap', whereby the counsellor is the authority and the patient is the vessel of received wisdom. Rather than a reliance on exhortation or persuasion there is, instead, an emphasis on exploration and curiosity about the patient's ambivalence towards change [6]. The interpersonal context is positive and conducive to change without coercion. The counsellor asks permission before providing information or advice. Counsellors must observe and manage their own expectations for the treatment, as the MI authors describe a session as 'a meeting of aspirations' [6, p. 34], which may diverge. A second core feature of MI is *evocation* or eliciting from the person indicators of self-directed motivation that can be explored and amplified for the sake of change. Patient *autonomy* is the third component of the MI spirit, such that patients are free to take or leave what is counselled. By making patient autonomy a central theme, MI explicitly acknowledges that change arises from within the person and is most lasting when it converges with the person's values, goals and aspirations. Patient autonomy, however, is not to be confused with interpersonal style, cultural practices of deference to authority or dependent personality features, as one does not forfeit autonomy even when the tendency or choice is to rely on others [14]. The counsellor can be autonomy-supportive even when patients are not able or willing to express their own ideas or wishes. These three elements of the spirit of MI focus on the timbre and therapeutic values embedded in MI. Next are described the principles that guide the practice of MI.

The four general principles of MI practice are: (i) *Express empathy*; (ii) *Develop discrepancy*; (iii) *Roll with resistance* and (iv) *Support self-efficacy* [6]. As noted earlier, a cornerstone of MI is the ability to apply reflective listening with accurate empathy. These features are considered vital in establishing a working therapeutic alliance, which is known to be important in the broader psychotherapy literature [15]. Acceptance of the person as she or he presents without condoning or agreeing is communicated through these empathic techniques. Judging, criticising and blaming are avoided. This is a paradoxical intervention in that the counsellor's communication of acceptance bolsters the individual's receptivity to change. The empathic counsellor validates the experiences and perspectives of the patient and normalises ambivalence, which is presented as a common source of being 'stuck' or 'in a rut'. The second MI principle entails *developing discrepancy* and diverges from non-directive counselling in that the intent is to resolve ambivalence in the service of positive change. Discrepancy is initiated and amplified by exploring with the patient how the current state of affairs contrasts with her or his own goals, aspirations or values. Individuals presenting for treatment of substance use problems may already be acutely aware of the discrepancies between their current behaviour and desired outcomes. MI will draw upon this 'motivational well (or supply)' and attempt to replenish it to support movement from the status quo.

The third principle, *roll with resistance*, entails consideration of the dynamics of MI in the moment when the counsellor may be entering into, or be perceived as such, a stance of advocating for change. This is a recipe for resistance in which the momentum for change reverses course as the patient argues against change – obviously an undesirable place to be in the change process! The 'rolling' part of managing resistance in MI proscribes directly confronting resistance; rather, one shifts to empathic listening and looks for opportunities to subtly reframe or direct the resistance towards a new momentum for change. The counsellor may also turn the problem back to the patient to engage her or him in the problem-solving. This sends a message that the patient is a capable, self-directed person and avoids the expert trap. Resistance also signals to the counsellor that the current approach should be adjusted to avoid interpersonal tension that can adversely impact the working alliance.

Finally, the fourth guiding principle in MI is to *support self-efficacy* regarding change. Self-efficacy is the person's belief that she or he can attain a certain outcome, such as quitting smoking. The concept of self-efficacy is a key component in most health behaviour change theories and exerts a powerful influence on motivation to change [16, 17]. One can be highly motivated to change behaviour, but if self-efficacy is low, the person is unlikely to succeed, that is 'I really want to stop marijuana, but I'm not so sure I can do it.' In MI, self-efficacy is supported not through advising patients in how they might succeed; rather, self-efficacy is strengthened in autonomy-supportive ways, including eliciting confidence talk, reviewing past successes, identifying personal strengths and supports and even providing information and advice, if the patient has expressed a wish to receive it. The four principles are the infrastructure for the practice of MI. Before this practice is illustrated further, the empirical support for the efficacy of MI is reviewed.

6.2 Processes and Techniques

Oncologic care offers unique and often multiple opportunities with patients to promote behaviour change that reduces health risks. The traditional medical model of patient care would seem in many ways hostile territory for the spirit of MI. An oncologist evaluating a new patient assesses the presenting problem, orders tests, provides a diagnosis and then treatment options, finalises a treatment plan and implements it, and conducts follow-up, maintenance or surveillance plans. Time spent in patient contact is constrained by economic and practical factors. Newly diagnosed cancer patients are often frightened, anxious, perhaps depressed or disoriented as they grapple with the unfolding and sometimes devastating picture of their condition, their prognosis and the immediate impact of cancer on their and loved ones' lives. This state of crisis, patient vulnerability and urgency can foster a default way of provider communication that is highly prescriptive and directive, and can reinforce unwittingly in patients a sense of loss of autonomy. Mental health providers may become susceptible to adopting this directive mode of counselling in response to the prevailing interactive style and demand characteristics of the milieu. On the other hand, to act only as a reflective listener would build rapport, but the practitioner would not necessarily address the presenting problem. MI moves beyond the directive and reflective or 'following' means of communication to include a third way of interacting – guiding [18]. Guiding is akin to tutoring or consulting in which the patient is the one who decides and uses the counsellor's proficiency to help make the best decision consistent with her or his goals and values. MI is said to be a refined type of the guiding communication style, but the developers of MI posit that in health care settings many presenting problems are best solved using a mix of the directive, reflective and guiding communication methods [18]. Presented in the following section is the translation of MI practice to medical settings. For examples or cases presented herein, no single individual is depicted; rather, generalised composite scenarios are presented without potentially identifying features so as to protect the confidentiality of individuals.

In adapting MI practice to health care settings the authors have addressed the contextual pull towards over-reliance on directive counselling by highlighting the strategy of *resisting the righting reflex* – the first of the four *RULE* strategies. The righting reflex is the powerful desire among health care providers to make things right, to heal and to prevent harm [18]. Although wanting to correct the mistakes and solve the problems of the ill and addicted is a praiseworthy intention, the challenge in MI is for the counsellor to pull back from trying to fix the problem. Why is this? Most substance abusers have some awareness that there are harms to what they are doing and live with ambivalence about their habit. If the counsellor takes the side of promoting abstinence, the natural response in addiction is to argue defensively that there is no serious problem or that the substance use brings benefits. The more patients verbalise and hear their own arguments for the status quo,

the less committed they are to change. It is the patient who ought to be making the change talk, not the clinician. This problem is illustrated below, with comments in parentheses indicating key elements in the dialogue.

COUNSELLOR: If you don't quit drinking your risk of oral cancer coming back is high. You are done with radiation and the cancer is gone, but your drinking is a problem. Alcohol is a known risk factor for this type of cancer. Isn't it time you stopped? (directive, confrontational)

PATIENT: I'm not an alcoholic! What's wrong with having a few beers after work? I get along with everyone, and I've never had a drunk-driving violation.

The second *RULE* practice strategy is to *understand your patient's motivations*. Be interested in the patient's reasons for change and how these fit with her or his values, goals and aspirations. In brief or single-session consultations, it may be best to ask patients why they would make a change and how they might do it. As noted earlier, the urgent medical context of cancer often elicits externally regulated motivation; thus, as the patient frames the change process in the session, *listening*, the third practice strategy, is important. Listening well is a complex clinical skill that many patients may not frequently encounter; thus, clinicians understandably worry that listening will only mire them in lengthy sessions. There is a risk for this happening; however, by setting an agenda first that acknowledges time constraints, thanking the person for information that helps you understand them and their concerns better, or assuring that in future encounters you hope to hear more, the clinician can gently manage this challenge. The fourth practice strategy is *Empower your patient*. Doing so increases self-efficacy for change by tapping into autonomous sources of motivation, such as protecting health and achieving cherished goals and aspirations. Patients are valued as having knowledge and internal resources, and hope is fostered by helping them see that they are the experts on how to make change work in their lives.

Below is an illustration of *RULE* strategies.

PATIENT: They said I needed to talk to you. I have to stop drinking, but I'm so stressed now, with surgery coming up in two weeks – it's the worst time for me to try to do that. Everyone is over-reacting.

COUNSELLOR: You are here today to talk about your drinking, and yet you are not sure that you can change it. We only have about 30 minutes today, so perhaps we can talk a bit about *why* you might want to stop drinking (set agenda, understand motivation, empower and develop discrepancy).

PATIENT: Well, my family is on my back and my doctor says I should stop if I want to get through surgery. I know it's strange, but I just don't want to!

COUNSELLOR: Right. Everybody seems to want you to stop, so it can make it hard to figure out what it is *you* want. If we called a time-out and everyone backed off a bit on the pressure, what do you think might happen? (listen, resist righting reflex and understand motivation).

In health care settings where interactions are often time-limited, a consultation may focus on preparing the patient to make a decision to undergo treatment of addiction or substance use or abuse in that setting or elsewhere. Setting an agenda at the beginning of a consultation is a strategy that clarifies the patient's expectations and puts forth the counsellor's as well. Using open-ended questions, affirming and supporting the patient, listening reflectively and summarising are good ways to engage the patient [6]. These tactics also set the stage for eliciting change talk – the evocation element of MI. There are several different ways to evoke change talk. One method that is particularly helpful is to use the 'importance ruler', in which the patient is asked to rate the importance of changing the presenting substance use behaviour using a 0-10 scale, with 0 being not at all important and 10 being extremely important. This can be done with a visual scale or by verbal description. The same scale can be used to indicate the level of confidence in the patient's ability to change the same behaviour, thereby providing a measure of abstinence self-efficacy. Note in the dialogue below that the counsellor encourages change talk by comparing the patient's rating to 0, not 10, as the latter would focus on deficits in readiness to change, rather than assets.

PATIENT: I would say I'm a '4', on how important quitting tobacco is for me.

COUNSELLOR: That's interesting – why did you put yourself at a 4, and not a 0?

PATIENT: Well, I think there could be a little something good about stopping smoking. My morning cough might not be as bad if I quit.

Another approach is to explore the disadvantages of the status quo.

COUNSELLOR: What worries you about your cocaine use? What's the downside?

PATIENT: I'm always worried about getting caught. A conviction will mean I lose my job. I just can't let that happen, because I would lose everything.

Optimism about change can be fostered by making use of the confidence rating the patient provided. Here, a patient provides a rating using the confidence ruler.

PATIENT: I'm not too confident – I would say a '5'.

COUNSELLOR: So moderately confident about getting sober – why did you put yourself at a 5, and not a 0?

PATIENT: I did quit for two weeks that time, which amazed me, but I went back to drinking when my buddies took me out to celebrate my birthday.

Evoking talk about intention to change can also help the patient contemplate abstinence.

COUNSELLOR: What would you be willing to try?

PATIENT: I'm not sure. Maybe start with what worked in the past, like not smoke in the house – only out on the patio. And when it's cold out, I just don't smoke as much.

Eliciting change talk is a critical element of MI, and when the patient voices change statements, how the counsellor responds is equally important. Perhaps the simplest way is to respond nonverbally to show interest, such as a head nod and eye contact, and also verbally with an invitation to elaborate, for example 'in what ways?' or 'how could you do it?' Reflecting change talk is another technique, but MI guides the counsellor to *selectively* reflect so that the change side of ambivalence is mirrored and amplified. Additionally, affirming change talk and linking change to values and goals deepens the commitment:

PATIENT: Now that I'm done with chemo, I just want to feel normal again. Yesterday, I had my first cigarette since I was diagnosed. I know, I know, I shouldn't have. Funny, it didn't taste as good as I had hoped it would, and I felt guilty. I haven't smoked since, but I'm not so sure I can stay away from my 'old friend'.

COUNSELLOR: So you were tempted, but the cigarette was a disappointment and made you feel uncomfortable (selective reflection; resists righting reflex).

PATIENT: Right – after about five puffs, I put it out. I could go back, I know, if I let myself, so I've got to try some things to avoid that.

COUNSELLOR: What are some of those strategies that would help you? (elicit elaboration)

PATIENT: Well, getting rid of all the cigarettes in the house. I found this one in a drawer, but more could be stashed away. The second thing is I could do is get back to walking daily. I have more strength now and the weather is warmer, so I can do that. Maybe my friend can join me and make it a chat session.

COUNSELLOR: Those sound like good ideas (affirm change talk). Was there anything else that kept you from picking up a second or third cigarette yesterday? Was there something you valued more than the cigarette? (understand motivation)

PATIENT: It seems all I want at that moment is to smoke. But I remember you asking me before why I wanted to be healthy! I thought you were nuts, but I saw that I wanted to live and be active – stay independent. I made a promise to my niece that I would quit. She loves her aunt and I love her so much. And she hates my smoking!

Managing resistance to change is a critical element to successful use of MI, and there are several strategies to 'roll with the resistance'. Among the most straightforward techniques is reflection, and using simple reflection is a low risk way to respond to resistance. Another approach is to amplify or exaggerate in the reflection with the intent that the patient pull back from the resistance and move towards the other side of the ambivalence. It is important that the amplified reflection be done in a supportive and matter-of-fact tenor and never with sarcasm, irony or irritation, as such inflections may evoke further resistance. A third approach is to mirror both sides of the ambivalence using 'and', while avoiding 'but', to appose the two sides. These techniques are demonstrated:

PATIENT: If my drinking bothers other people, that's just too bad! You and everyone else seem more concerned about a few drinks than my prostate cancer.

COUNSELLOR: It really bothers you that in the midst of your cancer so many are focused on your drinking (reflection).

PATIENT: Yes! Since I retired two years ago, enjoying a few cocktails has been a real treat – so I just don't get what the big deal is.

COUNSELLOR: So you don't see any reason for your doctor and family's concerns (amplified reflection).

PATIENT: Well, I do understand what they are saying and I don't want to become an alcoholic, either! Why don't they just let me handle this on my own?

Motivational Counseling

PROs of (substance use)	CONs of (substance use)
PROs of quitting (substance)	CONs of quitting (substance)

Figure 6.1 *Pros and cons of using and quitting a substance.*

COUNSELLOR: I am hearing that on one hand, you share their concerns about drinking too much alcohol, and, on the other hand, you are feeling pressured to make a change (double-sided reflection).

As noted earlier, exploring with the patient the pros and cons of using and quitting substances is a strategy that engages the patient and often provides rich material for developing discrepancy. Figure 6.1 shows a sample form used in the Tobacco Cessation Programme at Memorial Sloan-Kettering Cancer Center, with adaptation for any substance use. This form can be integrated into the initial consultation as a stimulus for discussion or provided as homework and explored together at the next session. By acknowledging that there are perceived benefits of substance use, the counsellor signals that a balanced approach will be used in helping the patient assess the presenting problem and the decision to quit or continue use. The tactic also minimises resistance while encouraging change talk.

6.3 Case Example

In the case presented, the pros and cons tool is used with Martha, a 52-year-old married woman who was diagnosed with early stage breast cancer, had a left mastectomy and adjuvant chemotherapy, and is now anticipating undergoing breast reconstruction. She had smoked a pack of cigarettes daily since age 19. She is employed as a professional investment banker, and she has two children, a 15-year-old son and a 17-year-old daughter. She only smokes in the outdoors, when driving her car and during working hours when possible. She reported that the plastic surgeon with whom she has consulted at the cancer centre has stated that she must quit smoking at least two weeks prior to the scheduled surgery date because of the greater risk of surgical complications, including failure of the breast reconstruction, due to nicotine's adverse effects on wound healing. Her surgeon referred her to the hospital's counselling centre to help her quit smoking.

COUNSELLOR: I understand that Dr. Smith referred you to the counselling center to talk about your smoking. We have 45 minutes today to talk about what you have in mind and how I might help. There are some background questions I will need to ask you, but I'd really like to hear first what you are concerned about – how *you* feel about coming here today? (agenda setting and open-ended questions)

PATIENT: Well, I have to quit smoking. That's what Dr. Smith says, if I want to have breast reconstruction. That makes me angry. If it were up to me, I would keep smoking. I know my cancer had nothing to do with my smoking.

COUNSELLOR: It's frustrating having to be here today and you're feeling pressured to quit. It's also hard to see the link between quitting smoking and your breast cancer (reflective listening and understanding motivations).

PATIENT: There is no link! I mean, he explained why he wanted me to quit – the reconstruction may fail if I don't quit. But I've got to tell you, I really do enjoy smoking. How would he know if I quit or not? How would *you* know?

COUNSELLOR: Well, it's true – the choice to quit is really yours. I am not the 'smoking police', and, frankly, I would not want to be (smiles)! You are an adult who has every right to make her own decisions, even if others might wish for different choices from you. What I hope we can do is learn more about how smoking fits in your life, what your goals are, and if you have some concerns about smoking at this time. Would you be willing to explore that? (reinforce autonomy, roll with resistance and ask permission)

PATIENT: Yes (sighs). I can't imagine giving up my 'best friend'. When I'm alone and needing to calm down from all that I've been through with breast cancer, I just feel so much better when I can put things in perspective. A cigarette helps me think things through and relax. At work, going out to smoke gives me a break, time to think and hang out with the other smokers. I need that!

COUNSELLOR: So there are three benefits of smoking that you have mentioned – keeping you company, helping you gather yourself to think and relax a bit and some socialising with other smokers. These are important to you, and it would be difficult giving these up. If we think about these benefits as the 'pros' of smoking, it may be worthwhile to also look at the downside or 'cons' of smoking. Here is guide we can use to keep track of these (see Figure 6.1). How would it be for you if you chose not to smoke? (listening, empathy and develop discrepancy)

PATIENT: Well, it would be hard – I think I would be a wreck for a few days, but I could take a break in the cafeteria or go out for fresh air. There's socialising at the coffee pot in the kitchen area on our floor. I guess I could do that, but it wouldn't be the same as a smoke.

COUNSELLOR: You would find ways to take a break – get some fresh air or get a cup of coffee inside without the temptation to smoke. It wouldn't be the same as smoking, and you could live with that. What about the cons of smoking – the things you don't like about smoking? (empower, support self-efficacy, reframe and develop discrepancy)

PATIENT: Well, I know smoking is bad for my health, that's obvious.

COUNSELLOR: Could you tell me what *specifically* you are thinking about when you say it's bad for your health? (eliciting)

PATIENT: My smoking had nothing to do with my breast cancer, but my father died at 65 of lung cancer – he was a heavy smoker – so I don't want that to happen to me. I am hoping to live well beyond that, although having had breast cancer I'm not so sure I will.

COUNSELLOR: Why is it important to you that you live longer? (understand motivation)

PATIENT: (*Patient looks surprised*) Why do I want to *live longer*? Well, I have two children who need me, and I want to see them graduate from high school, get through college, find good partners in life, and, I hope, make me a grandmother! That's why!

COUNSELLOR: So you are saying that if you protect your health, it will allow you to achieve some cherished goals – to be there for your children, to see them succeed in life and to hold that first grand-child in your arms (amplifies reflection and linkage of cons of smoking to intrinsic sources of motivation).

PATIENT: Right! I complain about those two teenagers all the time, but our whole world revolves around them and I wouldn't change that for anything. But I also want to be healthy for myself – to be able to travel when I retire, and for my husband and me to do so many things we have put off while we work and raise the kids. But what does this have to do with my smoking?

COUNSELLOR: Good point! So on the one hand you value what smoking provides you in the moment – relaxation, time to think – and, on the other hand, what you value most in life seems to be staying healthy for your kids and husband, your future, and your own goals and plans for that future (develop discrepancy and double-sided reflection).

PATIENT: That's true. When I want to smoke, I don't think about those things – being here for the kids and making sure I am around to see them through to when they have their families. But I sure plan to be around to see them deal with their own kids – and tell them 'I told you so!' (*Laughs*)

COUNSELLOR: Right, the best revenge is living! But somehow, when you are lighting up, this goal, this aspiration to be alive and thriving at age 65 and beyond is nowhere to be found. What do you think about that? (amplified reflection and develop discrepancy)

PATIENT: That bothers me (*falls silent*). If breast cancer has taught me anything, it's that life is precious.

COUNSELLOR: And your health seems to be the foundation of your dreams and aspirations. If you wanted to quit smoking, what are your thoughts about whether you could succeed? (amplify values and goals and elaborate change talk)

PATIENT: I did it before, when I was pregnant with each of my kids, but right after giving birth, I went back to it.

COUNSELLOR: How would your rate your confidence in your ability to quit smoking in the next few months. Let's assume a 0-10 scale, with 0 being no confidence at all, and 10 being the most confident you could imagine. What number between 0 and 10 would you choose? (evaluate and support self-efficacy)

PATIENT: I would put me at a six – after talking about this more, I feel I could do it, but I need help. I just have smoked so long, I know I need help.

COUNSELLOR: All right. We can help you. Besides help, is there anything else you would need to succeed? (elaborate change talk)

A key to understanding Martha's motivational dilemma is listening to her words to describe it: 'I *have* to quit smoking.' This and other externally focused words, such as 'must' or 'should' suggest ripe territory for exploring the nature of the patient's current motivation, which is likely to be extrinsic motivation highly regulated by external considerations, in this case, her plastic surgeon's request that she quit smoking. The task for the counsellor is to refrain from joining with the threat to autonomy, roll with resistance, and to help the patient explore her own values and goals as sources of motivation and forge linkages with efforts to quit smoking. This restores the locus of change to a more vibrant wellspring of motivation that may help her maintain abstinence well beyond the pressure point of breast reconstruction.

6.4 Evidence on Efficacy

The diffusion of MI or adaptations of MI into diverse intervention studies has been rapid since the early 1990s. Four meta-analyses of studies testing the efficacy of MI or MI adaptations across multiple problem behaviours have been published [19–22], with each successive meta-analysis examining, in order, 30, 72, 15 (only alcohol use studies were analysed) and 119 studies. A subsequent descriptive review of these meta-analyses summarised findings to facilitate their application in clinical practice [22]. Given these extensive analyses of MI interventions, a summary is presented. Meta-analyses showed a robust effect of MI interventions particularly in alcohol-related problems. MI treatments are superior to no treatment in tobacco use, marijuana dependence, and other drugs such as cocaine and heroin [22]. Effect sizes vary depending upon the comparison group and substance use outcome, but when compared to wait list or no-treatment groups, MI's average effect sizes were in the small to medium range. When MI is compared to active treatment groups, for example 12-step treatment or Cognitive-Behavioral Therapy (CBT), it is equally effective or more so. MI treatment duration, however, is typically shorter than comparison active treatments. When length of treatment was assessed in the meta-analyses, face-to-face time was about 100 minutes less (about two 50-minute sessions) than in the treatment-as-usual comparison conditions [22]. Thus, MI can be a cost-effective means of effecting behaviour change in alcohol, tobacco, and other substance abuse and dependence.

Despite finding an overall diminishing impact of MI treatment over time, the meta-analyses indicate that treatment effects can endure for at least one year after treatment, and two studies found effects of MI at two years [19, 23]. The evidence regarding format of MI treatment indicates that individual format is effective, with or without concurrent group-based MI, but group-based MI treatment alone lacks efficacy. It may be that the therapeutic alliance and the client-centred approach are diluted in group settings; thus, caution should be used in applying MI solely in group format. Another aspect of format is the application of MI as a pretreatment versus stand-alone treatment, as MI was initially developed as the former [5]. Three meta-analyses found support that MI worked best as a pretreatment in preparation for inpatient treatment or CBT, or with a standardised, problem-feedback component [19, 20, 23].

For which patient populations does MI work best? The meta-analyses found no differential effects of MI based on age or gender, suggesting that it works equally well across these demographic characteristics. Very little research has been conducted using MI with minors, and because of the strong cognitive elements of MI, it is likely that it would need to be adapted considerably for adolescents, and perhaps for young adults [24]. The meta-analyses also provide some support that MI may be more effective with ethnic and racial groups, for example Native Americans in the Southwest [20], possibly because the client-centred, non-confrontational communication style may be more compatible with cultural norms. This and other findings suggest that, if anything, MI may be especially effective with patients of certain minority groups. Since MI was formulated to work with clients resistant to change, it is not surprising that some data indicate that MI works best with those who are less ready for change [25, 26]. In summary, the extensive empirical evidence supports the efficacy of MI in treating diverse substance use problems and populations.

6.5 Service Development

Because of the complex nature of the philosophy and skill set of MI, effective practice is best achieved through formal training. Indeed, the authors specify eight stages of becoming proficient in MI [27]. The dissemination of MI is well supported by the Motivational Interviewing Network of Trainers, or MINT, an organisation dedicated to providing ongoing education internationally to clinicians, researchers and trainers [28]. MINT trainers offer interactive workshops designed for persons at different levels of expertise in MI, from beginners to advanced practitioners. Regarding who is eligible for training, notably, one meta-analysis of MI studies found that the degree and profession of the MI practitioner, for example undergraduate-, masters- or doctoral-level education, did not influence client outcomes [23]. Since all trial clinicians were trained in MI, this suggests that MI is a method that can be learned and applied effectively along a continuum of educational backgrounds.

6.6 Summary

This has been at best an introduction to the method of MI, and the reader is strongly encouraged to read the authors' texts and other writings in the references below, and to participate in formal training. The cancer context presents unique challenges to clinicians encountering substance use, abuse or dependence in their patients, but cancer also provides a compelling rationale for changing behaviour. Many cancer patients do stop smoking, alcohol use and other substances with little or no intervention from cancer care providers. It is critical that for those patients unable or unwilling to change their habit, clinicians appreciate their ambivalence about abstinence, even amidst this health threat, and have tools for guiding patients to explore their internal resources for change. MI has been presented as an evidence-based method for effecting change, and it is hoped that its use will enhance both cancer survivorship and substance use treatment outcomes.

Acknowledgements

This work was supported in part by NIH grants **R01CA90514**, **T32CA009461**, and **U54CA137788**, and the work of the members of the Tobacco Cessation Programme at Memorial Sloan-Kettering Cancer Center.

Mr. Christopher Webster's contribution in manuscript preparation is greatly appreciated.

References

1. Demark-Wahnefried, W., Aziz, N., Rowland, J. and Pinto, B. (2005) Riding the crest of the teachable moment: promoting long-term health after the diagnosis of cancer. *Journal of Clinical Oncology*, **23** (24), 5814–5830.

2. McBride, C.M. (2003) Teachable moments for promoting smoking cessation: The context of cancer care and survivorship. *Cancer Control*, **10** (4), 325–333.

3. Demark-Wahnefried, W., Peterson, B., McBride, C. *et al.* (2000) Current health behaviors and readiness to pursue life-style changes among men and women diagnosed with early stage prostate and breast carcinomas. *Cancer*, **88** (3), 674–684.

4. Bellizzi, K.M., Rowland, J.H., Jeffery, D.D. and McNeel, T. (2005) Health behaviors of cancer survivors: examining opportunities for cancer control intervention. *Journal of Clinical Oncology*, **23** (34), 8884–8893.

5. Miller, W.R. and Rollnick, S. (1991) *Motivational Interviewing: Preparing People for Change*, Ist edn, The Guilford Press, New York.

6. Miller, W.R. and Rollnick, S. (2002) *Motivational Interviewing: Preparing People for Change*, 2nd edn, The Guilford Press, New York.

7. Rogers, C.R. (1959) A theory of therapy, personality, and interpersonal relationships as developed in the client-centered framework, in *Psychology: The Study of a Science Formulations of the Person and the Social Contexts* (ed. S. Koch), McGraw-Hill, New York, pp. 184–256.

8. Yablonsky, L. (1965) *Synanon: The Tunnel Back*, McMillan, New York.

9. Yablonsky, L. (1989) *The Therapeutic Community: A Successful Approach for Treating Substance Abuse Disorders*, Gardner Press, New York.

10. Festinger, L. (1957) *A Theory of Cognitive Dissonance*, Stanford University Press, Stanford, CA.

11. Bem, D.J. (1972) Self-perception theory, in *Advances in Experimental Social Psychology* (ed. L. Berkowitz), Academic Press, New York, pp. 1–62.

12. DiClemente, C.C. and Velasquez, M.M. (2002) Motivational interviewing and the stages of change, in *Motivational Interviewing: Preparing People for Change*, 2nd edn (eds W.R. Miller and S. Rollnick), The Guilford Press, New York, pp. 201–216.

13. Deci, E.L. and Ryan, R.M. (1985) *Intrinsic Motivation and Self-determination in Human Behavior*, Plenum, New York.

14. Markland, D., Ryan, R.M., Tobin, V.J. and Rollnick, S. (2005) Motivational interviewing and self-determination theory. *Journal of Social and Clinical Psychology*, **24** (6), 811–831.

15. Martin, D.J., Garske, J.P. and Davis, M.K. (2000) Relation of the therapeutic alliance with outcome and other variables: a meta-analytic review. *Journal of Consulting and Clinical Psychology*, **68** (3), 438–450.

16. NCI (2005) *Theory at a Glance: A Guide for Health Promotion Practice*, National Cancer Institute, NIH Publication No. 05-3896.

17. Bandura, A. (1986) *Social Foundations of Thought and Action: A Social Cognitive Theory*, Prentice Hall, Englewood Cliffs, NJ.

18. Rollnick, S., Miller, W.R. and Butler, C.C. (2008) *Motivational Interviewing in Health care: Helping Patients change Behavior*, The Guilford Press, New York.

19. Burke, B., Arkowitz, H. and Menchola, M. (2003) The efficacy of motivational interviewing: a meta-analysis of controlled clinical trials. *Journal of Consulting and Clinical Psychology*, **71** (5), 843–861.

20. Hettema, J., Steele, J. and Miller, W.R. (2005) Motivational interviewing. *Annual Review of Clinical Psychology*, **1**, 91–111.

21. Vasilaki, E., Hosier, S. and Cox, W.M. (2006) The efficacy of motivational interviewing as a brief intervention for excessive drinking: a meta-analytic review. *Alcohol and Alcoholism: International Journal of the Medical Council on Alcoholism*, **41** (3), 328–335.

22. Lundahl, B. and Burke, B. (2009) The effectiveness and applicability of motivational interviewing: a practice-friendly review of four meta-analyses. *Journal of Clinical Psychology*, **65** (11), 1232–1245.

23. Lundahl, B.W., Kunz, C., Brownell, C. *et al.* (2010) A Meta-Analysis of Motivational Interviewing: Twenty-Five Years of Empirical Studies. *Research on Social Work Practice*, **20** (2), 137–160.

24. Baer, J.S. and Peterson, P.L. (2002) Motivational interviewing with adolescents and young adults, in *Motivational Interviewing: Preparing People for Change*, 2nd edn (eds W.R. Miller and S. Rollnick), The Guilford Press, New York, pp. 320–332.

25. Heather, N., Rollnick, S., Bell, A. and Richmond, R. (1996) Effects of brief counselling among male heavy drinkers identified on general hospital wards. *Drug and Alcohol Review*, **15** (1), 29–38.

26. Project MATCH, Project MATCH Research Group (1997) Project MATCH secondary a priori hypotheses. *Addiction (Abingdon, England)*, **92** (12), 1671–1698.

27. Miller, W.R. (2007) Eight stages in learning motivational interviewing. *Journal of Teaching in the Addictions*, **5** (1), 3–17.

28. MINT (Motivational Interviewing Network of Trainers. http://www.motivationalinterview.org/training/trainers.html Created by: Christopher C. Wagner, Ph.D. & Wayne Conners, M.Ed., Mid-Atlantic Addiction Technology Transfer Center, A CSAT Project (accessed 15 February 2011).

7 Narrative Therapy

Bo Snedker Boman

Departments of Oncology and Hematology, Roskilde Hospital, Roskilde, Denmark

7.1 Background

Narrative therapy denotes a number of psychosocial forms of intervention with individuals, couples, families, groups and organisations with a basis in narrative theories. The focus is on the narratives and the outlook and the vocabulary of the client which they bring to the therapy sessions. The focus is also on what influence or power or ability for marginalisation and debasement or dissatisfaction, these narratives and outlook and vocabulary have on the client themselves and the people they live with and among. Historically, narrative therapy was not created in a psycho-oncological context, but as a form of practice it is especially meaningful in the encounter with people with cancer and their network; primarily because it is concrete and straightforward and close to everyday existence in *its* outlook, and usually narrative therapy offers the client a sense of (again) being able to navigate a possibly chaotic life in which cancer and treatment and hospital admissions, and so on have become part of everyday life. Narrative therapy as a post-structuralist intervention form breaks away from many, more traditional forms of therapy and cannot immediately be integrated in other intervention forms. The epistemological premises of narrative therapy are too disparate from those of other forms of therapy for that. For a discussion of some of these aspects, please refer to [1]. More precisely, narrative therapy has a special focus on how identity is shaped by narratives: Who am I, and who will I be when certain narratives about me (now? e.g. as suffering from cancer) are given precedence over other narratives about me (e.g. as a caring father or a strong construction worker)? What happens to the identity of the cancer patient if the narratives of being a patient, dependent, medicated, powerless, helpless, and so on override the client's preferred narratives of being healthy or strong or happy or active, thus risking the client feeling marginalised in society and also within the cancer community which, at least in modern Western culture, primarily celebrate the winner, the survivor, the warrior?

The principal methodical definitions of narrative therapy have been made by Michael White, David Epston, Jerome Monk, John Winslade, Lorraine Hedtke, Jill Freedman and Johnella Bird (see [2–11]). Although, with regard to the clinical directions, naturally there are key differences in these authors, they all have their philosophical foundation in the works of Gregory Bateson, Michel Foucault, Jerome Bruner and Leo Vygotsky. The social-constructionist influence (and the influence from anthropology, sociology and comparative literature) is especially manifest, in that narrative therapy is not interested in the absolute truth, the normal, the authentic, the real, but rather the productive potential of the narratives that are given. Narrative therapy is not a part of an outright value nihilist project, but it is a form of therapy that insists on not simply consolidating the dictates of already dominating discourses of, for example the right ways of living with or dying of cancer.

7.1.1 Reservation

Consequently, in a sense, it is difficult to formulate a chapter on narrative therapy: as it is the objective of narrative therapy always and constantly to relate to factual and concrete aspects (unlike the at times somewhat academic psychological abstractions or simplified typologies of other psychotherapies) in the concrete encounter with the concrete client with precisely their narratives, the danger lies in this text being given the nature of a manual, thus removing itself from precisely the concrete aspects that narrative therapy seeks to meet and, unbiased, relate to.

7.1.2 Terminology

In narrative therapy it is essential to be continually and critically aware of the linguistic practice one brings as a professional. For this reason, in my daily work I refrain from using terms such as *client* or *patient* or *therapist*. For the sake of convenience, however, in this text I shall employ the term *client* about the person who has fallen ill with cancer, and *therapist* about the person who, over the course of one or more conversations, offers professional skills, experience and motivation. Often family members, friends, acquaintances, colleagues, other health professionals or other clients are invited along to the conversations in narrative therapy. These people are termed outsider witnesses, and I shall return to them later.

7.1.3 The Purpose of Narrative Therapy

In narrative therapy the therapist's primary objective is to orchestrate a meeting between a number of people, rather than being an expert on an (evidence based) psychological truth about, for example depression or anxiety. The therapeutic task is to provide the framework for a hopefully helpful and meaningful conversation between a client and a number of outsider witnesses and the therapist, in a manner that makes at least the client feel invited to adopt positions as more than just, for example tortured, lonely woman or depressive man with advanced lung cancer. This happens in order to not overlook or ignore the reason for the enquiry (anxiety, depression, anger, etc.) which de facto causes pain or insecurity or dread in the client's life; rather it is to challenge and explore a usually dominant and seldom positive perception in many people who involuntarily come into contact with a medically regulated and monocausal, essentialistically thinking health service: That 'the problem' (pain, depression, etc.) exists in itself and can be treated as such (as e.g. antibiotics against fever). In narrative therapy this notion is challenged by looking at, for example 'depression' as an external entity which, however, has been able to corrupt the client's life and possibly those of their family too. The ability of problems to give people the impression of their complete dominance first and foremost happens linguistically, most obviously in the use of adjectives. In narrative therapy the therapists seeks to privilege an intentional state understanding and avoid an internal state understanding, as the latter tends to

diminish the sense of personal agency and to discourage diversity [2].

7.1.4 Area of Application

The basic methods of narrative therapy can be employed in conversations with individuals, couples, families and groups. Michael White in particular offers elaborate descriptions of possible applications of the methods with children and young people. Inspired by narrative therapy Fredman [13] offers a detailed description of working with children and families in relation to illness and death and loss. White as well as Epston refer to narrative therapy as a playful approach to serious problems, and the experience of most practitioners is that narrative therapy through this playful approach often imbues conversations about even very serious subjects with a touch of levity and hope of change, giving the client a sense of security or drive or at least of not being excluded from their own life, which otherwise can be the impression left by cancer treatment. I employ narrative therapy in conversations with young and old cancer patients alike, with children and young people who are next-of-kin, in group therapy for people with cancer and in bereavement groups as well as (in adjusted form) when supervising nurses and doctors.

7.2 Processes and Techniques

Next I will describe some of the methods in a conversation that one can employ in narrative therapy. They are *externalising conversation, re-membering* and *responses from the outsider witnesses*. This is not an exhaustive account of narrative therapy but merely an introduction. In practice, in my experience, these methods are employed alternately. The starting point for a therapeutic conversation is usually that the client themselves has enquired or been referred by an oncologist, GP, nurse or the like, because something is wrong or inappropriate or painful and must be solved, helped, corrected, alleviated or accepted. In narrative therapy the referral is not regarded as merely a casual and now past event which has brought the client to the therapist's office.

When I receive a referral, I contact the client and introduce myself. I tell them what the referral says and ask the client if they wish to meet with me. If this is the case, I ask the client to consider if they want to invite along one or more friends or family members to our conversation. And I tell them that I would like to invite a psychology student or a nurse or some other professional, part of whose work is to learn more about life with cancer. Usually the client will show up with one or two friends or family members, and I often bring along a colleague or student.

At the beginning of a conversation, the question is asked, 'Whose idea was it that you and I meet?' *in order to illuminate which narratives about the therapeutic encounter have* already *been told. Or:* 'Who articulated which hope or which doubt before our conversation today?'

The client might respond, *'It was John, the doctor, who thought it would do me good to talk to someone about my situation of relapses of cancer, and so on.'*
This sort of phrase can be interpreted in many ways – and at least says something about the client's experience of a third party wanting the meeting between the client and the therapist. But the phrase is also a testament to a cultural convention which on the back of psychoanalysis has been prevalent in Western society for about a 100 years and which now (with the best of intentions, to be sure) has been repeated by the doctor upon the referral: Talking to someone is good, implicitly suggesting that not doing so is less good. In narrative therapy, however, it is considered a virtue to question conventions and not merely allow them to hold sway over people.

If the client responds as above, the next question is, 'Alright, how do you feel about what John, the doctor, says – that talking to someone is a good thing?'

The aim is not to tease the client or devalue the doctor's act but rather, with the aid of language, to set the client free and not have the client be positioned immediately on meeting the therapist as 'the problem describing client who, according to the doctor, is probably depressive and irascible and who now needs to talk to a professional'. In my experience, when asked this question, most clients will say that their experiences of talking about their situation are good, whereas others are given the opportunity to say that they would rather avoid the present conversation.

And if *the answer is affirmative, it makes a method oriented question possible:* 'Thanks for showing me the trust of coming here today – now tell me a bit about how you would like us to talk to each other. I can think of several ways of talking together. For instance would you prefer that I ask you a number of questions, or would you rather talk while I listen quietly, or something else entirely'

Again, the aim is the same: to place the client in the freest possible position in which as few conventions as possible determine the direction of the conversation, and instead to talk in a way that gives the client the greatest comfort.

At this point I position the other participants in the conversation. I tell the client's friends or family members and my colleague or student (the outsider witnesses) to pay attention to the conversation between the client and me. They can write things down as we go along, and I ask them to make sure they do not offer counsel, judgement or evaluations. I ask them to listen and preferably very intently – and I tell them that later I will ask them to reflect on some of the things they have heard.

With this introduction the client will usually begin to describe themselves and relatively soon probably also their difficulties. In this aspect narrative therapy hardly differs from other forms of intervention in its guidelines for the therapist: Listen to the client! In narrative therapy, however, it is important to listen to the *letter*. Now, what does that mean? As the therapeutic focus is the narratives that the client brings about themselves, it is key that the therapist notices *precisely* which words and expressions and intonations are employed by the client – and *himself uses* these words and expressions and intonations if he asks any questions.

In continuation of psychoanalysis, most psychological theories and psychotherapeutical methods throughout the twentieth century have dealt with mental phenomena as inherent in people. Everyday language supports this: 'The anxiety is within you' (as an infected appendix can be within you), 'I have low self-esteem' (as you can have low blood sugar) or 'he is full of rage' (as you can be filled up with food). In the rhetoric of many psychological theories, mental phenomena (good as well as bad ones) are internalised in the person.

A person with cancer whose doctor sees them as sad and hopeless is often described as *having* a depression – and symptoms (anger, resignation, agitation, etc.) in this regard are considered expressions of an inner, pathological state. Narrative therapy wholly recognises the agony of experiencing the world as sad and hopeless. But narrative therapy also seeks to challenge the notion that this is an inner state of a more or less abiding, so-called chronic nature. To simplify it, the client does not have a depression, but the depression has taken *hold of* the client, and it is the effects of this hold (as well as other things) that the client is now fighting and suffering under. This means that in theoretical and linguistic practice, a separation is inserted between the client and the depression. They are not identical as the adjective 'depressive' might lead the client and the therapist to believe. It is attempted to make the separation plain in a so-called *externalising conversation*.

A beneficial beginning to an externalising conversation could be a suggestion: 'Describe to me what you're struggling with these days.'

This suggestion will often lead to a series of narratives from the client about a number of circumstances of a painful nature in their life. The idea is that now the therapist just listens intently without judging or exposing his own normative perceptions of right and wrong or sad and awful or lovely and marvellous.

When the client has described what they are challenged by and struggling with, the next question in an externalising conversation is, 'What do you call what you're struggling with?' *or* 'Do you have a name or a term for what you have described to me?'

After this first step – called **naming** *– follows a series of questions such as* 'Why is this an apt name for what you're struggling with?', *and* 'Do you have other names for it?', *followed by* 'Has this been the term for it all along or has it changed in the process?'

In the conversation about naming, as a trained clinician with extensive knowledge about psychology and psychiatry, one must (at least temporarily) set aside one's own so-called diagnostic deliberations. If the client describes what she is fighting as 'the stupid anger', although as a therapist with a loyalty to the diagnostic system one would describe it as 'moderate depression' one allows the client's term to be the point of departure for the following conversation. One might say that the narrative therapist does not consider it his task to illustrate or even prove that he has access to special and exclusive words, a jargon, an argot for mental health workers.

Next step in an externalising conversation deals with the *effects* that, from the client's perspective, for example 'the stupid anger' has or has had or is feared to have on their life, possibly also including which effects 'the stupid anger' has or has had or is feared to have on other people in the client's life.

Often the description of the effects of, for example 'the stupid anger' concerns changes in behaviour, emotional life, thought, social relations, bodily conditions, understanding of self, and so on – and often a certain amount of sadness will accompany them. Thus, 'the stupid anger' is one cause among several of new narratives in the client's life: '*Usually I'm the strong one but that's no longer the case.*' In narrative therapy, narratives are said to have significance to the **identity conclusions** that people form about themselves: The narratives about 'the stupid anger' and its effects on the client, then, can cause them to conclude that '*I am weak*' or '*I have lost control*'.

In narrative therapy it is important to repeat the question, 'Has the problem other effects on your life?' *a number of times in order to contribute to a diverse description of the mostly unwanted changes that the client experiences in their life.*

Advancing too fast, one risks consolidating the usually monocausal model of explanation that the client has already employed, for example: 'The stupid anger' has had the effect that '*I constantly need my children around me*' or '*I cling to my children because I'm so afraid.*'

After the naming and the description of the effects, the client is encouraged to **evaluate the effects**: 'How do you feel about the fact that the stupid anger has had and seems still to have these effects on the lives of you and your family?'

Usually the evaluation leads to the client expressing their despair over the effects 'the stupid anger' has managed to have on the client's and family's lives: '*Well, I'm not happy about that*' or '*That's no good*' or '*Why, it's awful that these things affect my kids*'. It is through the evaluating questions that the therapist will usually have the chance to listen to the client's frustration or grief over a changed and often uncontrollable life situation.

And usually this is where the client will hear themselves express something that has not been told before. The therapist's question, 'So tell me: How do you feel about being sad that 'the stupid anger' ruins your nights?' *is often the question that marks it out from those of others, where the state 'angry' by definition is considered regrettable or unfortunate.*

In the fourth and final step in the externalising conversation – *justification* – the client is asked *why* she has evaluated thusly. In this manner **important values** in the client's life are introduced to the conversation: '*It's horrible because I want to be a good and loving mum, giving my children the opportunity* *to live their own lives.'* The aim of the externalising conversation can be said to be that, through an exploration of the effects of one or more problems on the client's life, it enables a conversation about what values and viewpoints the client brings with them in life and will probably go far to defend and which have now temporarily been corrupted by, for example 'the stupid anger'. In this manner an externalising conversation not only becomes a problem describing conversation but also a conversation about vital and important values in the client's life.

Note here that this step has nothing to do with positive psychology or solution focused method – because the externalising conversation takes its time in describing problems and the effects of problems and takes absolutely seriously what the client says, without seeking solutions. And talking about values on a general, existential level rarely offers solutions to concrete problems. The rationale is, through conversation, to bring the client into a position where hopefully it becomes manifest that complex aspects in their life have corrupted significant parts of the client's life. White [2] claims that it "(...) is quite common for this unravelling process to reveal the history of the 'politics' of the problems that bring people to therapy. This is a history of the power relations that people have been subject to and that have shaped their negative conclusions about their life and their identity" (p 27). 'The stupid anger', for example is stupid in that it seems to have the power to make the client be a mother in a different way than the one she prefers. White describes this as *the absent, but implicit*: Logically the client's preferred identity conclusions must be silently present in the current situation.

Note here that the externalising conversation does not necessarily make it easier for the client to be reconciled with their preferred way of living being temporarily or permanently suspended. However, a conversation which linguistically separates problem from naming from effects from evaluation from justification often gives the client an understanding of the complexity of the current situation, sometimes suggests a hope that change *might* be possible, and most importantly positions the client in a safe place: At the centre of the values which the client brings with them as particularly important in life and which usually have been significant (also) long before the cancer cropped up. Often these values have not been grabbed out of thin air or dropped from the sky, but are closely linked with narratives of the life lived and the experiences of the client in life, generally in the company of other people. These people and the narratives

about them can now be brought into the conversation, which is what the next section deals with.

7.2.1 Re-Membering

First, a short detour. In the psycho-oncological field, death, loss and parting are a possibly unpleasant but ineluctable part of the work – at least for the therapist who will often be invited into conversations concerning leaving or being left by people one cares for or does not like but which all the same one has been forced to spend a part of one's life with. Narrative therapy attempts to give voice to the general experience most adults have, more or less obvious to themselves: That the person we have become is influenced by those we have lived with or near or who have meant something to us generally – who have seen us, touched us or turned their back on us. That the narratives I have of myself are often influenced by who told what to whom about me when. Adults carry more or less obvious to themselves these narratives with them. And the connection to important people in my life can continue even when these people are no longer living. Whereas traditional psychoanalytic theory of drives (and a great deal of grief theoretical thoughts after Freud) often offers the view that so-called healthy handling of grief, for example of an adult woman who has lost her husband, is concerned with the gradual withdrawal of the libido and commitment to another relation, narrative therapy turns this schism upside-down. In his 1988 essay 'Saying Hullo Again', White [3] claims: 'It can be expected that (...) further grief work oriented by a normative model – one that specifies the stages of the grief process according to the saying goodbye metaphor – will complicate the situation further, rather than empower these persons and enrich their lives' (p 7).

I often pose these questions to dying clients, 'I wonder which stories about you will survive when your body is dead?', and 'Who would you like to remember what about you?', and 'Which stories about you wouldn't you mind dying with the body that has fallen ill?', etc.

As stated re-membering can also be employed in continuation of externalising conversations.

In a conversation with a client who has uttered how being a good and loving mother is valuable and important to her, I might ask: 'Who would have predicted your saying this today?', or 'Who would not be surprised to hear you say this?', *or* 'I wonder who inspired you to hold these things as valuable in your life?'

The client might respond, 'My mother', and the next question would then be, 'What does it mean to you that your mother would have predicted your saying this?'

The last question is the key one as it explores possible lines of connection between vital values in the client's life now and the people who have shaped the client up until now and who will possibly do so in the future.

7.2.2 *Responses from the Outsider Witnesses*

It is worth repeating that there are outsider witnesses present in the room during the conversation. Usually, after 30–35 minutes have elapsed, I will ask the outsider witnesses to converse with me while the client is entreated to listen and maybe jot down notes in the process. I subsequently pose the following questions more or less rigidly to the outsider witnesses:

1. 'What have you heard the client say? What grabbed you in what the client talked about?'

2. 'When the client says this, which values do you believe are present in the client's life?', and 'When saying things like that, what do you think one values in one's life?', and 'What are the important things to a person who talks like that?'

3. 'I wonder which skills the client possesses when he talks like that?', and 'What is the client capable of doing?'

4. 'What does this remind you of in your own life?', and 'Which of the narratives in your life do the client's narratives invoke?', and 'What resonates in you?'

5. 'So, what will you take with you today when you leave?', and 'What have you been encouraged by or become more aware of by listening to the client's narratives?'

The questions serve as a framework for what in narrative therapy must be considered crucial: That the client does not merely talk (talking cure) but is given a number of responses too. These responses from the outsider witnesses must not be patronising, advising, condescending or praising. Thus the outsider witnesses are supported in their respectful and sympathetic way of talking about the resonance which the client's

words and narratives have had. The assumption is that the outsider witnesses *have* been moved or enriched by listening to the client's struggles with life – and the assumption is that the outsider witnesses wish to and hopefully feel able to share their own life experiences with the client, the other outsider witnesses and the therapist. Based on my experience, this part of the conversation demands a *considerable* effort from the therapist: Partly because most outsider witnesses will be emotionally affected at this point in the conversation, and partly because many outsider witnesses will want to offer advice or even lecture the client about the reasonable, horrible or pointless aspects of their narratives. Naturally the outsider witnesses are allowed to show that they are emotionally moved (happy, sad, disappointed, sorrowful, etc.) but they cannot offer advice because the client did not ask the outsider witnesses for that! Whereas the outsider witnesses invited along by the client (family, friends, acquaintances) usually have no problems answering my questions and thus witnessing my client's narratives, for the outsider witnesses I have invited this often poses great difficulty.

To many nurses and psychologists and psychology students, talking about one's own experiences of problems in one's life is considered something of a violation of an historically handed down taboo. In particular, the fourth question above is considered difficult to answer. In many ways this question transgresses the traditional, deeply rooted limitations of what is given voice in a professional conversation. Note, however, that the question is not an invitation for the witnesses to relate their joys and sorrows in great detail. The reasoning behind the responses from the outsider witnesses is to give the client the experience that someone has listened to them carefully and thought about important values in the client's life and how this resonates in the outsider witnesses' narratives of a life lived – but no more. As a therapist the challenge lies in inviting outsider witnesses to generate thoughts of experiences through concrete examples – without these examples grabbing the focus of the conversation.

When the conversation between the outsider witnesses and me is over, I ask the client to comment on what has been said. At times the client decides not to say anything, but more often the client tells us that they have been very moved by the fact that people have listened so intently to the narratives they have offered. And usually the client says that it has been very significant and helpful to listen to the thoughts the outsider witnesses had about the resonance in their own lives of what the client has said.

In principle the conversation can continue like this for a while, giving the outsider witnesses a chance to speak up a second time. In my experience, however, at this point many clients and outsider witnesses are tired, and a more or less natural end to the conversation has been reached.

7.3 Case Example

Peter was 44 years old and worked as an upper-secondary school teacher. He had a child from his first marriage and two from his current relationship with a woman his age, Lisa. For some time he had felt generally unwell, had vague stomach pains, slept significantly more than usual and had trouble keeping up his running exercise because of fatigue. As he repeatedly found blood in his stool, he saw his GP. Finding the cause was frustrated by a series of administrative errors by his GP, and during the process his oldest child was seriously injured and admitted to hospital long-term. Peter was diagnosed with rectal cancer, was operated on, and a chemotherapeutical treatment was prescribed. In the conversations with the oncologist both Peter and Lisa took part, and it was noted in his records several times that Peter had many questions about his treatment, that he seemed irascible and abusive, while it was noted that Lisa cried profusely and talked a lot about alternative forms of treatment.

At one point during his treatment, Peter got a number of vague symptoms, and he was admitted in a severely febrile state to the oncological ward for observation. After some days on antibiotic treatment, a nurse asked about him and the well-being of his family. To this Peter responded that he did not care about his life, and that the family would be better served with him dead. During rounds he repeated these statements, and Peter accepted that the doctor referred him to me. The next day it had been arranged that Peter and Lisa as well as a psychology student, Thomas, came to my office. I started by welcoming them and clearly setting out the framework: (i) 75 minutes available; (ii) Thomas was introduced as an outsider witness with some special tasks, and Lisa was invited to adopt a similar position, which she accepted, 'as long as it is helpful to us'; (iii) I told them that during the conversation I would be taking notes that anyone who wished to could see.

Then I started interviewing Peter, and to begin with I was interested in hearing about his experiences of talking together in general and with so-called professionals like me in particular, and I modified my conversation accordingly. I told him what I knew from his records: That some people felt he was abusive, and that he was quoted as saying he did not care about his life.

At this point it was not intrinsically interesting to me whether Peter considered these observations to be true or not. So I told him, 'Peter, all these things are something that other people believe and have written. Tell me a bit about how you see the world. What are you struggling with at the moment?' Hesitant, Peter began talking about how annoying the fever condition and the hospital stay were, and via a number of the questions that belong to the externalising conversation, a certain (linguistic) distance was created between Peter and the so-called problems. He described doctors and nurses as ridiculous and incompetent and overly sensitive. He seemed especially irritated with the fact that many of the nurses were so considerate, almost motherly, in their treatment of him: 'I'm not a child, am I? What do they think they're doing? I don't want to feel something just for their sake'. I asked Peter, 'Why not?' and he responded with raised voice, 'Because I decide what to feel'. Here it maybe would have been obvious to ask Peter what he wanted to feel – but I was more interested in his identity conclusions, linked with his narratives about himself.

So my question was, 'What does it say about what is important to you, Peter, when you can say, 'Because I decide what to feel?' Peter hesitated slightly and then said, 'Well, I believe I set great store by deciding for myself and my own body – I guess I'm kind of the self-dependent type.' And further: 'And what does it mean to you to be 'kind of the self-dependent type?' And his response: 'Why, it means the world.' And the question: 'Alright, why is that?' And the response, now from a visibly affected man: 'Because if I can be the self-dependent type, I can take care of myself. And then I can take care of my children, and you need to be able to do that as a man.'

In principle the dialogue between Peter and me could have continued this way even longer. I wanted to carry out a scaffolding conversation in which the focus is on exploring Peter's intentions and values, ethics even – and so lead Peter on to 'safe ground'.

And then I asked Peter who inspired him to be a man in just this way – and his answer was immediate: 'My father did that. He was a good and proper man who always took good care of his family'. And then I told Peter, 'I'd like to hear more about him. Introduce him to me', whereupon Peter described his father in great detail.

It is important to stress that re-membering practice, which this is an instance of, not only permits florid descriptions of possibly deceased, central people in the client's life. The interesting thing is not how – in this case – his father actually was (an essentialist description). It is how Peter in the concrete situation constructs a description of his father (good and bad memories alike) and from that derives inspiration and support. Right here, right now. The idea is that through his description he remembers his father (remembering) and so includes him in his club of self-dependent men (re-membering). As a therapist, in my conversation with Peter, my starting point is not only to be interested in what is missing or is incomplete (deficit) or what is difficult (conflict), but also in what Peter wants and can do, despite of illness and his hospital stay (cf. the intentional state understanding). In psycho-oncological work, where loss and death by definition is more imme-diately present than in human life in general, it is a salient point to focus on intentionality and ability or skills. There are two reasons for doing this.

1. In connection with admittals where concrete prob-lems must be solved in a concrete way, health staff might risk treating the client as a case-study rather than a person, to an extent that they cease listening to what the client actually can and wants to do. In our conversation, Peter claimed that he wanted to be a man in a way in which he in his own way could take care of his three children. However, as stated, narrative therapy is concerned with concrete mat-ters, therefore I encouraged Peter to 'tell me about a time when you succeeded in being a man in just this way'.

2. The intentionality expressed in 'And then I can take care of my children, and you need to be able to do that as a man' (cf. above) logically must be an expression of what Peter wanted at that time and presumably in the future too. Cancer or other things might prevent Peter from being able to take care of his children in his way but despite its power it cannot prevent Peter from wanting it. In a palliative context this can generate meaningful conversations – and for Lisa probably it would be valuable to know about Peter's intentions in relation to the children.

I now told Peter that I would like to bring the outsider witnesses, who so far have only listened, into our conversation. He accepted this, and I now asked first Lisa for her responses, and then Thomas, one by one. Lisa said what she took notice of, what this told her about what Peter's important values might be, which skills he might possess, and how his narratives resonated in her life. She added that she

had had the opportunity to listen without being able to interrupt – and that she had been given food for thought. Thomas too answered the first, second and third question and then came to a halt. I asked him the fourth question and he answered that he did not know what to say: 'You know, I've never been ill. And I don't have any kids.'

In narrative therapy there are now at least two paths to choose. One can end the conversation with Thomas and return to Peter. Or as a therapist one can help Thomas talk about the resonance made by Peter's narratives – knowing full well that Thomas is not ill and has no children. The assumption is that despite these differences there must be a resonance, something that has been moved, in Thomas' life. Thomas then says that in connection with his father's illness some years previously, he wished to take care of his father – but circumstances made it very difficult for him in practice. Thomas and I then talked about experiences of wanting to but not always being able to – and about the grief which Thomas felt in connection to this relationship.

In conclusion Thomas thanked Peter for reminding him of these thoughts about wanting to and being able to, and said, 'My dad certainly had his own way of being a man, and now Peter has inspired me to think about how I can be a man in my own way.' I then returned to Peter and told him, 'If you want to, you can comment on what Lisa and Thomas have said – what grabbed you about it?' Peter was silent for a while and then said that it had been very meaningful for him to listen to Lisa and Thomas: What they had heard and what resonance they had felt. He felt it particu-larly significant that the conversation and the responses from the outsider witnesses had made it plain to him that he was fighting for something rather than against something. I asked him, 'Alright, what does it mean to you that you are fighting for something rather than against something?' 'Why', he interrupted, 'there's a huge difference. I'm not just a troublesome and abu-sive patient – I'm a man with something at stake in my life, and I need to tell the nurses that, so they won't think I'm mad at them.'

Before the conversation was finished, I asked Peter if he wanted the verbatim notes I had made during the conversation. Peter accepted them and left with Lisa. A week later they both turned up, mostly because 'We didn't want you to think we don't keep our appoint-ments.' I thanked them for having come and asked them about their lives without presupposing that they wished to continue down the path from last week's conversation.

7.4 Evidence on Efficacy

As of yet there are only a limited number of studies of the effect of narrative therapy [12]. There are several reasons for this. Partly, narrative therapy is still a relatively young form of practice, and only quite shortly before his death in 2007 did White formulate a theoretically and methodically consistent, coherent theory of narrative therapy [2]. But, probably more importantly, narrative therapy as such is a critique of a structuralist frame of understanding which places great emphasis on monocausal, globally valid effect measurements. As a post-structuralist system of concepts and methods, narrative therapy is first and foremost interested in the local and concrete meaning. Nonetheless it is likely that in future years we shall see effect measurements of narrative therapy too.

7.5 Service Development

Without discussion narrative therapy including responses from the outsider witnesses takes time. As stated it is demanding to the therapist and some training with regular outsider witnesses (nurses, students, etc.) is recommended. So is some consideration of the effects on the outsider witnesses of being included but yet not part of a conversation. In any aspect of narrative therapy as a therapist paying attention to one's own language is crucial in order not to take a power position when this has no reason and when this is not being helpful to the client. It is the experience of many practitioners of narrative therapy that this is not as easy as it sounds!

7.6 Summary

In narrative therapy the client and the therapist and a number of outsider witnesses work with the problems and struggles along with the intentions and values in the client's life, in psycho-oncology primarily related to cancer and treatment. The therapist focuses on the narratives and identity conclusions of the client and eagerly seeks to pay attention to his own language, avoiding the use of an internal state understanding. Three methods are described: Externalising conversations, re-membering and responses from the outsider witnesses. Via a case-study the benefits and difficulties of listening and responding to the client and the outsider witnesses are discussed.

References

1. Polkinghorne, D. (2004) Narrative therapy and postmodernism, in *The Handbook of Narrative and Psychotherapy. Practice, Theory, and Research* (eds L.E. Angus and J. McLeod), Sage Publications, Thousand Oaks, pp. 53–68.
2. White, M. (2007) *Maps of Narrative Practice*, W W Norton & Company, New York.
3. White, M. (1989) Saying Hullo Again: the incorporation of the lost relationship in the resolution of grief, in *Selected Papers* (ed. M. White), Dulwich Centre Publishing, Adelaide, pp. 5–18.
4. Epston, D. (2008) *Down Under and up Over: Travels with Narrative Therapy*, Karnac, London.
5. Monk, G., Winslade, J. and Crocket, K. *et al.* (eds) (1997) *Narrative Therapy in Practice. The Archaeology of Hope*, Jossey-Bass, San Francisco.
6. Winslade, J. and Monk, G. (2000) *Narrative Mediation. A New Approach to Conflict Resolution*, Jossey-Bass, San Francisco.
7. Hedtke, L. and Winslade, J. (2004) *Re-membering Lives. Conversations with the Dying and the Bereaved*, Baywood, New York.
8. Freedman, J. and Combs, G. (1996) *Narrative Therapy: The Social Construction of Preferred Realities*, Norton, New York.
9. Bird, J. (2000) *The Heart's Narrative. Therapy and Navigating Life's Contradictions*, Edge Press, Auckland.
10. Bird, J. (2004) *Talk That Sings. Therapy in a New Linguistic Key*, Edge Press, Auckland.
11. Bird, J. (2006) *Constructing the Narrative in Super-Vision*, Edge Press, Auckland.
12. Etchison, M. and Kleist, D.M. (2000) Review of narrative therapy. *Family Journal*, **8**, 61–67.
13. Fredman, G. (1997) *Death Talk. Conversations with Children and Families*, Karnac Books Ltd, London.

8 Dignity Therapy

Harvey Max Chochinov[1,2] and Nancy A. McKeen[3]

[1]CancerCare Manitoba, Winnipeg, Manitoba, Canada
[2]Department of Psychiatry, University of Manitoba, Winnipeg, Canada
[3]University of Manitoba, St. Boniface General Hospital, St. Boniface, Manitoba, Canada

8.1 Introduction

Dignity Therapy is a patient-affirming psychotherapeutic intervention designed to address existential and psychosocial distress in people who have only a short time left to live. It is unique in that it aims to improve the quality of life in terminally ill patients by encouraging them to reflect on important or memorable life events. The dignity therapist helps patients to recall events from their lives, along with important thoughts, feelings, values, as well as their life accomplishments. Patients are invited to share their hopes and dreams for loved ones, pass along advice or guidance to the important people in their lives and how they wish to be remembered.

Dignity Therapy has multiple benefits. For dying patients themselves, it can promote spiritual and psychological well being, mitigate suffering and engender meaning and purpose. In some instances, it helps people prepare for death or provides them comfort in the time they have remaining. For family survivors, Dignity Therapy can help ease bereavement by giving them a document that expresses the feelings and thoughts of their departed loved one.

In this chapter, we introduce the basic tenets and techniques of Dignity Therapy, review its development, underlying themes and processes and the data supporting its efficacy. To take the basic concepts presented in this chapter and incorporate them into practice will require further training and deliberate practice; however, readers will become familiar with the basic concepts of dignity, dignity-conserving care and Dignity Therapy, in the context of caring for people with life-threatening and life-limiting illnesses.

8.2 Background of Dignity Research

Although dignity has been given a high profile in discussions on palliative care and decision-making at the end-of-life, the issue of people seeking out assistance in ending their lives brought it to greater prominence. The concept of dying with dignity is often invoked as a key rationale for physician-assisted-suicide and euthanasia [1–3], and loss of dignity is often cited by physicians as the reason their patients sought a hastened death [4, 5]. This identification of dignity as a putative justification for hastening death underscores its importance. Few would argue that patients nearing death deserve care and compassion. As such, it is important to emphasise that in spite of dignity's unfortunate associations with assisted death, the construct of dignity can also provide invaluable guidance on how to improve the quality of life for patients nearing end-of-life [6, 7].

An empirically informed understanding of how considerations of dignity might shape care for the dying arose within a targeted programme of palliative care research [8]. One of the first research challenges was how to define dignity.

8.2.1 Defining Dignity

Until recently, the concept of dignity lacked definitional specificity; its meaning could be construed in different ways, depending on the varying perceptions of physicians and caregivers, close relatives or patients themselves [9–11]. Dignity is defined as the quality or state of being worthy, honoured or esteemed [12]. This definition conveys the notion of the inherent respect due to patients who are preparing for death [13–15]. For patients, a sense of dignity means feeling that they are respected and worthy of respect, despite the physical decline and psychological distresses their illnesses bring.

The concept of dignity is not limited, however, to ideas about self-respect and self-worth. It also includes notions of being able to maintain physical comfort, autonomy, meaning, spiritual comfort, interpersonal connectedness and belonging in the face of impending death [16–18]. A fractured sense of dignity, in contrast, is associated with feelings of degradation, shame and embarrassment and is linked to depression, hopelessness and desire for death [19].

From a broader perspective, dignity addresses the notion that all human beings have intrinsic worth. While a sense of dignity may be internally mediated and intrinsic to one's sense of self, dignity may also be constructed through our evaluations of social interactions [20, 21]. In that regard, dignity may be understood as a reciprocal process, in that it is nurtured and supported by the personal relationships that exist between people, and depends upon feedback from others to stay robust throughout life [22]. These aspects of dignity are derived not only from patients themselves, but from those around them, including physicians, family and caregivers. In this sense, dignity in palliative care is a function of the attitudes and behaviours communicated by others.

Empirical research into dignity has provided key data, demonstrating how a deeper understanding of dignity and dignity-related distress has helped to meet the needs of patients approaching the end-of-life. It has provided an empirically based *Model of Dignity*, focused primarily on end-stage cancer and outlining the dimensions of distress that have dignity-related implications [15]. This model has yielded both practical guidance for holistic, quality, dignity-conserving, end-of-life care [15, 19, 23–25] and provides the theoretical foundation for the development of Dignity Therapy.

8.2.2 The Model of Dignity

The empirical study of the concept of dignity began with a qualitative study designed to clarify the meaning of patient dignity and describe sources of distress that could infringe upon a sense of dignity for dying patients [15]. As part of a semi-structured interview, patients were asked how they understood and defined the term dignity and what experiences or issues supported or undermined their own sense of dignity.

Fifty men and women with terminal cancer (age range 37–90 years) with two to three months to live were interviewed and audio-taped.

Each patient's sense of dignity was explored, using the following questions: (i) In terms of your own illness experience, how do you define the term dignity? (ii) What supports your sense of dignity? (iii) What undermines your sense of dignity? (iv) Are there specific experiences you can recall in which your dignity was compromised? (v) Are there specific experiences you can recall in which your dignity was supported? (vi) What would have to happen in your life for you to feel that you no longer had a sense of dignity? (vii) Some people feel that life without dignity is a life no longer worth living. How do you feel about that? (viii) Do you believe that dignity is something you hold within you, and/or is it something that can be given or taken away by others? [15] Concepts were defined and refined, and an empirical model emerged, which reflected the concept of dignity as derived from the perspective of dying patients themselves (see Figure 8.1).

Three major categories were identified from the qualitative analysis: (i) illness-related concerns, (ii) a dignity-conserving repertoire and (iii) a social dignity inventory. These categories refer to experiences, events or feelings, where dignity or lack of dignity becomes a relevant concern within the course of patients' approaching death. Each category contains several themes and sub-themes, which form the foundation of a model for understanding dignity in the dying [9, 15]. The Model of Dignity is not hierarchical, so that any one or more of its elements may apply within individual circumstances.

8.2.3 Illness-Related Concerns

These derive from the illness experience itself and can impinge on the patient's sense of dignity. Within this category are two broad issues: level of independence and symptom distress. *Independence* is determined by the patient's ability to maintain cognitive acuity and a functional capacity to perform tasks of daily living. Many patients fear loss of independence at the end-of-life [26]; however, being dependent is made easier when caregivers are knowledgeable and considerate, and with whom patients have a relationship based on mutual respect and trust [27]. *Symptom distress* includes both physical and emotional distress and presents a profound challenge to the patient. Symptom distress has two existential sub-themes in the dignity model: (i) uncertainty (i.e. distress associated with uncertainty regarding one's health) and (ii) death

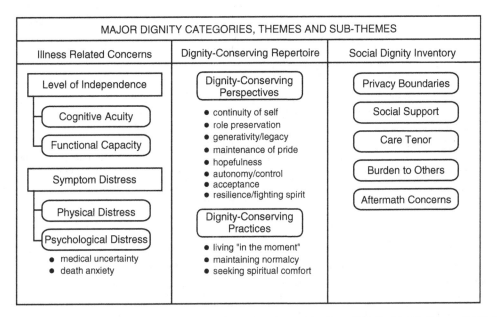

Figure 8.1 *Empirical dignity model*. Reprinted from *Social Science & Medicine*. Chochinov HM, Hack T, McClement S, Kristjanson L, Harlos M (2002). Dignity in the terminally ill: a developing empirical model, **54**: 433–443, with permission from Elsevier.

anxiety (i.e. fear associated with dying or anticipating death). These kinds of concerns are influenced, not only by the progression of the disease and how it is managed, but also by the way that caregivers and others perceive and respond to the patient as an individual [28].

8.2.4 Dignity-Conserving Repertoire

This incorporates aspects of patients' psychological and spiritual landscape that influence their sense of dignity [9]. There are two major themes, dignity-conserving perspectives and practices; these focus on the patient's own attitudes and behavioural responses to the illness. The concept of *dignity-conserving perspectives* refers to internally held, personal characteristics, attributes or world views that can strengthen an individual's sense of dignity. Eight sub-themes emerged, including: (i) continuity of self (the sense that one's identity remains intact in spite of the illness); (ii) maintenance of pride (the ability to retain positive self-regard or self-respect in one's own eyes); (iii) role preservation (the ability to function in usual social roles in a way congruent with prior-held views of self identity); (iv) hopefulness (the ability to see life as enduring or as having sustained meaning or purpose); (v) generativity/legacy (the ability to reflect on one's past life with a sense of satisfaction and the desire to leave something lasting to the next

generation – something that might transcend death); (vi) autonomy/control (a subjective sense of control or having a choice over life circumstances); (vii) acceptance (the ability to acknowledge changing life circumstances) and (viii) resilience/fighting spirit (the mental fortitude to overcome illness-related concerns and optimise quality of life). *Dignity-conserving practices* are part of the patient's coping repertoire, and they are the personal approaches or techniques that patients use to sustain their sense of dignity. Three elements were identified: (i) living in the moment (focusing on immediate issues and not worrying about the future), (ii) maintaining normalcy (continuing with routine activities) and (iii) seeking spiritual comfort (finding solace in one's religious or spiritual belief system) [9, 10, 29].

8.2.4.1 Generativity

The theme of generativity is derived from Erikson's life stages of psychosocial development [30] and warrants particular mention in the context of Dignity Therapy. Erikson described developmental challenges that all individuals must master, in order to negotiate successfully through the psychosocial tasks of adulthood. Generativity embodies the idea that as people age, they gain a sense of accomplishment and pride from their ability to contribute or give back to society and help guide future generations. Part of the contentment and satisfaction comes from the person's ability to reflect back on life with a sense of having created a legacy, a lasting personal account of who they are and what they value. For patients near the end-of-life, a therapeutic intervention mindful of generativity would need to facilitate the creation of something that captures the essence of who people are and what they feel, and it would include something that can be passed on to others. Dignity Therapy supports generativity by having the therapist create a carefully edited transcript, which encapsulates the things patients would want known by those they are about to leave behind. This generativity document is a vital component of Dignity Therapy.

8.2.5 Social Dignity Inventory

This part of the model refers to the quality of social interactions with others and how they enhance or detract from a patient's sense of dignity. Five primary themes were identified, including: (i) privacy boundaries (the level of intrusion into one's personal environment when receiving care or support), (ii) social support (the presence of a caring community of friends, family or health-care providers), (iii) care tenor (the attitude others display when interacting with the patient), (iv) burden to others (the distress engendered by having to rely upon others for personal care or management) and (v) aftermath concerns (worries about the burden that one's death will impose on others) [9].

8.2.5.1 Care Tenor

One aspect of the social dignity inventory that has a profound influence on a patient's sense of dignity is the care tenor. This conveys the idea that dignity depends on the positive attitude, active listening, empathy and compassion of health-care practitioners and on the degree to which health-care providers respect, value and appreciate patients as whole persons [19]. Clinicians who carry out Dignity Therapy, for example must be genuine and enthusiastic partners within the collaborative effort it takes to accomplish a therapeutic effect. Every patient has a unique story to tell; feigned interest is readily transparent, and nothing is more encouraging to a storyteller than an engaged listener [23]. However, while therapists try to discern what patients are thinking or feeling, patients try to read subtle clues provided by their therapist: '*Am I an interesting patient? Are you interested in what I have to say? Am I doing this right? How does my story compare to others you've heard?*' If patients feel that they are failing or

disappointing the therapist, the experience of personal disclosure will start to feel demeaning, leading to disillusionment and therapeutic disengagement [24].

Our model provides a sound empirical rationale and guidance for how to pursue this therapeutic approach, which targets dignity as a viable and achievable outcome. It provides an overarching framework that can guide physicians, patients and families towards defining objectives and therapeutic considerations fundamental to end-of-life care. The model helps facilitate care options, such as Dignity Therapy and encompasses the broad range of physical, psychological, social, spiritual and existential aspects of the patient's end-of-life experience [9, 10, 15].

8.3 The Conduct of Dignity Therapy: Processes and Techniques

Dignity Therapy formalises the creation of a legacy document, which aims to summarise value and underscore the meaning in the patient's life [9, 23]. Focusing on themes that are affirming can engender a connection with an individual's core sense of self. Creating a legacy document that can be read and shared by successive generations reinforces the notion of generativity.

8.3.1 Targeted Patient Groups

While palliative patients with cancer have taken part more than any other disease group, Dignity Therapy is now being piloted in patients with neurodegenerative disorders (such as muscular dystrophy and amyotrophic lateral sclerosis), end-stage renal disease and the frail elderly.

- **Who should be approached to take part in dignity therapy?** The criteria for eligibility to participate include the following: (i) anyone who is facing life-threatening or life-limiting circumstances; (ii) anyone interested and motivated to take part; and (iii) the patient must be able to speak the same language as the therapist and transcriptionist.

- **Who should not participate in dignity therapy?** Exclusion criteria should include the following: (i) anyone who is too ill and not expected to live more than about two weeks, corresponding to the usual time it takes to complete the protocol (it is prudent to ask the patient how they would like the transcript handled should they feel too ill to complete their review of it). (ii) A lack of cognitive ability, for example delirium, clouded consciousness or cognitive impairment, any of which can result in a product tainted by a false representation of self.

8.3.2 Dignity Therapy Question Framework

The following questions form the basic framework of Dignity Therapy and provide patients with appropriate openings to broach these delicate and often poignant areas of inquiry [9, 23, 29].

1. Tell me a little about your life history; particularly the parts that you either remember most, or think are the most important?

2. When did you feel most alive?

3. Are there particular things that you would want your family to know about you, and are there particular things you would want them to remember?

4. What are the most important roles you have played in your life (family roles, vocational roles, community service roles, etc.)? Why were they so important to you, and what do you think you accomplished within those roles?

5. What are your most important accomplishments, and what do you feel most proud of? Alternately, what do you take pride in?

6. Are there particular things that you feel need to be said to your loved ones, or things that you would want to take the time to say once again?

7. What are your hopes and dreams for your loved ones?

8. What have you learned about life that you would want to pass along to others? What advice or words of guidance would you wish to pass along to your (son, daughter, husband, wife, parents and other(s))?

8.3.3 Administration of Dignity Therapy, with Case Examples

Dignity Therapy invites patients to engage in a conversation, addressing issues or memories that they deem important or that they would want recorded for their surviving loved ones. The role of the therapist, besides guiding and enabling the process, is to imbue the therapeutic interaction with a sense of dignity. This means that patients must feel accepted, valued and honoured.

8.3.4 Step 1: Identify Patients Who Might Benefit from Dignity Therapy

As previously discussed, knowing when and when not to apply Dignity Therapy is very important. Suffering often takes place in silence and is sometimes covert. Psychosocial, existential and spiritual distress can be much less obvious than physical symptoms, although no less overwhelming for patients. Our assumptions about the suffering of another *must always* be tested against the patient's own subjective experience. The appearance of physical comfort does not necessarily mean that someone is at peace with themselves. Dignity Therapy may be applied in those who express severe distress or none whatsoever. It can be a welcome opportunity for anyone who wishes for a way to enhance meaning, purpose or well-being in their final months, weeks or days of life.

8.3.5 Step 2: Introduce Dignity Therapy to the Patient and Family

The choice of words used to begin will depend upon the patient's insight and openness in talking about their medical circumstances. Patients will often offer clues through the language they use, for example '*I know I don't have much time left*; *I think I might be nearing the end*; *I know I'm dying*.' However, the therapist should never assume full prognostic awareness and must listen carefully to how patients describe their circumstances. It is a mistake to assume that words like 'palliative', 'terminal' or 'death and dying' are safe to use, without some prior indication from the patient. Importantly, stating that Dignity Therapy is an intervention for those near the end-of-life, or for patients who are terminally ill or with a limited life expectancy, is a poor way to begin. It is not the role of the dignity therapist to disclose prognostic information.

A typical introduction may go something like this:

Your doctor/nurse told me that you might be interested in Dignity Therapy. I thought I would stop by and tell you a bit about it and answer any questions you have. Dignity Therapy is a 'talking therapy' that has been specially designed to help people who are living with significant medical challenges. It can help people cope with their illness and improve how they feel about themselves and their quality of life. It can also have benefits for family members. Dignity Therapy usually only takes a session or two and would give you a chance to talk about the things that are most important to you, things that you want to share with those closest to you, things you want to say. We record these conversations and edit them, and return a final summary to you. Most people find the experience very meaningful, and they find comfort in knowing that the document is for them and their loved ones.

8.3.6 Step 3: Answer Any Questions the Patient Might Have

Here are some common questions that therapists get with exemplar responses:

1. **Why do you think dignity therapy works?**

   It was developed for people who are quite ill and feel that who they are and the activities that helped to define them have started to fade. It can give people a sense that they still have something important to do. It gives people a chance to address any salient issues, including looking after people they care about, by creating a very personal document that they can share.

2. **What kinds of questions will you ask me?**

   I have an outline of questions that ask about what you would like others to know about you, and if are there words or thoughts you would like to share. I will leave you the questions, so you can think about how you might like to answer them, or think about other things you would rather talk about. There are no questions that you must answer. This is your therapy and the document that we will be creating will belong to you. I want you to feel free to talk only about the things that you want to talk about; if I ask you something you'd rather not talk about, we will simply move on.

Therapy sessions are structured so that patients can offer areas of important content spontaneously, or they can use the question framework to help them elicit areas for reflection. Some patients will choose to reflect on their life history and early development. Others want to provide advice to their children or grandchildren. Some present a careful chronological account of their life; others focus on special events that they consider memorable, formative or important.

3. **What if I get tired, start feeling too unwell to continue or I don't know what to say?**

   If you are tired or need a break, just say so and we will stop. I'll not go any longer than 45 minutes to an hour at most. I will be here to help you make this work. I will try and think of the right questions and give you all the cues and encouragement you need to get your story told. We are quite skilled at helping people and knowing when you might

need some guidance and direction, so that you can complete your Dignity Therapy.

The therapist structures the intervention for patients who lack the capability to do this by inserting prompts, pointing out possible connections and injecting energy to facilitate full and meaningful responses.

4. **Is it OK to have someone with me while the interview is taking place?**

   Some people do it on their own because it feels more private, more comfortable and makes it easier to share personal thoughts, feelings and recollections. Other people prefer to have someone else with them. Whichever choice works best for you will likely work best for the therapy.

5. **Why does it have to be tape recorded; what if I don't feel comfortable with that?**

   People can feel a bit uncomfortable with the tape recorder at the beginning, but usually, within a few minutes, you will forget about the recording entirely. The recording is important so that we can transcribe the conversation and use it to create your generativity document. If there is something we've missed, we can add it; if there is something there that you don't like, we can fix it. I will help you correct even the tiniest of errors. At the end of this process, I want you to feel completely happy with what you have done.

The generativity document can provide tangible and lasting testimony of a patient's most important thoughts and memories, preserved for those they will leave behind. This document, with the help of the therapist, serves as a record of their life, edited to capture the essence of who they are. Patients are given a copy for them to keep and share with anyone they wish.

As a 58-year-old woman with metastatic breast cancer said after completing her Dignity Therapy one week before her death, *'I may not be a famous person, and not many people will remember my name, but my sons (holding the edited document) will have this.'*

While some patients may not require much guidance or coaxing, others may feel overwhelmed, unless they are provided with extensive assistance and explicit direction from the therapist, whose purpose is to help them articulate the essence of who they are or what they want to say. The therapist's role is therefore absolutely critical.

8.4 The Therapist's Role

1. **The therapist must assume a dignity-affirming stance at all times, for all patients and under all circumstances**

   It is imperative that patients feel respected and valued in the therapeutic process. The therapist needs to be comfortable with existential issues, silences and emotions that can range from joy to sorrow.

2. **The therapist must be a highly engaged, active listener**

   The process can be likened to accompanying a rather unsteady person, attempting to walk along a chosen path. By active listening, the therapist ensures that even the most unsteady will be kept safe from falling.

3. **The therapist must be prepared to engage and guide the patient**

   Patients who are very ill and near the end-of-life can lack the energy and intuition to organise or sequence their responses effectively. The therapist strikes a balance between open-ended questions and imposing more structure. As a rule of thumb, the more fatigued or disorganised the patient, the more structured the questioning. The ideal exchange occurs when the patient is asked a question that generates an engaged and energised response.

4. **The therapist and the patient can look through a metaphorical photo album**

   A simple, but effective way to elicit detail is to use a photo-album metaphor: *'Imagine that you and I are looking at a picture book of your life. Tell me, in as much detail as you like, about some of the pictures we might see.'* One elderly gentleman indicated how important his career as a newspaperman had been, but gave few details. The therapist invited him to elaborate with the following, *'When you look back over your career as a newspaperman, are there particular moments, pivotal milestones or key accomplishments that you remember?'* The question is broad, and yet invites the patient to share more detail about the importance of his career.

5. **The therapist should be mindful that patients will disclose different kinds of stories**

Some patients will recall a life well lived and convey expressions of gratitude for various blessings. Patients may thank loved ones or describe how specific individuals enriched their lives. Others may recall personal tragedy, injustice, regrets or previous failures. One might think these disclosures are counter-therapeutic, but patients may want to 'set the record straight' towards the end-of-life, explaining their shortcomings, seeking forgiveness or in some cases, unburdening themselves. The most difficult and problematic stories therapists will hear are those that have the potential to harm the recipient(s) of the generativity document. One woman, for example described a deeply conflicted relationship with her son. They had not resolved many longstanding issues and in describing her 'hopes' for her son, she stated, *'He's a bum and a free-loader.'* The harshness of these words can amount to a permanent accusation, reprimand or assault, against which there is no defence and no possible retort. The therapist's role is to remind the patient that their words, once delivered, could have a lasting impact. She might say something like, *'If these were the last words you could say to your son, are they the ones you would want to leave him with, or might there be others you would want him to remember you by?'* In this case, the patient cried, stating she would want to tell him how much she loves him, wishing she could hold him, and, laughing by now, saying, *'He ought to get a job!'* If there is some doubt, the therapist can check in with the patient thus, *'You are raising some pretty difficult issues about your (family member) . . . how do you think they will feel hearing this? Have you ever discussed this with them before? Is this something you would consider talking about face to face?'*

6. **The therapist should help the patient provide clarity about the details of their stories**

   Patients often make assumptions in sharing their thoughts, without offering the detail needed for clarity. Simple questions like, *'How old were you at this time?'* can make it easier for the therapist to both follow the patient's train of thought and know how to direct the patient, should they start to wander. Rather than trying to achieve historical completeness, questions should elicit focused detail about pertinent life experiences. If a patient, for example comments that he *'never had a problem with my children'*, he may not wish to say anything further. However, the therapist might test this assumption: *'Are there some special memories of your children that you would like to talk about?'* There should be a high degree of collaboration to ensure that the patient feels engaged, involved, encouraged and nurtured.

7. **The therapist should follow the patient's affect**
As a rule of thumb, following the patient's emotional energy will serve the therapist well in making therapeutic decisions about what areas to include. For example, in one case, an elderly gentleman had demonstrated little energy or enthusiasm about his early life. However, when provided the opportunity to do so, he spoke quite readily about his marital problems, subsequent divorce and the unravelling of his early family life. He felt the document might provide an apology to his ex-wife and an explanation to their two, now adult, children.

8. **The therapist should give the patient permission to withhold recollections**
Sometimes, following the affect or emotional energy will lead to issues or memories that the patient finds too sad or difficult to tell. Unlike some forms of psychotherapy, which may try and guide patients through their conflicted feelings or offer interpretations to address this seeming resistance, Dignity Therapy does neither. The therapist must respect the patient's healthy defences, even when doing so precludes taking an 'uncovering' or 'interpretive' approach, thus facilitating the telling of the stories that the patient wants told.

9. **The therapist should pace the therapy to best match the patient's abilities**
Be mindful of pacing and keeping track of time, so that all questions within the framework can be broached.

10. **The therapist should leave some time for a debriefing with the patient**
At the conclusion of the therapy, it is fitting to take a moment to debrief. *'How was that for you? Are you pleased with how things went? Was that more tiring than you anticipated? I noticed that some parts were quite emotional – was that hard for you?'* Patients may provide some insights about the manuscript, which might help inform the editing process: *'I shouldn't have said that;*

I may not have said enough about my other daughter.' In most instances, the debriefing will be short and positive. However, should the patient have some misgivings or anxieties about what transpired, it is best to find out sooner, rather than having them worry about it until their next appointment. Be sure to thank the patient for the honour and privilege of being able to listen to and share this special time with them.

Box 8.1 provides an overview of the model.

Box 8.1 Summary of the Dignity Therapy Protocol Schedule

- Identify appropriate terminally ill patients who wish to take part in the therapy.
- Assist and guide the patient through the Dignity Therapy interview.
- Offer one to two therapy sessions, no longer than an hour each, within a one to three day interval.
- Transcribe conversations within two to three days of the final interview.
- Edit the transcript, about a 3- to 4-hour task, within the next one to three days.
- Revisit the patient when editing is complete and read them the entire manuscript.
- Make any necessary corrections to the document within 24–48 hours.
- Provide the patient with a hard copy of the final approved document.
- Patients may share or bequeath the document to anyone they choose.

8.5 Evidence of the Efficacy of Dignity Therapy

The first clinical trial of Dignity Therapy ran between 2001 and 2003, and was comprised of 100 patients [23]. The majority of these participants had end-stage cancer. Their median survival time, from the first point of contact to the time of death, was 51 days. To evaluate the efficacy of Dignity Therapy, participants completed questionnaires covering a wide range of physical, psychological and existential issues and concerns.

In this clinical trial, measures of suffering and depression showed significant improvement. Measures of dignity, hopelessness, desire for death, anxiety, will to live and suicide all showed favourable changes, and patients who reported higher initial levels of despair were more likely to benefit. Patients who found Dignity Therapy helpful were more likely to report that their lives had meaning, that they had a heightened sense of purpose and will to live, and that they had lower levels of suffering [23].

Ninety-one percent of patients reported feeling satisfied or highly satisfied with Dignity Therapy; 86% reported that the intervention was helpful or very helpful; 76% indicated that it heightened their sense of dignity; 68% indicated that it increased their sense of purpose; 67% indicated that it heightened their sense of meaning and 47% reported an increased will to live. Those who believed that Dignity Therapy had helped or would help their families were more likely to experience life as meaningful and purposeful and reported a greater will to live and less suffering [23]. For family members, 78% reported that the generativity document helped them during their time of grief and that it would continue to be a source of comfort [31]. Based on the results of this first study, the salutary effects of the model and its viability as an end-of-life intervention were wholly supported.

8.6 Service Development

There are resource implications for any psychosocial or palliative care programme, wanting to offer Dignity Therapy as a clinical service. For training and new practitioners, provision must be made for ongoing supervision and feedback. The feasibility of introducing Dignity Therapy depends on the availability of key support services. First, a transcriptionist is needed to transcribe the interview recording. After typing, some time (typically 3–4 hours) is needed for the therapist to edit the interview. Editing entails converting the original dialogue into a polished generativity narrative (e.g. remove colloquialisms, correct time sequences and eliminate material not intended for generativity purposes). Both transcription (within two to three days of the interview) and editing (within two to four days of the transcription) of the narrative must be accomplished in a timely way, before the patient becomes too ill or cognitively impaired to complete the protocol. The therapist's time commitment includes the interview (about 1 hour), the editing (about 3–4 hours), and the follow-up visit to confirm and finalise the document (about 1 hour), for a total time commitment for the therapist of about 5–6 hours.

The monetary cost of Dignity Therapy deserves mention. The time therapists spend with patients, in most circumstances, will be covered within existing resources, which provide for psychosocial care. However, additional costs for transcription services (1–3 hours of typing, depending on the length of the interview) and editing costs must also be factored in. Relative to the cost of most palliative chemo- or radiation therapy, these costs are indeed minor. Bearing in mind the evidence supporting the benefits of Dignity Therapy and its potential for multi-generational impact, finding the necessary resources will mean identifying modest new funding and, just as challenging, overcoming a dominant bias that psychosocial interventions, even those that work, should cost nothing whatsoever.

The therapist should also periodically take the time to debrief the transcriptionists, by asking them about their experiences of carrying out their work. The content of therapy is often quite emotional; even emotionally neutral material can resonate in ways that are quite poignant, given the circumstances of persons conveying their thoughts. People chosen for this task must have the emotional maturity to handle these disclosures and be offered opportunities to share their responses.

8.7 Conclusion and Future Directions

Following a skillfully guided, semi-structured interview with a patient, the typed transcript is edited to provide patients and their loved ones with a generativity document. These documents recount details of their lives, heart-felt thoughts, concerns, outlooks, passions and wishes. Generativity documents have the ability to offer dying patients a sense that the essence of who they are will be preserved and will provide a source of comfort for those they are about to leave behind. The rationale for many palliative care interventions is to make the sufferer less aware of his or her suffering. Dignity Therapy, on the other hand, allows patients to bolster their sense of meaning and purpose, while reinforcing a continued sense of worth, within a framework, that is supportive, nurturing and accessible, even for those close to death.

Future investigations into the efficacy of Dignity Therapy will examine its benefits in a randomised controlled study. By comparing Dignity Therapy to other forms of psychosocial end-of-life care, we can determine how helpful it is, its cost-benefit ratio, how it improves quality of life and the patient's sense of dignity relative to other forms of support. Because generativity is a life task facing everyone, it is possible that Dignity Therapy may prove helpful amongst a broad range of patients, beyond just those with cancer. Feasibility studies, addressing the applications of Dignity Therapy amongst other populations facing life threatening or life limiting conditions, are well underway.

We have much to learn about this exciting method of helping patients bring genuine closure to their lives.

Acknowledgements

The authors wish to acknowledge members of the Dignity research team, including Drs Susan McClement, Linda Kristjanson, Thomas Hack, Tom Hassard, Mike Harlos and research nurses Katherine Cullihall, Beverley Cann and Miriam Cohen. Funding sources for this work include the Project on Death in America, the American Foundation for Suicide Prevention, the Canadian Cancer Society and the National Cancer Institute of Canada. Dr Chochinov holds a Canada Research Chair in Palliative Care, with funding from the Canadian Institutes of Health Research. Finally, we are indebted to patients and families who have contributed to these studies.

References

1. Ganzini, L., Nelson, H.D., Schmidt, T.A. *et al.* (2000) Physicians' experiences with the Oregon death with dignity act. *The New England Journal of Medicine*, **342**, 557–563.
2. Sullivan, A.D., Hedberg, K. and Fleming, D.W. (2000) Legalized physician-assisted suicide in Oregon – the second year. *The New England Journal of Medicine*, **342**, 598–604.
3. Quill, T.E. (1994) Physician-assisted death: progress or peril? *Suicide and Life-Threatening Behavior*, **24**, 315–325.
4. Meier, D.E., Emmons, C.A., Wallenstein, S. *et al.* (1998) A national survey of physician-assisted suicide and euthanasia in the United States. *The New England Journal of Medicine*, **338**, 1193–1201.
5. Van Der Maas, P.J., Van Delden, J.J., Pijnenborg, L. and Looman, C.W. (1991) Euthanasia and other medical decisions concerning the end of life. *Lancet*, **338** (8768), 669–674.
6. Chochinov, H.M., Tataryn, D., Clinch, J.J. and Dudgeon, D. (1999) Will to live in the terminally ill. *Lancet*, **354** (9181), 816–819.
7. Schroepfer, T.A. (2006) Mind frames towards dying and factors motivating their adoption by terminally ill elders. *The Journals of Gerontology. Series B, Psychological Sciences and Social Sciences*, **61**, S129–S139.
8. Chochinov, H.M. (2003) Defending dignity. *Palliative and Supportive Care*, **1** (4), 307–308.
9. Chochinov, H.M. (2002) Dignity-conserving care – a new model for palliative care: helping the patient feel valued. *The Journal of the American Medical Association*, **287** (17), 2253–2260.
10. Chochinov, H.M., Hack, T., Hassard, T. *et al.* (2004) Dignity and psychotherapeutic considerations in end-of-life care. *Journal of Palliative Care*, **20** (3), 134–142.
11. McClement, S.E., Chochinov, H.M., Hack, T.F. *et al.* (2004) Dignity-conserving care: application of research findings to practice. *International Journal of Palliative Nursing*, **10**, 173–179.
12. Merriam-Webster Dictionary (2005) Merriam-Webster Online Dictionary, Merriam-Webster Online, Springfield, MA.
13. Kade, W.J. (2000) Death with dignity: a case study. *Annals of Internal Medicine*, **132** (6), 504–506.
14. Pannuti, F. and Tanneberger, S. (1993) Dying with dignity: illusion, hope or human right? *World Health Forum*, **14**, 172–173.
15. Chochinov, H.M., Hack, T., McClement, S. *et al.* (2002) Dignity in the terminally ill: a developing empirical model. *Social Science and Medicine*, **54**, 433–443.
16. Chochinov, H.M. and Cann, B.J. (2005) Interventions to enhance the spiritual aspects of dying. *Journal of Palliative Medicine*, **8** (Suppl. 1), s103–s115.
17. Enes, S.P. (2003) An exploration of dignity in palliative care. *Journal of Palliative Medicine*, **17** (3), 263–269.
18. Proulx, K. and Jacelon, C. (2004) Dying with dignity: the good patient versus the good death. *The American Journal of Hospice and Palliative Care*, **21** (2), 116–120.
19. Chochinov, H.M., Hack, T., Hassard, T. *et al.* (2002) Dignity in the terminally ill: a cross-sectional, cohort study. *Lancet*, **360** (9350), 2026–2030.
20. McClement, S.E. and Chochinov, H.M. (2006) Dignity in palliative care, in *Textbook of Palliative Medicine* (eds E. Bruera, I. Higginson, C. von Gunten and C. Ripamonti), Edward Arnold, New York, NY, pp. 100–107.
21. Pullman, D. (2004) Death, dignity, and moral nonsense. *Journal of Palliative Care*, **20**, 171–178.
22. Street, A.F. and Kissane, D.W. (2001) Constructions of dignity in end-of-life care. *Journal of Palliative Care*, **17** (2), 93–101.
23. Chochinov, H.M., Hack, T., Hassard, T. *et al.* (2005) Dignity therapy: a novel psychotherapeutic intervention for patients near the end of life. *Journal of Clinical Oncology*, **23**, 5520–5525.
24. Chochinov, H.M. (2004) Dignity and the eye of the beholder. *Journal of Clinical Oncology*, **22**, 1336–1340.
25. Hack, T.F., Chochinov, H.M., Hassard, T. *et al.* (2004) Defining dignity in terminally ill cancer patients: a factor-analytic approach. *Psycho-Oncology*, **13**, 700–708.
26. Johnston, B. and Smith, L.N. (2006) Nurses' and patients' perceptions of expert palliative nursing care. *Journal of Advanced Nursing*, **54**, 700–709.
27. Eriksson, M. and Andershed, B. (2008) Care dependence: a struggle toward moments of respite. *Clinical Nursing Research*, **17**, 220–236.
28. McKechnie, R., MacLeod, R. and Keeling, S. (2007) Facing uncertainty: the lived experience of palliative care. *Palliative and Supportive Care*, **5**, 367–376.
29. Chochinov, H.M. (2006) Dying, dignity, and new horizons in palliative end-of-life care. *CA: A Cancer Journal for Clinicians*, **56**, 84–103.
30. Erikson, E.H. (1950) *Childhood and Society*, Norton, New York.
31. McClement, S., Chochinov, H.M., Hack, T. *et al.* (2007) Dignity therapy: family member perspectives. *Journal of Palliative Medicine*, **10**, 1076–1082.

9 Written Emotional Disclosure

Robert Zachariae and Mikael Birkelund Jensen-Johansen

Psychooncology Research Unit, Department of Oncology, Aarhus University Hospital and Department of Psychology, Aarhus University, Aarhus, Denmark

9.1 Background

Like other significant stressful life events, a cancer diagnosis can be traumatic [1] by challenging the individuals' preexisting mental models of themselves and the world and question the core beliefs they hold about the future [2, 3]. This view is supported by the growing literature indicating that even after successful treatment, cancer diagnosis and treatment may continue to be a source of considerable distress [4–9].

A common assumption in theories of adjustment to traumatic events is that healthy adjustment occurs through repeated confrontation with the thoughts and memories of the trauma, which will assist the individual interpret the event, in this case the cancer, in a meaningful, coherent framework [10, 11], which eventually will lead to the ability to think about the traumatic event without inducing emotional distress. According to Horowitz [12], the cognitive processing of a traumatic event is characterised by two complementary aspects: (i) *intrusion*, that is involuntary intrusive thoughts and images about the event and (ii) *avoidance*, that is voluntary attempts to avoid thinking about the event. In this theoretical framework, intrusive thoughts are viewed as possessing an inherently adaptive quality as they are believed to be stimulated by the individual's need to master the trauma and integrate the trauma-related thoughts and memories into his or her mental model. However, intrusive thoughts can be highly distressing, and temporary use of various avoidance coping strategies is necessary to avoid being emotionally overwhelmed. On the other hand, if used excessively, avoidance strategies may interfere with the cognitive processing needed to resolve the trauma.

9.1.1 Emotional Expression and Non-Expression

One way of engaging in deliberate processing of a traumatic event is by expressing one's emotions regarding the traumatic event, and several lines of evidence suggest that both the ability and the opportunity to express emotions play a role in adjusting to stressful experiences such as cancer and cancer treatment. A large number of studies over the years indicate that while emotional expression may not be beneficial at all times, a general tendency to cope with stressful events through emotional non-expression may be detrimental to adjustment, and – reversely – that emotionally expressive forms of coping are associated with improved psychological adjustment, lower levels of emotional distress and improved quality-of-life. For example, in a study of women with breast cancer, Stanton and colleagues found that compared to those low in emotional expression, women who coped through expressing emotions about cancer had fewer medical appointments for cancer-related morbidities, experienced enhanced physical health and vigour and reduced distress during the next three months, when controlling for other potentially confounding variables [13]. Likewise, Schmidt and Andrykowski found that women who tended to be less aware of and tend less to their emotional states exhibited higher levels of distress [14]. In addition, women with high levels of emotional control in response to a diagnosis of breast cancer have been shown to be considerably more distressed than women showing lesser tendency to restrain their emotions [15]. That emotional non-expressive coping strategies may not only be detrimental in the short run, but also predict long-term maladjustment, has been shown in a study by Hack and colleagues indicating that women who respond to their breast cancer diagnosis with cognitive avoidance in the form of passive acceptance and resignation are at significant risk for poor long term psychological adjustment [16]. Such findings suggest that coping strategies involving lower levels of emotional restraint and higher levels of emotional expression may be important to the process of adjusting to the stressors associated with cancer diagnosis, treatment and survival [17]. It should be noted, however, that not all studies show negative associations between disclosure and psychological adaptation and trauma. For example, a prospective study failed to verify that the extent to which bereaved persons disclosed their emotions and talked about their loss to others was associated with better adjustment to the loss [18], and another study even found evidence of improved long-term adaptation associated with non-expression during bereavement [19], indicating that emotional expression should not be considered universally beneficial.

9.1.2 Social-Cognitive Processing Theory

Having the ability to identify and express feelings may not suffice if the social environment is unreceptive. The social-cognitive processing theory [3] suggests that when people experience *social constraints* on their expression of stress-related emotions and thoughts, for example when they perceive their spouse or other significant person to be unwilling to listen to their concerns, this can adversely affect their coping behaviours and psychological adjustment [20]. In a study of prostate cancer patients [21], the perception of others to be unreceptive to attempts to talk about their cancer-related concerns, that is higher levels of perceived social constraints, was related to increased avoidance in thinking and talking about cancer, which in turn was associated with increased distress. Furthermore, the association between intrusive thoughts about cancer appeared to be more strongly related to mental health in men with high levels of social constraints. The negative influence of social constraints on well-being has found support in subsequent research, both in studies with breast [22] and gastrointestinal cancer patients and their spouses [23]. Generally, the available research suggests that the way couples communicate, for example whether one or both partners avoid talking about cancer-related concerns, can either facilitate or reduce relational

intimacy and thereby influence both the patient's and partner's level of psychological distress [24].

9.1.3 Traits and Behaviours Associated with Inhibited Emotional Expression

Another explanation for the variability in the responding of individuals to the same stressor could lie in differences in their disposition to express emotions. Over the years, several theoretical models of emotional dysregulation in the form of *emotional inhibition* or *non-expression* have been developed, spanning from the early psychodynamic models of emotional inhibition as a defence mechanism [25], where excessive preventing of emotions to be consciously acknowledged and expressed are seen as resulting in psychological symptoms (neurosis) or physical symptoms, for example conversion hysteria [26], to more recent models of repressive coping [27] and alexithymia [28, 29].

In a conceptual model of the process of emotional expression, Kennedy-Moore and Watson [30] describe several steps at which inhibition of this process can occur. In response to a potential emotion-inducing stimulus, the process of emotional expression or non-expression begins with the individual's pre-reflective reactions including bodily reactions. Depending on the individual's distress threshold, he or she becomes aware of the reaction, labels it as emotional, and evaluates the response with regard to personal values and goals and the present context. At the next step, emotional inhibition may occur if the pre-reflective reactions are triggered but do not become conscious to the individual due to coping- or defence-mechanisms, either as a general disposition or due to the specific situation. One such dispositional coping- or defence mechanism has been defined as *repressive coping* [27]. It has been proposed that negative influences on health of defensiveness, repressive coping and other non-conscious types of emotional inhibition may stem from maladaptive consequences of the lack of behavioural motivation produced by the lack of emotional awareness or from the biological stress resulting from the psychophysiological effort associated with emotional inhibition [31]. At the next step in the process, inhibition of emotional expression may take place because the individual lacks the skills to process emotions. At this stage, emotional non-expression does not result from lack of conscious emotional experience, but from the inability to accurately label and interpret emotions, which in turn may lead to maladaptive behaviour in the face of stress. This type of emotional inhibition is closely associated with the term alexithymia, which was developed on the basis of clinical observations that psychosomatic patients generally appeared to be emotionally non-expressive [28, 29]. Alexithymia is generally viewed as a relatively stable trait, a view that has found support in twin studies suggesting that a considerable degree of the variation in the scores on an alexithymia scale is related to genetic factors [32]. However, a second type of alexithymia has also been suggested as a more transient state triggered by somatic illness or other severe stressors [33]. Finally, consciously experienced emotions that are accurately labelled and interpreted may still not be expressed but consciously suppressed. Depending on the belief systems, values and attitudes of the individual and the interpreted appropriateness in the particular context, the individual may choose to express or suppress his or her emotions. In summary the expression of emotions may be disrupted at different stages of emotional processing levels, and emotional non-expression may be seen as the result of more or less stable dispositions, as transient states triggered by specific situations, and a conscious choice based the evaluations of the individual in the specific context.

9.1.4 Written Emotional Disclosure

Disclosure is a core aspect of psychotherapy [34], and many psychotherapies use techniques aimed at promoting identification, exploration and expression of stress-related thoughts and feelings [35]. Although there are several ways of expressing emotions, one mode that has recently been linked with positive health outcomes is writing [36]. While writing has long been viewed as having the potential to increase well-being, it is primarily the early research conducted by Pennebaker and Beall [37–39] which has lent scientific credibility to expressive writing as a psychotherapeutic process by showing in a number of studies that individuals writing about a personal trauma have better health outcomes than individuals writing non-emotionally about a non-traumatic topic. Most studies examining effects of written emotional disclosure, that is 'expressive writing intervention' or EWI, have used a relatively straightforward procedure, in which the participants are instructed to write about their deepest thoughts and feelings about a traumatic event, preferably thoughts and feelings they have not previously talked about to others.

9.2 Evidence on Efficacy

9.2.1 Effects Found in Healthy and Clinical Samples

Over the years, findings from a growing number of controlled trials have suggested a wide range of benefits of EWI in both healthy and clinical participants. In the first meta-analysis of 13 studies of EWI published between 1986 and 1998, Smyth [40] found a moderate overall effect size for healthy participants (Cohen's $d = 0.47$). In a later meta-analysis of nine studies of various clinical populations, Frisina and colleagues [41] found a more modest effect ($d = 0.19$), and in a more recent meta-analysis of 29 studies focusing on effects of EWI on health care utilisation, Harris [42] found a modest effect size for healthy samples (Hedges $g = 0.16$), but not for samples of participants with medical conditions or samples screened for psychological conditions. In the latest available meta-analysis of 146 studies of emotional disclosure, Frattaroli and colleagues [43] found an even smaller overall effect size ($d = 0.15$), indicating a general effect devaluation over time when more studies, both published and unpublished, are included. The largest statistical significant effect size was found for subjective impact of the intervention ($d = 0.31$), while the effects were smaller for physiological function (e.g. immune parameters) ($d = 0.11$), self-reported physical health (e.g. symptoms) ($d = 0.11$), psychological health (e.g. distress, depression) ($d = 0.07$) and general functioning (e.g. work absenteeism, social relationships) ($d = 0.07$). This meta-analysis included both studies of clinical and healthy populations as well as several different settings and different modes of emotional disclosure intervention, for example both written and oral emotional disclosure methods. Although the overall effect found ($d = 0.15$), is usually referred to as 'small' [44], it may still represent a non-trivial effect. An effect of $d = 0.15$ thus corresponds to 54% of an intervention group experiencing a beneficial effect compared to only 46% in a control group [45].

9.2.2 What Works in EWI?

It has been stated that 'expressive writing has health benefits, but no one really knows why' [46]. Most theories on the mediating mechanisms of psychological intervention could also be made to fit as explanations of EWI as a therapy. However, over the years, a number of EWI-specific mechanisms have been suggested and are repeatedly mentioned in the literature. In line with the previous theoretical work on psychosomatics and emotional inhibition, Pennebaker originally suggested *emotional disinhibition* to be the primary mechanism of change in expressive writing [47]. This hypothesis was primarily derived from the first studies showing fewer physical illnesses over time in EWI participants compared to fact-writing controls [37], as well as other positive physical and psychological health-related outcomes like improved immune function [48] and better adjustment to college [49]. This interpretation was seen as supported by the early finding of lower skin conductance levels in participants who completed EWI [50], where low skin conductance levels have been viewed as indicating 'letting go' or disinhibition, while high skin conductance levels have been associated with 'holding back' or inhibition, as utilised in polygraph or 'lie detector' tests. Repeatedly confronting the trauma should allow for habituation to the associated thoughts, thereby reducing the chronic autonomic arousal chained up by holding back the traumatic experience. Other studies, however, show evidence to the contrary. It has for example been shown that writing about stressful events that one has already disclosed to others are as likely to produce beneficial results as writing about events that one has not disclosed previously [51]. Furthermore, writing emotionally about imaginary traumas has been found to produce similar results to writing about experienced traumatic experiences [52]. The assumption that writing must involve coping with a traumatic event to be beneficial is also challenged by the results of a study showing that participants writing about their 'best possible future self' experienced physical benefits equal to those who wrote about a traumatic experience [53].

More recent theories have focused on how emotional expression may facilitate cognitive adaptation to the stressful or traumatic experience through *cognitive processing or restructuring* of stressful memories, which – in turn-could lead to positive emotional and biological changes [54]. If, as suggested by Janoff-Bulman [2], the emotional distress experienced following a traumatic event is primarily due to the perceived discrepancies between preexisting schemas and the meaning associated with the traumatic event, the act of converting emotions into spoken or written language and a coherent narrative may serve to change the way the person organises, behaves and thinks about the trauma [55]. Once this process of cognitive integration is complete, individuals should exhibit a reduction in their distress as well as less frequent intrusive thoughts about the traumatic experience. Support for the cognitive restructuring hypothesis has been provided in several studies. For example, in a reanalysis of data from three previous studies, Campbell and Pennebaker found evidence that flexibility in the use of common words when writing about traumatic memories were predictive of beneficial physical health outcomes [56]. Another study comparing effects of instructions to write about stressful experiences in a fragmented format and instructions to construct a coherent narrative revealed beneficial effects only in the narrative writing group when compared to neutral writing controls [57]. That health benefits are mediated by cognitive restructuring is further supported by findings of associations with increased use of causal- and insight-related words across the writing sessions [58, 59]. The true causal nature of these associations is, however, difficult to evaluate, and cognitive or linguistic changes have also been found in the absence of psychological or physical health benefits after EWI [60–62].

Exposure provides a third possible mechanism [63]. In brief, the original traumatic experience may serve as an unconditioned aversive stimulus (UCS) that elicits an unconditioned response (UR) in the form of distress. In the learning process, as other previously neutral stimuli are paired with the UCS, they become conditioned stimuli (CS) that elicit distressing emotional responses as conditioned responses (CRs). Being instructed to write several times about stressful experiences may allow the participant to be repeatedly exposed to aversive stimuli that previously have been avoided, thereby allowing for the extinction of the conditioned associations between thoughts about the stressful or traumatic experience and the negative emotional response [55]. In addition, by overcoming a person's tendency to inhibit distressing memories and thoughts, written disclosure may assist appropriate processing or restructuring of emotional material. However, the results concerning exposure as a mechanism in EWI are mixed. Some studies have found reduced symptoms of post-traumatic stress in the form of intrusive thoughts following EWI, [64, 65], while others have found no evidence [61, 66]. Likewise, some have found reduced avoidance [64, 65], some have found no effects [18, 67], while others have found increased avoidance after EWI [52, 57]. As reviewed by Sloan and Marx [63], there may be several reasons for the mixed results, including insufficient statistical power and differences in sample characteristics. With respect to the latter, they suggest that EWI may work best for participants with low to moderate levels of symptomatology, and may even increase distress in those with more severe symptoms. Studies also vary with respect to whether participants have been restricted to write about specific events, for example their cancer, or have been allowed to write about a topic of their own choice, and it is suggested that freedom of choice in writing topic may enhance the likelihood of finding an effect.

Finally, according to the social-cognitive processing theory [3], expressive writing could be hypothesised to aid psychological adjustment to stressful experiences by improving relationships and *increasing social support*. The ultimate purpose of language is to communicate ideas and thoughts to other people. When a person talks – or writes – to other people about their experiences, it alerts them to his or her psychological state and thereby maintains his or her social ties to them [68]. By overcoming tendencies to avoid distressing thoughts and behaviours and by assisting the person in expressing his or her emotions in a more comprehensible and more socially acceptable manner, the participant's partner or other relations may become more willing to listen and to provide emotional support, which could reduce stress and promote psychological and physical health. Although there is some support for this hypothesis [68, 69], the possibility that effects of EWI can be mediated by changes in social interactions is clearly in need of further research.

9.2.3 For Whom Does EWI Work?

While the literature generally suggests that EWI can be beneficial in terms of both increased psychological and physical health, the results are not unambiguous, and there are both null-findings and negative findings in terms of worsened symptoms after EWI. In the review by Frattaroli [43], which also includes studies that do not adhere strictly to the Pennebaker writing paradigm, a number of possible moderating factors were investigated. When exploring within-study effects, participants with poorer health and higher levels of stress were more likely to benefit from the disclosure intervention, and studies in which participants were required to have a physical health problem has significantly larger effect sizes for self-reported health than studies where this was not an eligibility criterion. Between-study comparisons also revealed that the more recent the traumatic event, the larger effect size.

It is also possible that individual traits and behaviours related to emotional expression moderate the effects of EWI. In the first meta-analysis, Smyth [40] found that studies with a higher proportion of men had larger effect sizes than studies with a higher proportion of women, and proposed that men may benefit more from experimental disclosure because they tend to be less likely than women to naturally disclose information as a result of traditional sex roles. While the most recent meta-analysis [43] did not reveal any moderating effect of gender, it is still possible that individuals who are less inclined to disclosure due to social or cultural factors could benefit more from a structured, formalised disclosure intervention. In contrast, it has been suggested that when individuals either do not consciously acknowledge negative emotions, for example as in emotional repression, or are unable to identify and differentiate their feelings, as when high in alexithymia, they may be less likely to benefit – or even experience worsening – from emotional disclosure [70]. The moderating influence of emotional repression has only been investigated in very few studies, and there is therefore only tentative evidence that repressive copers will benefit less than non-repressors [71, 72]. The inability of alexithymic persons to understand their own feelings and psychological states may interfere with the task of identifying a stressor to disclose, labelling their emotions and gaining insight and understanding about their feelings and about the event that they are disclosing. While no overall moderating effect was found in seven experimental disclosure studies which had included a measure of alexithymia [43], most of these studies have not focused specifically on the role of pre-disclosure emotional inhibition. In contrast, support for emotional coping as a potential moderator of effects of EWI has been found when the writing tasks have been tailored to the individuals' preferred coping strategy [73, 74]. The results indicated that health benefits were more likely to occur when individuals inclined to cope through emotional approach were induced to deal with their emotions, and – in contrast – that individuals low in emotional approach coping gained benefits when instructed to look forward with a positive attitude.

9.2.4 Influence of Writing Instructions and Setting

Moderating effects have also been found of various aspects of the disclosure instructions and setting [43]. For instance, the available evidence suggests significantly greater effects on psychological health outcomes when participants disclosed at home versus in a controlled setting, or when they disclosed in a private room versus in a group setting. Greater effects were also found for both psychological and

| Table 9.1 | Expressive writing intervention studies with cancer patients | | | | | | | |

Authors/year	N	Cancer	Writing topic, schedule	Control	Manipulation check	Outcomes	Combined effect size Cohen's d^a	p
Walker *et al.* [61]	39	Breast	Cancer, daily	Non-writing	–	A	–0.09	0.80
Stanton *et al.* [77]	60	Breast	Cancer, weekly	Neutral writing	+	A, C, D	0.20	0.45
Rosenberg *et al.* [78]	30	Prostate	Free, not rep.	Non-writing	–	A, B, C	0.28	0.46
De Moor *et al.* [67]	37	Renal	Cancer, weekly	Neutral writing	–	A, B, C	0.39	0.26
Zakowski *et al.* [79]	104	Prostate, gynecology	Cancer, daily	Neutral writing	+	A	0.05	0.81
Cepeda *et al.* [80]	234	Mixed	Cancer, weekly	Non-writing	–	B, C, E	0.00	1.00
Gellaitry *et al.* [81]	104	Breast	Cancer, daily	Non-writing	–	A, C, E	0.08	0.80
Jensen-Johansen, M., Christensen, S., Valdimarsdottir, H. *et al.* 2010a, 2010b (unpublished manuscripts)	507	Breast	Free, weekly	Neutral writing	+	A, C	0.10	0.29
Psychological health (seven studies)	–	–	–	–	–	A	0.03	0.638
Physical health (six studies)	–	–	–	–	–	C	0.14	**0.038**
Combined outcomes (eight studies)	–	–	–	–	–	A–E	0.08	0.208

^{a}The combined effect sizes across outcomes were taken either from already published meta-analyses or, or if more recent and not included in these, independently calculated. Effect sizes were combined using random effects models. Separate analyses were conducted for the outcomes of psychological and reported physical health which were included in a sufficient number of studies.
A, psychological health; B, physiological function; C, reported physical health; D, subjective benefit of intervention; E, quality-of-life/general functioning.

self-reported physical health outcomes when disclosure sessions lasted at least 15 minutes compared to less than 15 minutes, and when the intervention included at least three sessions versus fewer than three sessions. Generally, it did not seem to be important whether the sessions were administered daily or weekly. When instructions were more directed, for example giving specific examples, greater effects were found for self-reported physical health than when no specific instructions were given, and studies which specifically instructed participants to disclose an event that they had not previously discussed with others also showed greater effect sizes. Due to too few studies where participants had been instructed to write about positive events, it was not possible to analyse the influence of the emotional valence of the topic. Furthermore, the mode of disclosure: hand-written, typed or oral, did not appear to moderate the effects.

9.2.5 Expressive Writing with Cancer Patients

So far, only a few studies of written emotional disclosure have included cancer patients. A systematic review of the literature revealed seven published studies in addition to a large study conducted by our group, currently awaiting publication. These eight studies and their results are summarised in Table 9.1. The remaining trials of emotional disclosure with cancer patients have used verbal rather than written disclosure (e.g. [75, 76]). The studies have assessed several outcomes, including *psychological outcomes* such as cancer-related distress, *physiological outcomes* such as changes in various immune parameters, different reported *physical health* outcomes, including self-reported somatic symptoms, pain, sleep quality and medical appointments. Generally, the studies focusing on EWI with cancer patients failed to find significant main effects of EWI. The numbers of patients included in the studies, however, were generally small, which could account for the negative findings.

As the previously published meta-analyses have not focused separately on studies with cancer patients, we conducted a preliminary meta-analysis of the eight currently available studies. The individual and combined effect sizes are shown in Table 9.1. The results indicate a significant effect of written emotional disclosure on self-reported physical health, with the combined effect size (Cohen's $d = 0.14$) being slightly larger than that found for self-reported physical health across healthy and clinical samples in the most recent meta-analysis by Frattaroli ($d = 0.11$). In contrast, the combined effect on psychological health did not reach statistical significance and was smaller ($d = 0.03$) than that reported by Frattaroli ($d = 0.07$). The numbers of studies with cancer patients examining general functioning, physiological functioning and subjective impact of the intervention were not sufficient for meta-analysis.

In four studies, non-writing patients were used as control groups, rather than patients instructed to write about a neutral topic, as required by the Pennebaker expressive writing paradigm. Omitting a neutral-writing control group makes it difficult to evaluate whether effects are due to the specific elements of written emotional disclosure, rather than non-specific factors related to being in an intervention group as such. When analysing only the four studies using a neutral writing control group, the effect on reported physical health ($d = 0.23$) remained statistically significant, while there continued to be no significant effect for psychological outcomes ($d = 0.04$). Four studies had used four writing sessions, three studies had used three sessions and the remaining study had included a group with three sessions and a group with only one session. Four studies had employed writing sessions spaced a week apart, while three studies used daily sessions. In the last study, the sessions depended on clinic visits. While the results did not reach statistical significance, studies with four sessions had a larger combined effect size ($d = 0.16$) than studies with three sessions ($d = 0.06$), and weekly sessions yielded a larger effect size ($d = 0.09$) than daily session ($d = 0.03$).

Adherence is a potential concern in studies of EWI, particularly in home-based studies. In home-based studies, the issue of non-adherence is often dealt with by having research assistants contacting the participants by telephone before and after each writing session. Furthermore, several experimental EWI studies have included a manipulation check by asking the participants after the session how personal they considered their writing to be and to what degree they had expressed emotions in their writing. Another method is to assess positive and negative mood immediately before and after each writing session. The research indicates that EWI is usually followed by immediate increases in negative mood, especially after the first writing session, and lack of such changes could be an indicator of non-adherence. Studies which had

included a manipulation check tended to show a greater effect ($d = 0.10$) than studies which had not ($d = 0.06$).

Taken together, the results of the available studies with cancer patients support the results of previous meta-analyses indicating larger effects of EWI on self-reported physical health than on psychological health in clinical samples. The effect sizes found are generally small. One reason could be that patients willing to participate may be experiencing fewer symptoms, and that this may introduce a 'floor effect', making it more difficult to reduce these symptoms even further. Again, it should be noted that even small effect sizes could be considered of clinical relevance, especially considering the low costs associated with EWI.

9.3 Target Patients

9.3.1 Which Cancer Patients Are Likely to Benefit?

While the effects of EWI, especially for psychological outcomes, appear to be limited for cancer patients taken as a whole, some patients may be more likely to benefit than others. Among the few possible moderating factors examined so far are avoidance, emotional inhibition, social constraints and the choice of writing topic. In the study by Stanton and colleagues, a moderating effect was found of cancer-related avoidance, suggesting that writing focusing especially on benefit finding and positive emotions in relation to cancer was more effective in women high in avoidance, while the traditional writing instructions, asking the participants to focus on their deepest thoughts and feelings concerning breast cancer was more effective in women low in avoidance. With respect to emotional repression, the few previous studies with non-cancer samples suggest that repressive copers may be less able to recognise and acknowledge stressful experiences and to access the emotional memories of the experience, making it less likely that they, compared to non-repressors, will benefit from a written emotional disclosure procedure [71, 72, 82]. In contrast to most previous findings, our study (Jensen-Johansen, M., Christensen, S., Valdimarsdottir, H. *et al.* 2010b, unpublished manuscript) indicated that patients in the EWI group identified as repressive copers reported fewer somatic symptoms nine months after the intervention, compared to repressive copers in the control group, who reported an increase in somatic symptoms. One explanation could be that the more private nature of the written disclosure task is better suited for repressive copers. In non-cancer samples, participants with high scores on alexithymia, that is difficulties identifying and/or describing feelings, have been found both to benefit less [29] and more [82] from EWI. In our study (Jensen-Johansen, M., Christensen, S., Valdimarsdottir, H. *et al.* 2010b, unpublished manuscript), EWI participants with high scores on the difficulties describing feelings subscale showed *both* increased number of medical appointments and increased report of somatic symptoms after the intervention. The mixed results concerning alexithymia are difficult to interpret, but could suggest that the moderating influence of alexithymia may depend on other factors, for example the type of traumatic event and the level of post-traumatic distress, and more research is clearly needed.

As reviewed above, the social-cognitive processing theory of adjustment to stressors [3] suggests that when people perceive significant others to be unwilling to listen to their concerns, this can adversely affect their coping behaviours and psychological adjustment [20]. It is therefore possible that EWI may be more beneficial for patients experiencing high levels of social constraints by giving them an alternative opportunity to express their emotions, thereby buffering the negative influence of social constraints. This hypothesis is supported by the results of a study by Zakowski and colleagues [79]. Although they found no main effects of EWI on cancer-related distress, participants in the control group with high levels of social constraints had the highest levels of distress, while patients in the EWI with high social constraints had levels of distress comparable to those of patients with low levels of social constraints. Likewise, in our study, we found a reduced number of medical appointments after the intervention in the EWI group among patients reporting high levels of social constraints (Jensen-Johansen, M., Christensen, S., Valdimarsdottir, H. *et al.* 2010b, unpublished manuscript). If reduced health care utilisation can be interpreted as a proxy of improved health, then the results may be interpreted as supporting the hypothesis that EWI can buffer the negative influence of social constraints.

Most studies with cancer patients have been restrictive with respect to the writing topic, and have only allowed the participants to write about their cancer. Patients high in cancer-related avoidance or with a tendency to repressive coping may, if given a choice, prefer to write about other topics than their own cancer in order to avoid distress. It may also be more beneficial for individuals with depression or tendencies to ruminate not to dwell on concerns about their cancer,

as they may be unable, without sufficient support, to cope efficiently with highly emotional thoughts and negative emotions within the short time-frame of EWI. Furthermore, for some patients, the cancer diagnosis and treatment may not be the most stressful or traumatic experience, and – if given a choice – they might have chosen to write about an experience more relevant to them at the particular point in time. Our own study (Jensen-Johansen, M., Christensen, S., Valdimarsdottir, H. *et al.* 2010a, unpublished manuscript) is the only study so far, which has specifically examined the influence of the choice of writing topic. While there generally were no differences at baseline, women in the EWI group who chose to write about their cancer reported an increased number of medical appointments following intervention compared to controls (Jensen-Johansen, M., Christensen, S., Valdimarsdottir, H. *et al.* 2010b, unpublished manuscript). How to interpret this result depends on whether medical visits should be considered a proxy for improved health or the opposite.

9.3.2 Summarising the Evidence

Although emotional expression may not be beneficial under all circumstances, and under certain conditions even intensify distress and interfere with active coping [30], there is still considerable evidence to suggest that a general tendency to cope through emotional non-expression will reduce the chance of adjustment to traumatic events such as cancer. In addition, emotionally expressive forms of adjustment have generally been found associated with improved psychological adjustment and lower levels of distress. EWI is a relevant, brief and potentially cost-effective intervention aimed at helping individuals adjust to traumatic events. Systematic reviews reveal that EWI is associated with beneficial effects on both psychological well-being and physical health-related outcomes such as somatic symptoms and health care utilisation. While this appears to be particular true for studies with healthy participants [40], significant effects have also been found for studies with clinical samples [41, 43], although not for all types of outcomes [42]. In line with the findings for clinical populations in general, the results of the relatively few available studies with cancer patients suggest a potential beneficial effect of EWI on reported physical health-outcomes such as medical appointments, pain and other somatic symptoms, while the effects on psychological health outcomes were small and non-significant.

While the individual studies generally fail to show a main effect of EWI in cancer patients, results of the individual studies suggest several potential moderating effects, indicating that some patients, for example those experiencing *high* levels of social constraints and those with *low* levels of emotional repression or alexithymia, could be more likely to benefit than others. Some delivery methods and instructions may also be more efficacious than others. The current evidence indicates, for example, larger effects for studies with writing sessions conducted at home or in a private room and studies with at least three writing sessions that lasted at least 15 minutes. The effects found appear to be similar for different types of written disclosure, that is hand-written versus typed, and when comparing written and oral disclosure, for example over the telephone, the available results show no differences. As written disclosure is likely to be more cost-effective, this supports the use of written disclosure. Due to the limited number of studies, it is yet unclear whether the writing topic should be restricted to the cancer experience, and who will benefit from specific instructions to focus on positive emotions and benefit-finding. Although research on the mechanisms of EWI is still limited, there is some evidence to suggest that participants who are able to write a more coherent narrative will benefit more.

9.3.3 Efficacy versus Effectiveness

When interpreting the results, it is important to acknowledge that the currently available evidence for EWI in general and for cancer patients in particular is almost entirely based on *efficacy* studies, attempting to maximise the *internal* validity, that is the confidence that the observed associations between the independent variable (emotionally expressive writing vs. control – in most cases non-emotional writing) and the outcome is causal. In contrast, there is currently no clear evidence to support the *effectiveness* of EWI, that is whether the effects found in tightly controlled efficacy studies can be *generalised* to the clinical setting under real world conditions.

The self-selection of participants into the studies is one of several factors that may influence the validity of efficacy studies [83]. On the one hand, non-participants may be less motivated and have less confidence that the intervention is helpful for them, which could lead to overestimation of the effect. On the other hand, patients with more psychological problems and more severe trauma may decline to participate, which may contribute to the pre-selection of well-functioning participants, who are less likely to benefit from the intervention. Effectiveness could also depend on the type of instructions given. In randomised clinical trials, the golden standard when investigating efficacy, the instructions are typically highly standardised, while in the real world therapeutic setting, the therapists have opportunity to alter instructions based on the feedback from the patients, thereby providing more individualised instructions with higher external validity. Given that EWI can be implemented in many ways, including to large populations at minimal costs, even relatively limited average effects have the potential to be very cost-effective.

9.4 Processes and Techniques

EWI can be implemented through individual face-to-face therapy or delivered through other methods, for example the Internet or printed workbooks.

9.4.1 Face-to-Face

Lange and colleagues have described implementations of EWI, both as a part of face-to-face psychotherapy and delivered through the Internet [84]. Based on the mechanisms believed to be crucial in adjusting to and overcoming traumatic events, their model for EWI in clinical practice consists of three phases: (i) self-confrontation, (ii) cognitive reappraisal and (iii) taking leave of the past.

In the self-confrontation phase, the therapist encourages the patient to describe the traumatic experience and explains the importance of self-confrontation in general and the use of writing assignments in particular. The therapist checks whether the patient is stable enough to meet the demands of self-confrontation, and if the therapist and patient agree, a contract is established. The therapist then gives the first instructions to write about the event. The patient is asked to write at a fixed place, at fixed times and for a fixed duration, and instructed to focus on the most painful elements and their deepest feelings. After each writing session, the therapist and the patient discuss the impact of the writing. If permitted, the therapist reads the written material. When the patient reports that the emotions have become less strong and that focusing on the writing has become difficult, the therapist instructs the patient to change the content of the writing and to focus on challenging dysfunctional thinking (e.g. shame, guilt, etc.) thereby promoting cognitive reappraisal. Finally, when the patient has completed all writing assignments, he or she is instructed to write a last letter or essay. This should be a dignified, immaculate product written in a way so that it can be read and understood by others, for example a spouse, although this person may not actually read it. The therapist reads the writing and may give suggestions to improve style and content. If the writing is not sent or given to another person, it may be sent in a symbolic way, for example by placing it in a box.

The clinical procedure described above was tested in a trial with patients referred from local physicians who had suffered from traumatic events. The effect in the group of patients who received the combination of both the self-confrontation and cognitive reappraisal elements described above was considerable with changes in avoidance and intrusive thoughts corresponding to large effect sizes (d = 1.1 and 1.4 respectively).

9.4.2 Internet-Based

The authors have implemented the above described intervention on an Internet-based platform, which included screening for post-traumatic stress symptoms and instructions corresponding to the three phases of self-confrontation, cognitive reappraisal phases and sharing and farewell. The participants are instructed to write twice weekly over a period of five weeks. In the middle of each phase, the therapist gives feedback and further instructions by e-mail. If the content of the writing indicates that the Internet-based therapy may not be appropriate, the participant may receive an e-mail followed by a telephone call to discuss other ways of treatment. An evaluation of the Internet-based EWI with 50 patients showed similar large effects on avoidance and intrusive thoughts as found in the therapist-delivered intervention (d = 1.66 and 0.96). It should be noted that previous experimental EWI studies differ by not including an active therapist involved in giving instructions and feedback.

9.4.3 Workbooks

Workbooks represent a third possible method of delivering EWI. Workbooks can be a cost-effective, mass-produced and easily repeatable method to deliver the intervention, which could be especially relevant for EWI. As suggested by L'Abate [85], workbooks can provide treatment plans that are more detailed and specific than verbally administered treatment plans, permit participants to take on more responsibility in their

change processes, extend the brief face-to-face therapy sessions, allows for reaching underserved populations, such as handicapped persons, and may be an efficient method of generalising the effects of an intervention in the larger community setting. A meta-analysis of 18 studies evaluating the effects of workbook-based interventions shows significant effects both for psychological health problems (d = 0.44) and physical health outcomes (d = 0.25) [86].

Recently, Pennebaker has provided a detailed example of a workbook approach to EWI with detailed instructions and exercises aimed at the lay person [87]. The core instructions are similar to those used in most research of EWI, and can serve as a framework for developing instructions and exercises for specific target populations, in this case cancer patients or survivors. Based on his experience with expressive writing, Pennebaker outlines the following general aims and guidelines: That people tend to benefit most from expressive writing when: (i) they acknowledge their emotions – both negative and positive – openly, (ii) when they are able to construct a coherent meaningful story of what has happened and how it is affecting them, (iii) when they are able to switch perspectives and view the traumatic event through the eyes of others and (iv) when they in their writing strive to find their 'own voice', writing to themselves rather than focusing on style. Furthermore, people are instructed only to deal with traumatic memories that bother them, and to avoid writing about issues that they no longer think about or are affected by. Further recommendations include a 20-minute minimum for each writing session, a minimum of four writing sessions, a fixed time and fixed private place to write, and writing continuously during each session. Finally, people are instructed that it is a normal reaction to experience an increase in negative feelings immediately after writing, especially after the first session.

In *writing session 1*, the person is instructed to write about and explore their deepest thoughts and feelings about a particularly traumatic event or emotional upheaval. *Writing session 2* involves instructions to continue to explore their thoughts and feelings about a traumatic event or emotional upheaval, this time *really* exploring their deepest thoughts and feelings, either about the same event or a completely different one. *Writing session 3* instructs the person to continue to write about their deepest thoughts and feelings, this time focusing on the emotions and thoughts about the event, that is affecting his or her life most right now, especially the issues about which he or her is particular vulnerable.

During *writing session 4*, the final session, the person is asked to stand back and think about the events, issues, thoughts and feelings that he or she has disclosed in the previous sessions. The person is instructed to try to tie up anything that hasn't been confronted, to focus on what has been learned, lost and gained as a result of the experience and to think about how the experience will guide his or her thoughts and actions in the future. After each writing session, people are instructed to reflect upon their writing experience and how it has affected them, for example what they feel after writing and to what degree the writing was valuable and meaningful to them.

Finally, after completing all four sessions, preferably after several weeks, the person is suggested to read what he or she has written, and to review the process by checking for changes, for example reduced psychological and physical symptoms. The person is also encouraged to analyse his or her writing and the changes in style, writing and content, and to review the writing in terms of some of the characteristics found in effective writing, including using negative emotions in moderation, using many positive emotions, constructing a coherent story through the writing process and changing the perspective from viewing the event mostly from the person's own perspective to being able to see the event in a broader perspective from different angles.

The above described instructions can relatively easily be altered to be used with cancer patients or cancer survivors. An example is given in the Appendix. Although session 4 includes suggestions to look at potential benefits and what has been learned from the experience, the instructions described above are relatively non-specific. As suggested by the findings of Stanton and colleagues [77], some individuals, in particular those using avoidance strategies to high degree, may benefit more from more detailed instructions to focus on benefit finding and positive emotions. One possibility is therefore to develop more individualised instructions, for example focusing on benefit-finding and positive emotions in session 3, to use with such patients.

9.5 Appendix: Sample Instructions for Expressive Writing for Cancer Patients and Survivors

The instructions below are a version of the standard EWI instructions [37] adapted to cancer patients (Jensen-Johansen, M., Christensen, S., Valdimarsdottir, H. *et al.* 2010a, 2010b, unpublished manuscript).

9.5.1 Day 1: Writing Instructions

This is the first of four days of emotional writing. Today, your goal will be to write about your *deepest thoughts and feelings* about the traumatic event or emotional distressing experience that affects you most. This can be your *cancer experience*, but it doesn't have to be. If there is another event or experience that has affected you more, you may chose to write about this experience or event. In your writing, let go and explore the events and how it has affected you. Don't worry about grammar or style. Remember that you are writing to *you*, and not anybody else.

If possible, explore thoughts and feelings that you have had difficulties sharing with others. As you write, you might begin to tie it to other aspects of your life. For example, how is it related to your relationships with your spouse or partner, your parents and other close relations? How is it related to the people you have most loved, feared and been angry at? How is it related to your current life situation, your work and your place in life in general? How is it related to who you were in the past, the person you are now and how you would like to be in the future?

Make sure that you will not be disturbed while you write. Remember that what you are writing is for *you* – not anyone else. Write continuously for 20 minutes. Do not stop writing during the 20 minutes. Remember that the goal is to really explore your deepest thoughts and feelings about the distressing experience, whether it is about your cancer or any other topic you chose to write about. When you have completed your writing, please go to the *Post-writing section*, where you will be asked a few questions about your writing.

_____

_____

_____

_____

_____

(Add more lines as needed)

9.5.2 Post-Writing Questions

Congratulations. You have now completed your first day of writing. Before putting your writing assignment down for today, please complete the following brief questionnaire. Write a number between 0 and 10 by each question, where the numbers mean:

0 1 2 3 4 5 6 7 8 9 10
Not at all   Somewhat   A great deal

1 To what degree did you express your deepest thoughts and feelings? _____
2 To what degree do you currently feel sad or upset?[a] _____
3 To what degree do you currently feel happy?[a] _____
4 To what degree was today's writing valuable and meaningful for you? _____

[a] *These general questions can be replaced by a more detailed mood assessment questionnaire, for example the Positive and Negative Affect Scale (PANAS)* [88].

The instructions for the following writing sessions are very similar to the instructions for Day 1 and continue to ask the person to write about his or her deepest thoughts and feelings about the traumatic event, but adds more detailed suggestions to write about how the event is affecting the person's life in general, and how the person might be responsible for some of the effects of the trauma (Day 2), to focus more specifically on how the person's thoughts and emotions may affect their life right now and how they are feeling as they write (Day 3), and by tying up loose ends and focusing on costs, benefits and what you have learned in the final writing session (Day 4). The instruction described in this appendix lets the person choose whether to write about his or her cancer or some other experience. If relevant, the instructions can be changed so as to instructing the person to focus on his or her experience with cancer.

9.5.3 Day 2: Writing Instructions

Today is the second day of the writing process. In today's writing, your task is to *really* examine your deepest thoughts and feelings. You may write about the same event as on Day 1 or a completely different one. While the instructions are similar to those of Day 1, try today to go deeper into your thoughts and feelings if possible. Try to link the distressing experience to other parts of your life and how it affects your way of thinking about the past. Also, try to explore how you may be partly responsible for some of the effects of the experience. Again, you may choose to write about your cancer, or a completely different experience. Write continuously for 20 minutes, and do not stop writing during the 20 minutes. When you have completed your writing, please go to the *Post-writing section*.

9.5.4 Day 3: Writing Instructions

You have now completed two writing sessions. After today, you will only have one more day to write and wrap up your story. It is, however, important to continue to explore your deepest thoughts and feelings about the topics you have been examining so far. You may write about the same events as on Day 1 and Day 2 or a different one. While the instructions are similar to those of Day 1 and 2, the goal today is to focus on how your thoughts and feelings about the experience affect your life right now. You may write about the same experience as on Day 1 and 2, but try to explore it from different angles and different points of view. What are you thinking and feeling as you write your experience? How has the event influenced your life and who you are? Make sure to write continuously for 20 minutes. When you have completed your writing, please go to the *Post-writing section*.

9.5.5 Day 4: Writing Instructions

This is the final day of the writing exercise. As previously, your goal is to explore your deepest thoughts and feelings about the issues and experiences that have been distressing for you. As you write, stand back and think about the events, issues, thoughts and feelings you have been writing about. As it is the last day of the exercise, try to wrap things up and complete your story and address any issues that you have not yet confronted. What are you feeling at this point in the process? What have you learned? What are your losses and gains as a result of the experience? How have they shaped you as a person? In what ways will your experiences guide your thoughts and actions in the future? Really let go, and be as honest with yourself as possible. Do your best to merge the entire experience into a meaningful story that you can take with you into the future. Write continuously for 20 minutes without stopping. When you have completed your writing, please go to the *Post-writing section*.

References

1. American Psychiatric Association (1994) *Diagnostic and Statistical Manual of Mental Disorders*, 4th edn, American Psychiatric Association, Washington, DC.
2. Janoff-Bulman, R. (1992) *Shattered Assumptions. Towards a New Psychology of Trauma*, The Free Press, New York.
3. Lepore, S.J. (2001) A social-cognitive processing model of emotional adjustment to cancer, in *Psychosocial Interventions for Cancer* (eds A. Baum and B.L. Andersen), American Psychological Association, Washington, DC, pp. 99–116.

4. Gallagher, J., Parle, M. and Cairns, D. (2002) Appraisal and psychological distress six months after diagnosis of breast cancer. *British Journal of Health Psychology*, **7**, 365–376.

5. Kissane, D.W., Clarke, D.M., Ikin, J. *et al.* (1998) Psychological morbidity and quality of life in Australian women with early-stage breast cancer: a cross-sectional survey. *The Medical journal of Australia*, **169**, 192–196.

6. Koopman, C., Butler, L.D., Classen, C. *et al.* (2002) Traumatic stress symptoms among women with recently diagnosed primary breast cancer. *Journal of Traumatic Stress*, **15**, 277–287.

7. Coyne, J.C., Palmer, S.C., Shapiro, P.J. *et al.* (2004) Distress, psychiatric morbidity, and prescriptions for psychotropic medication in a breast cancer waiting room sample. *General Hospital Psychiatry*, **26**, 121–128.

8. Christensen, S., Zachariae, R., Jensen, A.B. *et al.* (2009) Prevalence and risk of depressive symptoms 3-4 months post-surgery in a nationwide cohort study of Danish women treated for early stage breast-cancer. *Breast Cancer Research and Treatment*, **113**, 339–355.

9. O'Connor, M., Christensen, S., Jensen, A.B. *et al.* (2011) How Traumatic is Breast Cancer? Post-traumatic Stress Symptoms and Risk Factors for PTSD 3 and 15 Months After Surgery in a Nationwide Cohort of Danish Women Treated for Breast Cancer, Br J Cancer [E-pub ahead of print].

10. Horowitz, M.J. (1986) *Stress Response Syndromes*, 2nd edn, Jason Aronson, New York.

11. Greenberg, M. (1995) Cognitive processing of traumas: the role of intrusive thoughts and reappraisals. *Journal of Applied Social Psychology*, **25**, 1262–1296.

12. Horowitz, M.J. (1982) Stress response syndromes and their treatment, in *Handbook of Stress* (eds L. Goldberger and S. Breznitz), Free Press, New York.

13. Stanton, A.L., Danoff-Burg, S., Cameron, C.L. *et al.* (2000) Emotionally expressive coping predicts psychological and physical adjustment to breast cancer. *Journal of Consulting and Clinical Psychology*, **68**, 875–882.

14. Schmidt, J.E. and Andrykowski, M.A. (2004) The role of social and dispositional variables associated with emotional processing in adjustment to breast cancer: an internet-based study. *Health Psychology*, **23**, 259–266.

15. Iwamitsu, Y., Shimoda, K., Abe, H. *et al.* (2005) The relation between negative emotional suppression and emotional distress in breast cancer diagnosis and treatment. *Health Communication*, **18**, 201–215.

16. Hack, T.F. and Degner, L.F. (2004) Coping responses following breast cancer diagnosis predict psychological adjustment three years later. *Psychooncology*, **13**, 235–247.

17. Owen, J.E., Giese-Davis, J., Cordova, M. *et al.* (2006) Self-report and linguistic indicators of emotional expression in narratives as predictors of adjustment to cancer. *Journal of Behavioral Medicine*, **29**, 335–345.

18. Stroebe, M., Stroebe, S., Schut, H. *et al.* (2002) Does disclosure of emotions facilitate recovery from bereavement? Evidence from two prospective studies. *Journal of Consulting and Clinical Psychology*, **70**, 169–178.

19. Bonanno, G.A., Holen, A., Keltner, D. *et al.* (1995) When avoiding unpleasant emotions might not be such a bad thing – verbal-autonomic response dissociation and midlife conjugal bereavement. *Journal of Personality and Social Psychology*, **69**, 975–989.

20. Lepore, S.J., Silver, R.C., Wortman, C.B. *et al.* (1996) Social constraints, intrusive thoughts, and depressive symptoms among bereaved mothers. *Journal of Personality and Social Psychology*, **70**, 271–282.

21. Lepore, S.J. and Helgeson, V.S. (1998) Social constraints, intrusive thoughts, and mental health after prostate cancer. *Journal of Social and Clinical Psychology*, **17** (1), 89–106.

22. Cordova, M.J., Cunningham, L.L., Carlson, C.R. *et al.* (2001) Social constraints, cognitive processing, and adjustment to breast cancer. *Journal of Consulting and Clinical Psychology*, **69**, 706–711.

23. Porter, L.S., Keefe, F.J., Hurwitz, H. and Faber, M. (2005) Disclosure between patients with gastrointestinal cancer and their spouses. *Psychooncology*, **14**, 1030–1042.

24. Manne, S., Badr, H., Zaider, T. *et al.* (2010) Cancer-related communication, relationship intimacy, and psychological distress among couples coping with localized prostate cancer. *Journal of Cancer Survivorship*, **4**, 74–85.

25. Breuer, J. and Freud, S. (1978) *Studies on Hysteria*, Penguin Books, Harmondsworth.

26. Pennebaker, J.W. (1997a) *Opening Up: The Healing Power of Expressing Emotions*, Guilford Press, New York.

27. Weinberger, D.A. (1990) The construct validity of the repressive coping style, in *Repression and Dissociation* (ed. J.L. Singer), University of Chicago Press, Chicago, pp. 337–386.

28. Sifneos, P.E. (1973) The prevalence of alexithymic characteristics in psychosomatic patients. *Psychotherapy and Psychosomatics*, **22**, 255–262.

29. Taylor, G.J., Bagby, R.M. and Parker, J.D-A. (1997) *Disorders of Affect Regulation: Alexithymia in Medical and Psychiatric Illness*, Cambridge University Press, New York.

30. Kennedy-Moore, E. and Watson, J.C. (1999) *Expressing Emotion: Myths, Realities, and Therapeutic Strategies*, The Guildford Press, New York.

31. Traue, H.C. and Pennebaker, J.W. (1993) *Emotion, Inhibition and Health*, Hogrefe & Huber Publishers, Seattle, WA.

32. Jorgensen, M.M., Zachariae, R., Skytthe, A. and Kyvik, K. (2007) Genetic and environmental factors in alexithymia: a population-based study of 8,785 Danish twin pairs. *Psychotherapy and Psychosomatics*, **76**, 369–375.

33. Freyberger, H. (1977) Supportive psychotherapeutic techniques in primary and secondary alexithymia. *Psychotherapy and Psychosomatics*, **28**, 337–342.

34. Stiles, W.B. (1995) Disclosure as a speech act: is it psychotherapeutic to disclose? in *Emotion, Disclosure, and Health* (ed. J.W. Pennebaker), American Psychological Association, Washington, DC, pp. 71–91.

35. Smyth, J. and Helm, R. (2003) Focused expressive writing as self-help for stress and trauma. *Journal of Clinical Psychology*, **59**, 227–235.

36. Lepore, S.J. and Smyth, J. (2002) *The Writing Cure: How Expressive Writing Promotes Health and Emotional Well Being*, American Psychological Association, Washington, DC.

37. Pennebaker, J.W. and Beall, S.K. (1986) Confronting a traumatic event: toward an understanding of inhibition and disease. *Journal of Abnormal Psychology*, **95**, 274–281.

38. Francis, M.E. and Pennebaker, J.W. (1992) Putting stress into words: the impact of writing on physiological, absentee, and self-reported emotional well-being measures. *American Journal of Health Promotion*, **6**, 280–287.

39. Pennebaker, J. (1995) *Emotion, Disclosure, and Health*, American Psychological Association, Washington, DC.

40. Smyth, J.M. (1998) Written emotional expression: effect sizes, outcome types, and moderating variables. *Journal of Consulting and Clinical Psychology*, **66**, 174–184.

41. Frisina, P.G., Borod, J.C. and Lepore, S.J. (2004) A meta-analysis of the effects of written emotional disclosure on the health outcomes of clinical populations. *The Journal of Nervous and Mental Disease*, **192**, 629–634.

42. Harris, A.H. (2006) Does expressive writing reduce health care utilization? A meta-analysis of randomized trials. *Journal of Consulting and Clinical Psychology*, **74**, 243–252.

43. Frattaroli, J. (2006) Experimental disclosure and its moderators: a meta-analysis. *Psychological Bulletin*, **132**, 823–865.

44. Cohen, J. (1988) *Statistical Power Analysis for the Behavioral Sciences*, Lawrence Erlbaum Associates, Hillsdale, NJ.

45. Rosenthal, R. and Rubin, D.B. (1982) A simple, general purpose display of magnitude of experimental effect. *Journal of Education and Psychology*, **74**, 166–169.

46. King, L.A. (2002) Gain without pain? Expressive writing and self-regulation, in *The Writing Cure* (eds S.J. Lepore and J. Smyth), American Psychological Association, Washington, DC, pp. 119–134.

47. Pennebaker, J.W. and Susman, J.R. (1988) Disclosure of traumas and psychosomatic processes. *Social Science and Medicine*, **26**, 327–332.

48. Petrie, K.J., Booth, R.J., Pennebaker, J.W. *et al.* (1995) Disclosure of trauma and immune response to a hepatitis B vaccination program. *Journal of Consulting and Clinical Psychology*, **63**, 787–792.

49. Pennebaker, J.W., Colder, M. and Sharp, L.K. (1990) Accelerating the coping process. *Journal of Personality and Social Psychology*, **58**, 528–537.

50. Pennebaker, J.W., Hughes, C.F. and Oheeron, R.C. (1987) The psychophysiology of confession – linking inhibitory and psychosomatic processes. *Journal of Personality and Social Psychology*, **52**, 781–793.

51. Greenberg, M.A. and Stone, A.A. (1992) Emotional disclosure about traumas and its relation to health: effects of previous disclosure and trauma severity. *Journal of Personality and Social Psychology*, **63**, 75–84.

52. Greenberg, M.A., Wortman, C.B. and Stone, A.A. (1996) Emotional expression and physical health: revising traumatic memories or fostering self-regulation? *Journal of Personality and Social Psychology*, **71**, 588–602.

53. King, L.A. (2001) The health benefits of writing about life goals. *Personality and Social Psychology Bulletin*, **27**, 798–807.

54. Lepore, S.J., Greenberg, M.A., Bruno, M. *et al.* (2002) Expressive writing and health: self-regulation of emotion-related experience, physiology, and behavior, in *The Writing Cure: How Expressive Writing Promotes Health and Emotional Well-being* (eds S.J. Lepore and J.M. Smyth), American Psychological Association, Washington, DC, pp. 99–117.

55. Pennebaker, J.W. (1997b) Writing about emotional experiences as a therapeutic process. *Psychological Science*, **8**, 162–166.

56. Campbell, R.S. and Pennebaker, J.W. (2003) The secret life of pronouns: flexibility in writing style and physical health. *Psychological Science*, **14**, 60–65.

57. Smyth, J., True, N. and Souto, J. (2001) Effects of writing about traumatic experiences: the necessity for narrative structuring. *Journal of Social and Clinical Psychology*, **20**, 161–172.

58. Pennebaker, J.W. and Francis, M.E. (1996) Cognitive, emotional, and language processes in disclosure. *Cognition and Emotion*, **10**, 601–626.

59. van Middendorp, M.H. and Geenen, R. (2008) Poor cognitive-emotional processing may impede the outcome of emotional disclosure interventions. *British Journal of Health Psychology*, **13**, 49–52.

60. Batten, S.V., Follette, V.M., Hall, M.L.R. *et al.* (2002) Physical and psychological effects of written disclosure among sexual abuse survivors. *Behavior Therapy*, **33**, 107–122.

61. Walker, B.L., Nail, L.M. and Croyle, R.T. (1999) Does emotional expression make a difference in reactions to breast cancer? *Oncology Nursing Forum*, **26**, 1025–1032.

62. Park, C.L. and Blumberg, C.J. (2002) Disclosing trauma through writing: testing the meaning-making hypothesis. *Cognitive Therapy and Research*, **26**, 597–616.

63. Sloan, D.M. and Marx, B.P. (2004) Taking pen to hand: evaluating theories underlying the written disclosure paradigm. *Clinical Psychology-Science and Practice*, **11**, 121–137.

64. Klein, K. and Boals, A. (2001) Expressive writing can increase working memory capacity. *Journal of Experimental Psychology. General*, **130**, 520–533.

65. Schoutrop, M.J., Lange, A., Hanewald, G. *et al.* (2002) Structured writing and processing major stressful events: a controlled trial. *Psychotherapy and Psychosomatics*, **71**, 151–157.

66. Lepore, S.J. (1997) Expressive writing moderates the relation between intrusive thoughts and depressive symptoms. *Journal of Personality and Social Psychology*, **7**, 1037.

67. de Moor, C., Sterner, J., Hall, M. *et al.* (2002) A pilot study of the effects of expressive writing on psychological and behavioral adjustment in patients enrolled in a Phase II trial of vaccine therapy for metastatic renal cell carcinoma. *Health Psychology*, **21**, 615–619.

68. Pennebaker, J.W. and Graybeal, A. (2001) Patterns of natural language use: disclosure, personality, and social integration. *Current Directions in Psychological Science*, **10**, 90–93.

69. Slatcher, R.B. and Pennebaker, J.W. (2006) How do i love thee? Let me count the words: the social effects of expressive writing. *Psychological Science*, **17**, 660–664.

70. Lumley, M.A. (2004) Alexithymia, emotional disclosure, and health: a program of research. *Journal of Personality*, **72**, 1271–1300.

71. Esterling, B.A., Antoni, M.H., Kumar, M. *et al.* (1990) Emotional repression, stress disclosure responses and Epstein-Barr viral capsis antigen titers. *Psychosomatic Medicine*, **52**, 397–410.

72. Lumley, M.A., Tojek, T.M. and Macklem, D.J. (2002) Effects of written emotional disclosure among repressive and alexithymic people, in *The Writing Cure – How Expressive*

Writing Promotes Health and Emotional Well-being (eds S.J. Lepore and J.M. Smyth), American Psychological Association, Washington, DC, pp. 75–96.

73. Austenfeld, J.L. and Stanton, A.L. (2008) Writing about emotions versus goals: effects on hostility and medical care utilization moderated by emotional approach coping processes. *British Journal of Health Psychology*, **13**, 35–38.

74. Austenfeld, J.L., Paolo, A.M. and Stanton, A.L. (2006) Effects of writing about emotions versus goals on psychological and physical health among third-year medical students. *Journal of Personality*, **74**, 267–286.

75. Sandgren, A.K. and McCaul, K.D. (2007) Long-term telephone therapy outcomes for breast cancer patients. *Psychooncology*, **16**, 38–47.

76. Graves, K.D., Schmidt, J.E., Bollmer, F. *et al.* (2005) Emotional expression and emotional recognition in breast cancer survivors: a controlled comparison. *Psychology and Health*, **20**, 579–595.

77. Stanton, A.L., Danoff-Burg, S., Sworowski, L.A. *et al.* (2002) Randomized, controlled trial of written emotional expression and benefit finding in breast cancer patients. *Journal of Clinical Oncology*, **20**, 4160–4168.

78. Rosenberg, H.J., Rosenberg, S.D., Ernstoff, M.S., Wolford, G.L., Amdur, R.J., Elshamy, M.R. *et al.* (2002) Expressive disclosure and health outcomes in a prostate cancer population. *Int J Psychiatry Med*. **32**, 37–53.

79. Zakowski, S.G., Ramati, A., Morton, C. *et al.* (2004) Written emotional disclosure buffers the effects of social constraints on distress among cancer patients. *Health Psychology*, **23**, 555–563.

80. Cepeda, M.S., Chapman, C.R., Miranda, N., Sanchez, R., Rodriguez, C.H., Restrepo, A.E. *et al.* (2008) Emotional disclosure through patient narrative may improve pain and well-being: results of a randomized controlled trial in patients with cancer pain. *J Pain Symptom Manage*, **35**, 623–31.

81. Gellaitry, G., Peters, K., Bloomfield, D. and Horne, R. (2010) Narrowing the gap: the effects of an expressive writing intervention on perceptions of actual and ideal emotional support in women who have completed treatment for early stage breast cancer. *Psychooncology*, **19**, 77–84.

82. Baikie, K.A. (2008) Who does expressive writing work for? Examination of alexithymia, splitting, and repressive coping style as moderators of the expressive writing paradigm. *British Journal of Health Psychology*, **13**, 61–66.

83. Smyth, J. and Catley, D. (2002) Translating research into practice: potential of expressive writing in the field, in *The Writing Cure – How Expressive Writing Promotes Health and Emotional Well-being* (eds S.J. Lepore and J. Smyth), American Psychological Association, Washington, DC, pp. 199–214.

84. Lange, A., Schoutrop, M., Schrieken, B. *et al.* (2002) Interapy: a model for therapeutic writing through the internet, in *The Writing Cure – How Expressive Writing Promotes Health and Emotional Well-being* (eds S.J. Lepore and J.M. Smyth), American Psychological Association, Washington, DC, pp. 215–238.

85. L'abate, L. and Kern, R. (2002) Workbooks: tools for the expressive writing paradigm, in *The Writing Cure – How Expressive Writing Promotes Health and Emotional Well-being* (eds S.J. Lepore and J. Smyth), American Psychological Association, Washington, DC, pp. 239–255.

86. Smyth, J. and L'abate, L. (2001) A meta-analytic evaluation of work-book effectiveness in physical and mental health, in *Distance Writing and Computer-Assisted Interventions in Psychiatry and Mental Health* (ed. L. Labate), Ablex, Westport, CT, pp. 77–90.

87. Pennebaker, J. (2004) *Writing to Heal – A Guided Journal for Recovering from Trauma and Emotional Upheaval*, New Harbinger Publications, Oakland, CA.

88. Watson, D., Clark, L.A. and Tellegen, A. (1988) Development and validation of brief measures of positive and negative affect: the PANAS scales. *J Pers Soc Psychol*, **54**, 1063–1070.

Section B

Group Models
of Therapy

10 Supportive-Expressive Group Psychotherapy

Catherine C. Classen[1] and David Spiegel[2]

[1]Department of Psychiatry, Women's College Hospital, University of Toronto, Toronto, ON, Canada
[2]Stanford University School of Medicine, Stanford, CA, USA

10.1 Introduction

Supportive-Expressive Group Psychotherapy (SEGT) was designed and evaluated in the crucible of existential threat among women with metastatic breast cancer. Its use has since been extended to those with primary breast and other cancers. It is an intensive, weekly group psychotherapy that addresses fundamental existential, emotional and interpersonal problems facing cancer patients.

10.2 Theoretical Background and Themes

The fundamental domains covered by this model include confronting existential issues, promoting emotional expression and optimising social support.

10.2.1 Existential Concerns

While cancer is an assault on one's body, it is also an attack on one's psyche, threatening one's sense of self and the future. The more uncertain the future, the more valuable it becomes. Cancer activates the 'ultimate concerns of existence', which Yalom describes as isolation, meaning, freedom and death [1]. These fundamental concerns fill the cancer patient with dread and yet also present an opportunity. Our aim is to have SEGT turn this existential crisis into an opportunity to reconstruct one's present life and enrich the meaning of the future.

Cancer is an isolating experience. The patient is horrified at the diagnosis, and so are those who care about the patient. Suddenly a chasm is created that separates the once healthy person from those around them, who are also forced to face their own existential anxiety. This chasm is difficult to bridge. The need for connection is heightened and yet the ability to feel connected is greatly diminished. Patients often feel that no one can truly understand what they are going through. The patient might feel the need to protect others from their pain. Similarly, loved ones may feel unable to share completely how they feel out of a belief that their needs are not important at a time like this. This lack of mutual sharing further exacerbates the sense of isolation. This, in turn, amplifies death anxiety, because one of the ways in which we comprehend the meaning of nonbeing is aloneness. Social isolation comes to be experienced as a harbinger of death. Yalom's description of the existential conflict of isolation is 'the tension between our awareness of our absolute isolation and our wish for contact, for protection, our wish to be part of a larger whole' [1, p. 9]. For the cancer patient, being in a group with other cancer patients can be a powerful antidote to the feeling of isolation.

Cancer confronts the patient with the prospect of a foreshortened future and in so doing can raise questions about meaning. As Yalom states, 'If we must die, if we constitute our own world, if each is ultimately alone in an indifferent universe, then what meaning does life have?' [1, p. 9]. This is a bleak question and yet inevitable. The expression of this question can come in many forms. For the cancer patient it might be 'Why me? Why now?' Some might ask 'What did I do to get cancer?' Or, 'What is this teaching me about myself, about my place in the world, about what matters to me?' All these questions express the struggle to make meaning out of cancer.

Handbook of Psychotherapy in Cancer Care, First Edition. Edited by Maggie Watson and David W. Kissane.

The existential concern of freedom is about having to manage the reality of living in the absence of structure – of groundlessness. The patient is faced with the fact that we must choose how to live, that we 'create' our lives. Cancer forces the patient to redefine or reconstruct themselves and their place in the world. Cancer affects body image and sense of self and the patient must find a way to navigate these changes. Patients must choose the extent to which they will allow cancer to affect their way of being in the world. Will they choose to 'put it behind' them and carry on as though nothing has changed? Or, will they make some conscious changes in their lives?

Undoubtedly, the most profound of the existential concerns is facing the prospect of death [2]. For many, this may be the first direct confrontation with their own mortality. What had been an abstract idea, or at least an idea the person was able to hold at bay, is now 'in your face' as some patients have described it. One woman described it as having the sword of Damocles hanging over her. The terror of death is activated regardless of whether it is early stage and curable or it is late stage and the patient has only weeks or months to live.

10.2.2 Emotional Expression

Unfortunately, there is a common belief in popular psychology that it is important to have a 'positive attitude' if you have cancer, to be upbeat no matter what and avoid, suppress or even deny 'negative' emotions. Yet cancer inevitably summons the darkest of emotions – fear, anger, sadness. Many cancer patients and their families are caught in the 'prison of positive thinking', feeling that giving in to these emotions is the equivalent of yielding to the cancer itself [3]. Negative feelings about cancer are inevitable. It is natural to be afraid, angry and feel pain and sadness over what is happening and how it affects one's loved ones. The challenge often lies in whether, how and when to express those emotions. Some patients will consciously and actively struggle with whether or not to share their negative feelings. For others, the feelings will go underground.

Research suggests that verbally describing a difficult emotional experience can lead to greater life satisfaction [4]. Pennebaker's work on expressive writing has demonstrated a range of psychological and physical health benefits from writing about emotionally difficult experiences [5] and we argue that similar benefits apply to verbal communication of the emotional challenges of cancer. SEGT significantly reduces suppression of emotion and enhances emotional self-efficacy.

10.2.3 Social Support

Social support is vital to our emotional and physical wellbeing. In 1979, Berkman and Syme [6] demonstrated the link between social relationships and mortality. The risks associated with insufficient social support have been clearly shown to be equivalent to those from smoking or high serum cholesterol levels [7]. A recent systematic review examined the role of social support on disease progression and found evidence for a relationship between social support and breast cancer; although the evidence was less convincing for other types of cancers or studies with a mix of cancers [8]. The availability of social support also has a positive influence on cancer patients' subjective well being [9, 10]. Cancer patients high in perceived social support are more likely to experience post-traumatic growth [11]. A lack of social support is associated with a desire for a hastened death among patients in palliative care [12].

10.3 Goals of Supportive-Expressive Groups

There are several broad goals that we strive for in SEGT groups. These include enhancing mutual support, greater openness and emotional expression, improved social and family support, the integration of a changed sense of self and body image, more active coping skills, improving the doctor/patient relationship, detoxification of dying and death and a reordering of life priorities [13]. While the degree of importance of each of these goals for individual patients will depend on the unique needs of the patient, in general, all goals have some relevance for all group members.

10.3.1 Mutual Support

A fundamental goal is that the group becomes a place where members experience the support of one another and build strong new bonds of emotional support. Creating a safe and supportive environment is critical to the success of a group. Members should feel that the group is a place where they can bring their concerns and feelings and can count on being heard, understood and supported. Knowing that this resource is both available and reliable helps to reduce the sense of isolation that can come with the diagnosis and has a buffering effect on the stress of cancer [14]. Furthermore, they are in a position to see their own problems from the perspective of observing them in others they have come to like and respect, and to give as well as receive help. This enhances self-esteem and builds confidence in coping with cancer.

10.3.2 Greater Openness and Emotional Expression

Enhancing a patient's ability to be open about his or her experience, including openly expressing emotions, is a central goal of this treatment. Not uncommonly, patients are concerned about expressing their emotions for fear of being a burden or of showing their weakness [15]. Patients believe they should be strong and able to cope. They strive to maintain a 'positive attitude', which many think means denying concerns and only expressing optimism. This can consume a lot of energy, often to ill effect.

The aim of SEGT is to help cancer patients express all concerns and emotions, whether positive or negative. We especially encourage the expression of difficult emotions such as fear, anger and sadness. Being able to share these in a place where they do not have to worry about protecting others is a powerful benefit of a support group. Finding that the group can tolerate these emotions gives the patient the courage to be more open and expressive with loved ones, and thereby enhances intimacy.

10.3.3 Improved Social and Family Support

A terrible consequence of cancer is that it can distance the patient from family and friends at a time when they are most needed. This is not to say that family and friends do not rally; they do. The problem is that they often do not know how or what kind of support to give [16, 17]. Additionally, the patients' loved ones also suffer and are in need of support, but feel they must put their needs aside so as not to burden the patient [18, 19]. Altogether, this can create the paradoxical situation of greater disconnection at a time when connection and support is what everyone needs.

There are similar levels of psychological distress for patients and their caregivers [20, 21]. Improving support in both directions reduces distress for each [22]. Thus, we aim to improve communication, and reduce barriers created by fear and concern, so that patients make full use of their support system [23].

10.3.4 Integration of a Changed Self and Body Image

Cancer and its treatment is an assault on a patient's sense of self and body image. Side-effects such as fatigue, disfigurement, sexual dysfunction, pain, weight change, infertility and hair loss radically alter self and body image [24–27]. The patient may also find that he or she is no longer capable of engaging in familiar activities and must adjust to significant role changes. These changes can pose a major challenge to self esteem [28].

Sharing with others can help put these changes into perspective and normalise the experience. It provides an opportunity to process what has happened, make sense of it and integrate the experience into a more coherent and stable sense of self. Grieving what was lost and accepting what has changed enables the patient to create a new perspective of self and body. Observing such effects in other members helps to put these changes into perspective.

10.3.5 Improved Coping Skills

Cancer brings a vast array of new situations and problems. Patients must learn to navigate the health care system, make treatment decisions and deal with the consequences of treatment. They must deal with the impact on relationships with family, friends and co-workers. Often they feel unprepared, ill-equipped and struggle to cope.

Our goal is to help patients improve and expand their repertoire of coping skills. These include facing stress-inducing situations directly, gathering more information, altering their perspective on the problem, finding an aspect they can actively do something about, express rather than suppress emotion and enhance their social contact and support. Group members are a major resource for learning about and trying out new coping strategies. Good copers are excellent role models for others and inspire change.

10.3.6 Improved Doctor-Patient Relationship

The patient's relationship with his or her doctor is vital, but often ambivalently-held. The doctor is the bearer of bad news, the source of hope, the conduit of dreaded treatments, and holds authority, knowledge and power. However, via the Internet, patients have access to more information. Through a more consumerist approach to medicine, there is more 'doctor shopping' and demanding of specific treatments. Doctors find their job arduous. With a heavy patient load, many are emotionally taxed and must find a way to provide responsible care while being time efficient. Many physicians manage this through bypassing emotional cues from patients [29, 30], which can exacerbate distress. Altogether, these ingredients are a recipe for an unhealthy doctor-patient relationship [31].

A goal of SEGT is to help patients develop a collaborative relationship with their doctors. With greater understanding and awareness of their needs, patients can problem solve effective ways of communicating, develop a partnership and ensure shared decision-making.

10.3.7 Detoxify Death and Dying

A central goal is to help patients face their fears about death. These may include whether it will involve a long and painful physical deterioration, the idea of non-being, the process of dying, loss of autonomy or the impact their death will have on their loved ones [32].

Being consciously or unconsciously gripped by anxiety and fear about dying adversely affects a person's ability to embrace life and live it fully. By helping the patient tolerate thoughts of death and dying, we have in a sense 'detoxified' these thoughts; their potency and ability to detract from living has been diminished [33]. We hope to help patients live more fully in the present for whatever time they have left. Powerful and constructive meetings around the bedside of dying members help the group face what they most fear, provide comfort to the dying and in return receive strength and wisdom from those who are close to death, but still making choices and living their lives fully.

10.3.8 Reorder Life Priorities

One positive outcome of having cancer is that it can be the impetus for patients to reevaluate their lives and reprioritise. Reconsidering such priorities is a way to discover fresh meaning, which then diminishes distress [34, 35].

10.4 Target Groups of Patients for Whom It Is Appropriate

SEGT was originally developed for metastatic breast cancer patients [36, 37] and most research has been conducted in this setting. However, it is an appropriate treatment for all cancers because the diagnosis of cancer activates strong emotions and fears regardless of the type and stage of the disease. Fears of death and dying do not differ across stage or time since diagnosis [32]. The degree to which a patient is preoccupied by these concerns and prepared to discuss them with the group depends on personality style, availability of social support, life circumstances, and so on.

10.5 Processes and Techniques

Careful planning and preparation is recommended prior to starting an SEGT group. Each prospective member should be met with individually to assess suitability and to prepare him or her for the group. This involves getting a sense of their personal history, cancer story, current life situation including support system and any concerns they might have about participating. We recommend describing the philosophy and rationale for SEGT so that patients understand that the group is a place to share what they cannot share elsewhere and so they are also prepared to listen to others. Rules around attendance, confidentiality, arriving on time and mutual respect should be explained so as to create a safe and secure environment. Unlike most psychotherapy groups, there are no prohibitions against socialising outside of group as building patients' support system is a goal of SEGT. However, they are encouraged to be attentive to any issues that may arise through out-of-group contact and to bring them back to the group if they pose concern.

We suggest starting with 10–12 members, which allows for any attrition or absence due to illness. An optimal size for a working group is eight to nine members. The more advanced the cancer, the more members you should include to ensure an optimal number each week. Although groups are closed (that is drop-ins are not permitted), new members can be judiciously brought into the ongoing groups as attrition occurs due to illness. Be careful about the timing of bringing in new members so that a message is not conveyed that ill or deceased members are easily replaced. Sometimes having new members join in twos increases their sense of mutual support. Ongoing recruitment to replace members who die or leave is desirable for long-term groups of members with advancing disease.

A time-limited group for early stage disease is advised; we have offered 12-week groups. Some patients have considered this too brief, while others were satisfied with the length.

Groups meet weekly for 90 minutes and are unstructured. Topics of conversation are allowed to emerge naturally. The therapist's role is to guide the discussion such that the underlying existential concerns are identified, latent emotions expressed and support is provided.

There are five main therapeutic strategies. These include: (i) maintain the focus on cancer, (ii) facilitate emotional expression, (iii) encourage supportive interactions, (iv) focus on concrete, personal issues and (v) facilitate active coping.

10.5.1 Maintain the Focus on Cancer

Maintaining the focus on cancer may seem an obvious treatment strategy; however, it is not always easy. Both patients and group leaders can sometimes find themselves discussing noncancer-related issues rather than attending to the fear and anxiety that lurks beneath the surface. When patients are spending an extended period of time discussing issues that appear unrelated to cancer, we encourage the therapist to consider the following questions: How might this topic be related to living with cancer or is there something else going on in the group that the members are avoiding? Depending on the answer, the therapist can then make an intervention to refocus the discussion. In some situations, it may be wise to recommend additional outside support if a given patient's needs and concerns extend beyond what the group can offer.

10.5.2 Facilitate Emotional Expression

Facilitating emotional expression is at the core of SEGT. Cancer evokes a multitude of feelings and there are few places where patients can express them fully while feeling supported and understood. Patients are often reluctant to express their feelings out of a fear of being overwhelmed or overwhelming others. Yet no thought or feeling is too frightening or dangerous to express. When the material appears overwhelming, help patients explore it in manageable doses.

Some patients may have limited awareness of key feelings or discount their importance. There are underlying feelings with any discussion. Sometimes these are obvious; at other times, not. The therapist should be alert to any emotion and encourage its expression. One golden rule is to 'follow the affect', directing the course of the discussion along lines of pursuing and developing emotion rather than completing stories. Asking the group for their feelings in response to hearing someone speak will facilitate emotional expression. When discussions become abstract or there is a sudden shift from a difficult to an easier topic, there are often underlying feelings that need to be expressed. Facilitating emotional expression generally leads to a productive examination of existential concerns. Another golden rule is to chase any expression of ambivalence – powerful feelings usually underlie these [38].

10.5.3 Facilitate Supportive Interactions

It is essential that the group be a place where patients feel supported. Typically, this is something that naturally evolves as the group matures. However, early on in the life of any group, it may be important for the therapist to encourage supportive interactions through modelling support. This modelling is important as not all members will understand the most effective ways of providing support.

One common approach to providing support is through giving advice. Although this is meant to be supportive, it frequently misses the mark. This form of support is common early in the life of a group and it is important that therapists quickly intervene to educate the group about more effective ways of providing support. For example, a therapist might say the following: 'Janice, I can see that you are wanting to be helpful to Meredith and it's great to see your expression of caring. Meredith, I'm wondering whether this suggestion is what you need from us right now?' This intervention acknowledges Janice's good intention and also gives Meredith an opportunity to reveal what kind of support would prove most helpful. Occasionally, advice will be appropriate but, more often than not, the member simply needs to be heard and understood.

Another issue found in the early phase of a group is that support is not offered when it is needed. Such a situation is a good time for the therapist to model support. It can be helpful to ask the member 'Is there anything that you need from the group right now?' Or, 'Would it be helpful to get some feedback from the group?' Alternatively, the therapist can turn to the group members and say, 'I'm wondering what it is like to hear Diane tell us about what she is dealing with right now?' Such an invitation typically evokes a supportive response.

10.5.4 Focus on Personal, Concrete Issues

A strategy that patients often use to manage their anxiety about cancer is to speak about it in abstract and impersonal ways. This is a way of appearing to deal with an issue while not truly addressing it. When this happens, the patient should be invited to speak more personally and specifically about the issue. Consider the following example where a patient reacted to hearing that another member's cancer had recurred: 'Life is just so unfair and cancer is so rampant. There's nothing you can do about it. You can fight for the doctors to listen to you and to help you, but there's no control over the situation. If there was just something we could do to make it better for her and for the world. I get frustrated and angry that the medical community can't come up with an answer'. In order to get the member to speak more directly about what this news has stirred up in her, the therapist might ask 'Sophie, I hear your concern for Betty and that you are upset over how little control we have over this disease. How is Betty's news making you feel right now about your illness?'

Focusing on the here-and-now is an optimal way to help members speak personally and more concretely about their concerns. For instance, ask 'What is happening inside you right now? Are there feelings, thoughts or memories that are coming up?' Answering this question can open up a discussion that directly addresses their concerns.

10.5.5 Facilitate Active Coping

A coping style we encourage is one that is active and problem-focused. When confronted with a potentially lethal disease, it is not uncommon for patients to feel helpless. No matter how difficult it might seem or how helpless or powerless the person might feel, we encourage patients to find at least one thing they can do to better manage the situation. We want to help patients identify their needs so that they can devise a plan of action to meet them. No matter how small that act, the ability to take action gives patients a greater sense of power and control and contributes to a sense of hope and optimism.

A specific coping tool we teach is self-hypnosis [39]. This exercise is conducted at the end of every session with an emphasis on managing pain [40] and consolidating what has been discussed during the session. A detailed description on using this technique can be found in our book, *Group Therapy for Cancer Patients: A Research-based Handbook of Psychosocial Care* [3].

10.6 Case Example

In a longstanding metastatic breast cancer group, one of the members, Brenda, has complained about the mixed messages she has been receiving from her doctors. The members rally to support her by offering advice about how to get what she needs from her doctors. The therapist notices that Brenda seems to be suppressing a strong emotion and intervenes. This shifts the nature of the discussion and reveals the underlying concern. This segment has several teaching points including: the importance of facilitating emotional expression; examples of defensive strategies members use to manage their discomfort with existential concerns; that encouraging active coping can sometimes be premature and how uncovering and attending to

the underlying concern can open up opportunities for greater support and connection within the group.

BRENDA: I'm just uncomfortable with this situation.

MEMBER A: But this is something that's just developed, right? Why would you have said something sooner if it wasn't that way sooner? Don't blame yourself.

MEMBER B: Don't blame yourself.

MEMBER A: And don't worry about their *feelings*, they're working for *you*!

This is spoken with strong emphasis as Member A tries to change how Brenda is thinking and feeling about the situation with her doctors. Brenda responds below in a passive and defeated voice.

BRENDA: I know that. I know that.

MEMBER C: I think one problem you've had was the trainee doctor – that seems to be more of the caretaker – had an opinion about this option over here and then your doctor came in later and said, 'No, I don't want to do that, I want to do this.' Wasn't that it? That was the dilemma there? And you haven't been able to sit both of them down and figure out why are they ... why is there a conflict and if there is a conflict, how?

MEMBER A: But if your doctor came in and said, 'No, I want to do this', and you didn't at the time say, 'Oh, but the fellow said this and why are you ... ?'

BRENDA: No, you see it never happened that way.

MEMBER A: You didn't have a chance to say that to him?

BRENDA: No, and since this shift occurred, I've not had the opportunity ... He was gone on one occasion. And, the next occasion ... I just didn't have the opportunity to see him ... And Thursday we had to change ...

MEMBER A: What do you want Brenda?

Here we see that Member A is realising that Brenda is not responding to her advice and tries a different tactic. However, this member is so desirous of having Brenda take charge of the situation that she quickly reverts back to giving advice.

BRENDA: (Sighs in response to Member A's question.)

MEMBER A: Do you want them both there together so you can hash this out?

BRENDA: I almost wish that. I almost wish that. (Said again in a passive and defeated voice.)

MEMBER A: Then why don't you go in and make an appointment today and say, 'I want to make an appointment with doctor so-and-so and doctor whatever-the-fellow-is and I want to see them together...'

BRENDA: I feel like they're having a difference of opinion as far as... and that makes me uncertain.

MEMBER A: ... and what's the soonest we could get them together. Say this.

MEMBER B: Yeah, just say it.

MEMBER A: Just call and say I want to talk to both of them at the same time. And I want to do it – you know – if not today, tomorrow.

BRENDA: Tomorrow's Thursday

MEMBER A: *Do it! Do it!* ... They'll both be there tomorrow. *Do it!*

Group member A is desperate to get Brenda to engage in this active coping strategy. The sense of urgency in her voice is so strong that she seems to be thinking that she can almost will Brenda to act solely by her tone of voice. During this exchange, the therapist sees Brenda's passive rejection of advice but, more importantly, that Brenda seems full of emotion. Clearly, the focus on active coping is premature and the therapist decides to intervene. What follows is a shift in Brenda's emotional state as she expresses what is on her mind.

THERAPIST: I'm wondering if I could interject here. I'm aware of all this energy and intense desire that the group has to be helpful to you, Brenda. And at the same time, I have the sense that you're sitting on a lot of feeling. I keep seeing different emotions pass across your face. I'm wondering if you could tell us what you're feeling.

BRENDA: Well... I guess that... I know for the first time I really... I've begun to lose hope. And I thought I'd never ever do that. It's just that I've felt so rotten and so, you know, weak. And, they've run all sorts of tests and... I have a strong heart... The lungs are clear. But, it's a rotten liver and, um,... I'm been just really down today, and I just... I just... Anyway, um... My kids are coming... (tears) I'm sorry... and um, I guess I just want to make it through.

At this point the therapist wonders whether Brenda is suggesting that she might not live long enough to see her children. The therapist hopes to have Brenda say this directly and so nudges her to say more.

THERAPIST: You want to make it through?

BRENDA: You know, until they are here, until they come.

MEMBER A: When are they coming?

BRENDA: The 22nd!

Brenda's elaboration does not address her concern that she will die before her children arrive. The therapist intervenes again with a more explicit question so that this issue will be addressed directly in the group. Following this intervention, there is a dramatic shift in the group.

THERAPIST: You're afraid you might not last?

BRENDA: Yeah.

MEMBER A: Really?

MEMBER B: Is that why they're coming? There's some urgency they need to come?

BRENDA: No... no, it was planned.

MEMBER A: Why do you think you might not last, Brenda? Oh Brenda, you're so precious.

BRENDA: We've all faced this.

MEMBER B: It's so obvious she has these feelings and she doesn't have any confidence in her doctors... that's compounding...

Several people talking at once.

MEMBER A: That's happened to other people in our group. Right at the crucial moment, their doctors flake out.

The fact that Brenda fears she will die in the near future is now directly in the room. This immediately activates everyone, such that suddenly members are talking over each other. We hear expressions of surprise and concern, expressions of affection, as well as intense anxiety. A striking indication of the intensity of the anxiety is that they shift into talking about Brenda in the third person. This is an unconscious strategy to distance themselves from Brenda and the pain of acknowledging they might lose her alongside the terror of acknowledging their own mortality. The therapist recognises that there is a lot going on in the group, but decides that the priority at that moment is to support Brenda. She cuts through the animated discussion to speak directly to Brenda.

THERAPIST: How can we help you, Brenda? Right now, how can the group help you?

BRENDA: Well, you know, I almost didn't come today because I felt so bad, but I mean... I always feel better when I come in here. And I want you all to know that this last year-plus-whatever has been incredible for me. All of you have contributed an enormous amount to me. Maybe I don't say it as well or as fluently, and stuff like that...

MEMBER B: You have contributed so much to us. You do all the time.

Helping Brenda to speak about her concern that she had little time left opened the door for her to receive support, words of affection and for her to tell the group how much they meant to her. This direct discussion of death along with the guidance of the therapist allowed for open expression of caring. In this way, it contributed to detoxifying death. Addressing death directly made it less frightening and reduced Brenda's sense of being alone with her fears.

10.7 Evidence for Efficacy of SEGT

Most efficacy trials have focused on metastatic breast cancer. There is clear evidence that SEGT has psychosocial benefits. It reduces mood disturbance, depression, traumatic stress symptoms, emotional control, and maladaptive coping, and improves quality of life [41–45]. Research on the use of hypnosis in SEGT has shown that it can substantially reduce the intensity of pain and suffering, although it does not reduce the frequency of pain [46, 47]. An examination of group process in metastatic breast cancer found that the expression of negative affect was associated with a healthier cortisol response [48].

Research on the efficacy of SEGT in improving mood and adjustment of women with primary breast cancer has been less clear. Although a nonrandomised trial provided preliminary evidence that 12-weeks of SEGT was beneficial for primary breast cancer patients [49], a multicentre randomized controlled trial failed to demonstrate clear-cut psychosocial benefits [50]. A nonrandomised trial for lesbians with primary breast cancer found that a 12-week SEGT reduced emotional distress, traumatic stress symptoms and improved coping [51]. However, there was also an unexpected reduction in instrumental and informational support [51]. A large (N = 303) randomised trial of 20 sessions of Cognitive-Existential Group Therapy developed with a similar focus on existential and interpersonal issues found lower anxiety and improved family functioning [52], with stronger outcome among groups led by experienced psychotherapists.

Four separate trials examined whether SEGT improves survival among metastatic breast cancer patients. The original trial of SEGT in the late 1970s, while not originally designed to address this question, found significantly longer survival [53]. Several attempts to replicate this finding have confirmed the emotional benefits, but not the increase in survival time [41, 44, 54]. A trial by our group found no overall increase in survival, but a significant interaction with women with estrogen receptor negative tumours which was not the case among ER positive women [55]. Recently, a randomised trial of group therapy for women with primary breast cancer that addressed similar themes with a more psychoeducational approach found significantly fewer relapses and longer survival [56].

SEGT has been adapted to other treatment modalities including teleconferencing and asynchronous web-based groups. One Australian nonrandomised trial for rural women with metastatic breast cancer utilised teleconferencing for those who could not attend in person, and found improvement in mood after one year [57]. A 12-week, semi-structured, web-based support group for primary breast cancer patients was developed based on SEGT principles, and in an RCT, significant improvements in depression, traumatic stress symptoms and perceived stress occurred [58].

10.8 Service Development

10.8.1 Recruitment

Although SEGT was initially based on groups that are homogeneous to disease type and stage, we believe this model has considerable flexibility. Some settings may not have a large enough patient population to form homogeneous groups and so it may be necessary to include a mix of disease types. However, if possible, we recommend that groups be homogeneous to stage of disease such that the group is either all early stage or advanced stage. However, this does not mean that someone in an early stage group should be ejected if their cancer advances. Ejecting such a person would only reinforce everyone's worst fears, which is to be utterly alone during the dying process. Leaders should foster a sense of commonality and equality, such that each person's problems are seen as being equally important, regardless of differences in age, prognosis or cancer type.

10.8.2 Facilitation

SEGT groups can be taxing and careful consideration should be given to issues related to facilitation. If resources allow, we recommend co-facilitation of SEGT groups. These should be professional co-leaders, ideally one with group psychotherapy experience and the other with knowledge about cancer. Two therapists enable one therapist to focus attention on the overt material in the moment, while the other therapist tracks and monitors the observing members and intervenes as needed. Perhaps more importantly, the co-therapists can be a source of support for each other. Existential concerns are universal and thus helping patients face their worst fears and concerns can take its toll on the therapist. Therapists must be alert to countertransference getting in the way of effective facilitation. Ongoing supervision or the ready availability of consultation is strongly recommended.

Recommended Reading

Kissane, D.W., Grabsch, B., Clarke, D.M., *et al.* (2004) Supportive-expressive group therapy: the transformation of existential ambivalence into creative living while enhancing adherence to anti-cancer therapies. *Psycho-Oncology*, **13**, 755–768.

Kissane and his colleagues provide their clinical reflections and recommendations for leading SEGT groups based on their experience in conducting a randomised clinical trial for metastatic breast cancer patients in Melbourne, Australia. This rich and thoughtful paper covers issues pertaining to forming groups, the stages of group development, therapist issues, group themes and anti-group phenomenon.

Spiegel, D. and Classen C. (2000) *Group Therapy for Cancer Patients: A Research-based Handbook of Psychosocial Care*.

This text provides an explication of supportive-expressive group therapy. It describes the rationale for SEGT groups, guidelines on how to form and facilitate these groups, how to work with existential themes, and how to manage group problems or challenging situations that may arise.

Yalom, I.D. (1980) *Existential Psychotherapy*, Basic Books, New York.

Yalom's accessible and illuminating textbook on existential psychotherapy provides a thorough grounding in the four 'ultimate concerns' and how to work with them in psychotherapy. Although the focus is on individual therapy, it provides a basis to address existential themes regardless of treatment modality.

Yalom, I.D. and Leszcz, M. (2005) *The Theory and Practice of Group Psychotherapy*, 5th edn, *Basic Books*, New York.

Yalom's seminal text on group psychotherapy, now in its fifth edition, is a comprehensive and authoritative guide for the novice and expert group therapist alike. This is a must read for all group therapists.

References

1. Yalom, I.D. (1980) *Existential Psychotherapy*, Basic Books, New York.
2. Becker, E. (1973) *The Denial of Death*, Free Press, New York.
3. Spiegel, D. and Classen, C. (2000) *Group Therapy for Cancer Patients: A research-Based Handbook of Psychosocial Care*, Basic Books, New York.
4. Keltner, D., Locke, K.D. and Audrain, P.C. (1993) The influence of attributions on the relevance of negative feelings to personal satisfaction. *Personality and Social Psychology Bulletin*, **19**, 21–29.
5. Pennebaker, J.W. and Chung, C.K. (2007) Expressive writing, emotional upheavals, and health, in *Handbook of Health Psychology* (eds H. Friedman and R. Silver), Oxford University Press, New York, pp. 263–284.
6. Berkman, L.F. and Syme, S.L. (1979) Social networks, host resistance, and mortality: a nine-year follow-up study of Alameda County residents. *American Journal of Epidemiology*, **109** (2), 186–204.
7. House, J.S., Landis, K.R. and Umberson, D. (1988) Social relationships and health. *Science*, **241** (4865), 540–545.
8. Nausheen, B., Gidron, Y., Peveler, R. and Moss-Morris, R. (2009) Social support and cancer progression: a systematic review. *Journal of Psychosomatic Research*, **67**, 403–415.
9. Hipkins, J., Whitworth, M., Tarrier, N. and Jayson, G. (2004) Social support, anxiety, and depression after chemotherapy for ovarian cancer: a prospective study. *British Journal of Health Psychology*, **9**, 569–581.
10. Pinquart, M. and Frohlich, C. (2009) Psychosocial resources and subjective well-being of cancer patients. *Psychology and Health*, **24**, 407–421.
11. Bozo, O., Gundogdu, E. and Buyukasik-Colak, C. (2009) The moderating role of different sources of perceived social support on the dispositional optimism – posttraumatic growth relationship in postoperative breast cancer patients. *Journal of Health Psychology*, **14**, 1009–1020.
12. Rodin, G., Zimmermann, C., Rydall, A. *et al.* (2007) The desire for hastened death in patients with metastatic cancer. *Journal of Pain and Symptom Management*, **33**, 661–675.
13. Classen, C., Diamond, S., Soleman, A. *et al.* (1993) *Brief Supportive-Expressive Group Therapy for Women with Primary Breast Cancer: A Treatment Manual*, Stanford University School of Medicine, Stanford, CA.
14. Cohen, S. and Wills, T.A. (1985) Stress, social support, and the buffering hypothesis. *Psychological Bulletin*, **98** (2), 310–357.
15. Servaes, P., Vingerhoets, A.J.J.M., Vreugdenhil, G. *et al.* (1999) Inhibition of emotional expression in breast cancer patients. *Behavioral Medicine*, **25**, 23–27.
16. Pistrang, N. and Barker, C. (1992) Disclosure of concerns in breast cancer. *Psycho-Oncology*, **1**, 183–192.
17. Lepore, S.J., Glaser, D.B. and Roberts, K.J. (2008) On the positive relation between received social support and negative affect: a test of the triage and self-esteem threat models in women with breast cancer. *Psycho-Oncology*, **17**, 1210–1215.
18. Kuijer, R., Ybema, J., Buunk, B.P. and DeJong, M. (2000) Active engagement, protective buffering, and overprotection. *Journal of Social and Clinical Psychology*, **19**, 256–275.
19. Manne, S., Dougherty, J., Veach, S. and Kless, R. (1999) Hiding worries from one's spouse: protective buffering among cancer patients and their spouses. *Cancer Research Therapy and Control*, **8**, 175–118.
20. Hodges, L.J., Humphris, G.M. and Macfarlane, G. (2005) A meta-analytic investigation of the relationship between the psychological distress of cancer patients and their carers. *Social Science and Medicine*, **60**, 1–12.

21. Youngmee, K., Wellisch, D.K. and Spillers, R.L. (2008) Effects of psychological distress on quality of life of adult daughters and their mothers with cancer. *Psycho-Oncology*, **17**, 1129–1136.

22. Manne, S., Ostroff, J., Fox, K. *et al.* (2009) Cognitive and social processes predicting partner psychological adaption to early stage breast cancer. *British Journal of Health Psychology*, **14**, 49–68.

23. Spiegel, D., Bloom, J. and Gottheil, E. (1983) Family environment of patients with metastatic carcinoma. *Journal of Psychosocial Oncology*, **1**, 33–44.

24. Helms, R.L., O'Hea, E.L. and Corso, M. (2008) Body image issues in women with breast cancer. *Psychology, Health and Medicine*, **13**, 313–325.

25. Fobair, P., Stewart, S.L., Chang, S. *et al.* (2006) Body image and sexual problems in young women with breast cancer. *Psycho-Oncology*, **15**, 579–594.

26. Lemieux, J., Maunsell, E. and Provencher, L. (2008) Chemotherapy-induced alopecia and effects on quality of life among women with breast cancer: a literature review. *Psycho-Oncology*, **17**, 317–328.

27. Bukovic, D., Silovski, H., Silovski, T. *et al.* (2008) Sexual functioning and body image of patients treated for ovarian cancer. *Sexuality and Disability*, **26**, 63–73.

28. Carpenter, J.S. and Brockopp, D.Y. (1994) Evaluation of self-esteem of women with cancer receiving chemotherapy. *Oncology Nursing Forum*, **21**, 751–757.

29. Detmar, S.B., Aaronson, N.K., Wever, L.D. *et al.* (2000) How are you feeling? Who wants to know? Patients' and oncologists' preferences for discussing health-related quality-of-life issues. *Journal of Clinical Oncology*, **18**, 3295–3301.

30. Eide, H., Quera, V., Graugaard, P. and Finset, A. (2004) Physician-patient dialogue surrounding patients' expression of concern: applying sequence analysis to RIAS. *Social Science and Medicine*, **59**, 145–155.

31. Stacey, C.L., Henderson, S., MacArthur, K.F. and Dohan, D. (2009) Demanding patient or demanding encounter?: A case study of a cancer clinic. *Social Science and Medicine*, **69**, 729–737.

32. Mehnert, A., Berg, P., Henrich, G. and Herschbach, P. (2009) Fear of cancer progression and cancer-related intrusive cognitions in breast cancer survivors. *Psycho-Oncology*, **18**, 1272–1280.

33. Spiegel, D. and Glafkides, M.C. (1983) Effects of group confrontation with death and dying. *International Journal of Group Psychotherapy*, **33** (4), 433–447.

34. Jim, H.S. and Andersen, B.L. (2007) Meaning in life mediates the relationship between social and physical functioning and distress in cancer survivors. *British Journal of Health Psychology*, **12**, 363–381.

35. Kernan, W.D. and Lepore, S.J. (2009) Searching for and making meaning after breast cancer: prevalence, patterns and negative affect. *Social Science and Medicine*, **68**, 1176–1182.

36. Yalom, I.D. and Greaves, C. (1977) Group therapy with the terminally ill. *American Journal of Psychiatry*, **134** (4), 396–400.

37. Spiegel, D. and Yalom, I. (1978) A support group for dying patients. *International Journal of Group Psychotherapy*, **28**, 233–245.

38. Kissane, D.W., Grabsch, B., Clarke, D.M. *et al.* (2004) Supportive-expressive group therapy: the transformation of existential ambivalence into creative living while enhancing adherence to anti-cancer therapies. *Psycho-Oncology*, **13** (11), 755–768.

39. Spiegel, H. and Spiegel, D. (1978) *Trance and Treatment: Clinical Uses of Hypnosis*, American Psychiatric Press, Washington, DC.

40. Spiegel, D. (1985) The use of hypnosis in controlling cancer pain. *CA Cancer Journal for Clinicians*, **35** (4), 221–231.

41. Classen, C., Butler, L.D., Koopman, C. *et al.* (2001) Supportive-expressive group therapy and distress in patients with metastatic breast cancer: a randomized clinical intervention trial. *Archives of General Psychiatry*, **58** (5), 494–501.

42. Spiegel, D., Bloom, J.R. and Yalom, I. (1981) Group support for patients with metastatic cancer. A randomized outcome study. *Archives of General Psychiatry*, **38** (5), 527–533.

43. Goodwin, P.J., Leszcz, M., Ennis, M. *et al.* (2001) The effect of group psychosocial support on survival in metastatic breast cancer. *New England Journal of Medicine*, **345** (24), 1719–1726.

44. Kissane, D.W., Grabsch, B., Clarke, D.M. *et al.* (2007) Supportive-expressive group therapy for women with metastatic breast cancer: survival and psychosocial outcome from a randomized trial. *Psycho-Oncology* **16**, 277–286.

45. Giese-Davis, J., Koopman, C., Butler, L. *et al.* (2002) Change in emotion-regulation strategy for women with metastatic breast cancer following supportive-expressive group therapy. *Journal of Consulting and Clinical Psychology*, **70** (4), 916–925.

46. Butler, L.D., Koopman, C., Neri, E. *et al.* (2009) Effects of supportive-expressive group therapy on pain in women with metastatic breast cancer. *Health Psychology*, **28**, 579–587.

47. Spiegel, D. and Bloom, J.R. (1983) Pain in metastatic breast cancer. *Cancer*, **52** (2), 341–345.

48. Giese-Davis, J., DiMiceli, S., Sephton, S. and Spiegel, D. (2006) Emotional expression and diurnal cortisol slope in women with metastatic breast cancer in supportive-expressive group therapy: a preliminary study. *Biological Psychology*, **73**, 190–198.

49. Spiegel, D., Morrow, G.R., Classen, C. *et al.* (1999) Group psychotherapy for recently diagnosed breast cancer patients: a multicenter feasibility study. *Psycho-Oncology*, **8** (6), 482–493.

50. Classen, C.C., Kraemer, H.C., Blasey, C. *et al.* (2008) Supportive-expressive group therapy for primary breast cancer patients: a randomized prospective multicenter trial. *Psycho-Oncology*, **17**, 238–447.

51. Fobair, P., Koopman, C., DiMiceli, S. *et al.* (2002) Psychosocial intervention for lesbians with primary breast cancer. *Psycho-Oncology*, **11** (5), 427–438.

52. Kissane, D.W., Bloch, S., Smith, G.C. *et al.* (2003) Cognitive-existential group psychotherapy for women with primary breast cancer: a randomised controlled trial. *Psycho-Oncology*, **12** (6), 532–546.

53. Spiegel, D., Bloom, J.R., Kraemer, H.C. and Gottheil, E. (1989) Effect of psychosocial treatment on survival of patients with metastatic breast cancer. *Lancet*, **2** (8668), 888–891.

54. Goodwin, P.J., Leszcz, M., Ennis, M. *et al.* (2001) The effect of group psychosocial support on survival in metastatic breast cancer. *New England Journal of Medicine*, **345** (24), 1719–1726.

55. Spiegel, D., Butler, L.D., Giese-Davis, J. *et al.* (2007) Effects of supportive-expressive group therapy on survival of patients with metastatic breast cancer: a randomized prospective trial. *Cancer*, **110**, 1130–1138.

56. Andersen, B.L., Yang, H.C., Farrar, W.B. *et al.* (2008) Psychologic intervention improves survival for breast cancer patients: a randomized clinical trial. *Cancer*, **113** (12), 3450–3458.

57. O'Brien, M., Harris, J., King, R. and O'Brien, T. (2008) Supportive-expressive group therapy for women with metastatic breast cancer: improving access for Australian women through use of teleconference. *Counselling and Psychotherapy Research*, **8**, 28–35.

58. Winzelberg, A.J., Classen, C., Koopman, C. *et al.* (2003) An evaluation of an internet support group for women with primary breast cancer. *Cancer*, **97** (5), 1164–1173.

11 A Short Term, Structured, Psychoeducational Intervention for Newly Diagnosed Cancer Patients

Fawzy I. Fawzy[1] and Nancy W. Fawzy[2]

[1]Department of Psychiatry and Biobehavioral Sciences, David Geffen School of Medicine at the University of California, Los Angeles
[2]School of Nursing at the University of California, Los Angeles

11.1 Introduction

As survival rates have improved with advances in medical care, the importance of psychosocial interventions designed to assist cancer patients in dealing with diagnosis and treatment has increased. Much research has been done that helps us to understand the psychological distress that patients with cancer and their families experience [1–3]. Several reviews and investigations associate cancer with high rates of emotional distress. One such review [4] demonstrated a high prevalence of major depression and an even higher occurrence of dysthymia and adjustment disorder with depressed mood in cancer patients. A meta-analysis of 58 studies involving the psychological sequelae of cancer diagnosis [5], found that rates of depression were significantly higher in patients with cancer as compared to a non-medical population. Zabora et al. [6] found that 35% of patients with cancer experienced a high level of distress that increased during the terminal phase of the illness. Similarly, Grassi et al. [7] revealed that 31% of patients with various primary cancer sites exhibited significant depressive symptoms. As high levels of emotional distress in medical patients are known to adversely affect survival, quality of life, compliance with treatment, duration of hospital stay and ability to care for oneself, the need for intervention is great and immediate [8].

Several critical reviews revealed the availability of a wide range of psychosocial intervention options for patients with cancer [9–14]. Over the years, the outcomes of psychosocial interventions have yielded improvements in both psychological and biomedical functioning (Table 11.1). Holland, in 1982, stated that the goals of these interventions ought to focus on decreasing feelings of alienation and isolation by talking with others in a similar situation, reducing anxiety and helplessness about treatments and assisting in clarifying misperceptions and misinformation. The added benefit of such interventions is that they encourage more responsibility to get well and compliance with medical regimens [15].

11.2 Theoretical Background and Themes of Our Psychoeducational Model

The four most common forms of psychosocial interventions for medically ill patients are education, behavioural training, coping skills training and supportive therapy. Examples of each of these intervention categories are reviewed here.

11.2.1 Education

Jacobs et al. [25] employed a purely educational intervention in a randomised study of patients with Hodgkin's disease. Three months later, the intervention group had increased their knowledge levels compared with the control patients. The intervention

Table 11.1	A sampling of early psychoeducational and behavioural intervention outcomes		
Outcomes	**Type of intervention**	**Results**	**References**
Psychological	Education and supportive therapy	Increased effectiveness in dealing with psychosocial problems	Gordon *et al.* [16]
	Education	Decreased depression	Pruitt *et al.* [17]
	Behaviour training	Decreased anxiety	Gruber *et al.* [18]
	Cognitive behaviour or supportive therapy	Decreased fear of progression, anxiety and depression	Herschbach *et al.* [19]
Physical	Behaviour training	Decreased anticipatory nausea	Arakawa [20]
	Education	Decreased pain intensity	de Wit *et al.* [21]
	Behavioural training and coping skills training	Decreased pain intensity, fatigue and sleep disturbance	Kwekkeboom *et al.* [22]
Combined	Supportive therapy	Decreased emotional distress and pain	Spiegel *et al.* [23]
	Education, behavioural training, coping skills training and supportive therapy	Decreased emotional distress Enhanced coping Increased immune parameters	Fawzy *et al.* [24] [66]

group also showed decreased anxiety and treatment problems as well as a trend for decreased depression and life disruption.

Gordon *et al.* [16] examined the effects of a programme of education combined with counselling on 157 patients with different types of cancer. Evaluations conducted three and six months after hospital discharge revealed that there was a decrease in depression, hostility and anxiety, as well as a greater return to activities of daily living and activities outside the home than with 151 patients in two control groups. Education alone failed to show the same benefits.

Pruitt *et al.* [17] randomised radiation therapy patients with mixed diagnoses to either a three-session intervention or a standard control group. The education consisted of information about radiation therapy and cancer, coping strategies and communication skills. Knowledge levels were unchanged in both groups, and depression was the only measure of affective state found to improve.

Ali and Khalil [26] assessed the effects of a psychoeducational intervention programme on reducing anxiety among a group of patients with bladder cancer. The experimental group showed significantly less anxiety at both three days post operation and just before hospital discharge compared to the control group.

Richardson *et al.* [27] randomly assigned newly diagnosed haematology patients to either a control group or one of three educational intervention groups. Using regression analysis, it was concluded that low severity of disease, assignment to an educational programme (anyone), plus high allopurinol compliance were predictive of increased survival in patients with newly diagnosed haematological malignancy.

Patient education not only offers diagnosis and treatment specific information to patients who may have misconceptions, no conceptions at all, and who may be hesitant to ask for such information, but may also enhance coping skills [28]. The literature shows that education alone may be helpful, but it appears that it is more useful as a component of a more comprehensive intervention [29].

11.2.2 Behavioural Training

Behavioural training utilises a variety of techniques including hypnosis, guided imagery or visualisation, relaxation training and biofeedback. Relaxation training and hypnosis have been described as effective in reducing nausea, emotional distress and physiological arousal following chemotherapy [30, 31].

Bridge *et al.* [32] conducted a randomised study to determine whether relaxation and imagery training could decrease the level of distress in Stage I and II breast cancer patients. The six-week intervention was divided into three groups: (i) a control group in which patients were encouraged to talk about themselves, (ii) a muscle relaxation group and (iii) a relaxation and guided imagery group. The second and third groups were given cassette tapes repeating the intervention instructions and told to practice once a day. At the end of the six weeks, there was significantly lower total mood disturbance in the intervention groups (with the relaxation and imagery group reporting less disturbance than the relaxation-only group) than in the control group.

Decker *et al.* [33] studied the impact of stress reduction by relaxation training and imagery in 63 radiation therapy patients. Significant reductions were noted in tension, depression, anger and fatigue. Results suggest that relaxation training substantially improves several psychological parameters associated with quality of life in patients undergoing radiation therapy for cancer.

Gruber et al. [18] randomly assigned breast cancer patients to either an immediate treatment group, which received relaxation, guided imagery and biofeedback training, or a delayed treatment control group. Results showed that anxiety levels reduced shortly after each group began the intervention.

Baider et al. [34] studied the effects of progressive muscle relaxation and guided imagery training on cancer patients. Notable improvements were found on the Brief Symptom Inventory and the Impact of Events Scale for all patients who completed the behavioural intervention. This improvement was maintained up to the six-month follow-up period. This supports the findings of other investigators who showed that psychological improvement was maintained long after the interventions were completed. In summary, all of these early behavioural studies improved psychosocial well-being.

11.2.3 Coping Skills Training

Coping skills training often consists of stress management, including problem solving and coping strategies and techniques. An important aim of the coping skills training is to increase the patient's awareness of what Weisman [1] termed the 'key ingredients of good coping': (i) optimism (the expectation of positive change), (ii) practicality (learning that options and alternatives are seldom completely exhausted), (iii) flexibility (changing strategies to reflect the changing nature of perceived problems) and (iv) resourcefulness (developing the ability to call on additional information and support to strengthen coping). Weisman et al. [35] developed Project Omega, which taught positive coping strategies as a way of diminishing stress and enhancing coping. It included learning an approach to problem solving, practicing the approach theoretically and applying the approach to personal problems via a series of pictures. They found highly distressed patients used fewer coping strategies, employed less effective ones, had more problems and concerns and achieved poor resolutions when attempting to solve critical illness-related concerns. The authors compared two interventions, one involving clarification, emotional expression and individual problem identification with the second, a cognitive skills training intervention. Both interventions were effective in reducing emotional distress during a six month follow-up period when compared to controls [36].

Berglund et al. [37] established a prospective randomised study with cancer patients who took part in a seven week rehabilitation programme. The intervention focused on 'starting again' and consisted of physical training, coping skills and information. Subjects in the experimental condition improved significantly in physical training, physical strength, fighting spirit, body image, sufficient information and decreased sleeping problems when compared to control patients. All three goals of the intervention were met and results indicated that the 'starting again' programme has many beneficial effects for cancer patients.

Hosaka [38] reported on an intervention that included psychoeducation, problem solving, psychological support, relaxation training and guided imagery. In comparing pre- and post-intervention scores, there was a decrease in all categories of negative emotions.

Cocker et al. [39] studied the effects of cognitive behaviour therapy that consisted of cognitive restructuring, relaxation, assertion training and self instructional coping methods. At the end of the three month intervention, depression scores improved.

Hershbach et al. [19] found a significant decrease in fear of progression as well as anxiety and depression over a one year period for 174 cancer patients randomly assigned to a four session cognitive-behavioural therapy or a supportive-experiential therapy versus 91 controls that showed only short term improvements.

These and other studies have elucidated the positive effects of coping skills training on the emotional states of cancer patients [40–42].

11.2.4 Supportive Therapy

11.2.4.1 Group Therapy

The stresses of having a disease such as cancer and the mode of its treatment create the need for emotional support. Support groups are frequently employed in psychosocial interventions. There is some evidence to suggest that social support groups are associated with better psychosocial adjustment to illness [16, 23, 24, 43–49].

Spiegel et al. [46] reported improved mood, increased coping and less fear in female patients with metastatic breast cancer who participated in group therapy once a week for a year when compared to randomly selected controls. The weekly discussion sections focused on practical coping problems associated with terminal illness, feelings and attitudes towards death, and interpersonal relationships with family, friends and physicians. Patients were assessed at four-month intervals for a one year period.

Cella *et al.* [50] detailed an eight-week support group for cancer patients in a local community. There was no random selection or a control group in this study. As expected, self-reported quality of life improved significantly by the final session, compared to reports completed at the start of the intervention. Community and peer support was noted by participants as the most helpful aspect of the programme and the group evaluations showed high satisfaction levels in all areas.

Cunningham *et al.* [51] compared two different formats of a brief, group psychoeducational programme for cancer patients. Patients were randomly assigned to either a standard (six weekly 2-hour sessions) intervention or a 'weekend-intensive' intervention group. At 19 weeks following the intervention, the two formats were found to have comparable effects on mood and quality of life. Quality-of-life improvement appeared to be somewhat greater for the standard six week intervention group.

11.2.5 Individual Therapy

There is some evidence for the value of one-on-one supportive counselling for patients with cancer. Linn *et al.* [52] randomly assigned 120 men with end-stage cancer to a supportive intervention or to a control condition. Patients receiving counselling showed significantly better quality-of-life scores at three months. Among those who survived, these differences held up through the one year follow-up.

A prospective randomised study by Greer *et al.* [53] found that adjuvant psychological therapy improved psychological distress among 174 cancer patients. The authors looked at anxiety, depression and adjustment in patients with primary diagnosis or first recurrence of cancer. Compared to the control patients, the experimental patients scored significantly higher in fighting spirit and significantly lower in anxiety, anxious preoccupation, helplessness and fatalism. Some of the effects were still observable at four month follow-up.

Moorey *et al.* [54] completed a one year follow-up of patients with cancer who had received individual adjuvant psychological therapy (i.e. a brief cognitive-behavioural treatment). The experimental patients exhibited less anxiety and depression than controls at one year following treatment.

Fawzy [55] investigated the efficacy of a psychoeducational nursing intervention to enhance coping and affective state in newly diagnosed malignant melanoma patients. At three month follow-up, patients in the intervention group demonstrated less

psychological distress and decreases in Brief Symptom Index somatisation and were using less ineffective 'passive resignation' coping strategies than the control group.

11.3 Target Groups of Patients and Evidence of Efficacy of the Structured Psychoeducational Group Intervention

11.3.1 Phase of Illness

The psychosocial struggles of cancer patients can be divided into four phases: diagnostic phase, initial treatment phase, recurrence phase and terminal phase [56, 57]. Within each phase lie normal/adaptive behavioural responses and abnormal/maladaptive behavioural responses. This intervention is appropriate for people who have been definitively diagnosed with cancer and who are in the treatment or initial recurrence phases. It is not appropriate for patients in the terminal phase of their cancer. Emotion-supportive therapies are more appropriate for this population [46, 58].

11.3.2 Efficacy

This intervention model was used for a group of newly diagnosed malignant melanoma patients who had undergone standard surgical treatment of their tumours (consisting of wide excision of the primary site and regional lymphadenectomy when indicated) [24]. Patients were assigned to either a control group receiving routine medical care or to an experimental group receiving the same kind of routine medical care plus the structured intervention model described.

11.3.2.1 Affective State

All the patients reported moderate to high levels of psychological distress at baseline comparable to other cancer patients. However, at the end of the six week structured group intervention, the experimental subjects ($N = 38$) exhibited significantly lower levels of distress than the control subjects ($N = 28$) (Figure 11.1) [24]. Six months following the intervention, the group differences were even more pronounced. The experimental group reported significantly lower levels of confusion, depression, fatigue and total mood disturbance, and higher levels of vigour on the Profile of Mood States (POMS) (Figure 11.2) [24]. Participation in the group intervention appeared to reduce the psychological turmoil associated with cancer diagnosis. At the one year

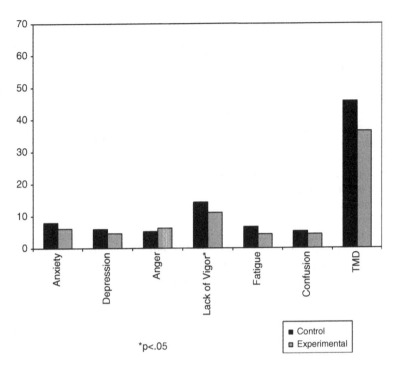

Figure 11.1 *Mean POMS scores at week six post structured psychoeducational and coping intervention for patients with early stage melanoma. TMD = Total Mood Disturbance.*

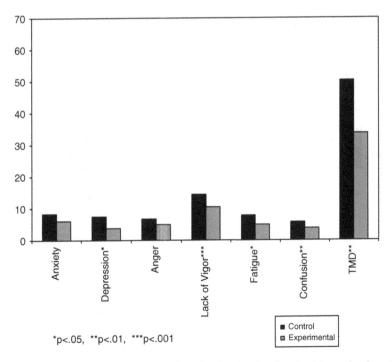

Figure 11.2 *Mean POMS scores at six months after structured psychoeducational and coping intervention for patients with early stage melanoma. TMD = Total Mood Disturbance.*

follow-up, the experimental group continued to show significantly lower confusion and higher vigour [59].

11.3.2.2 Coping Methods

Immediately following the six-week structured intervention, the experimental subjects showed significantly greater use of active-behavioural coping methods than the control subjects. In addition, the experimental subjects used significantly more active-positive, active-expressive, active-reliance, cognitive-positive and distraction coping strategies (Figure 11.3). Six months following the intervention, the experimental patients continued to use significantly more active-behavioural coping methods, as well as more active-cognitive coping methods than the controls (Figure 11.4) [24]. At the one year follow-up, active-behavioural and avoidance coping methods (specifically distraction) were significantly higher in the experimental patients compared to controls [59].

11.3.2.3 Affective State and Quality of Life

In both experimental and control subjects combined, quality of life was strongly negatively correlated with anxiety ($p = 0.0001$), depression ($p = 0.0001$), anger ($p = 0.007$), confusion ($p = 0.0001$) and total mood disturbance ($p = 0.0001$) at six months follow-up. As negative affective state decreased (through lower levels of anxiety, depression, anger, confusion and total mood disturbance), the quality of life of these patients increased [59].

11.3.3 Type of Cancer

This intervention model has been tested empirically and reported on in melanoma patients [24, 44, 55, 59, 60] and in Japanese women with breast cancer [38]. In addition, the authors have had 10 years of successful clinical experience using this model with melanoma, breast and prostate cancer patients.

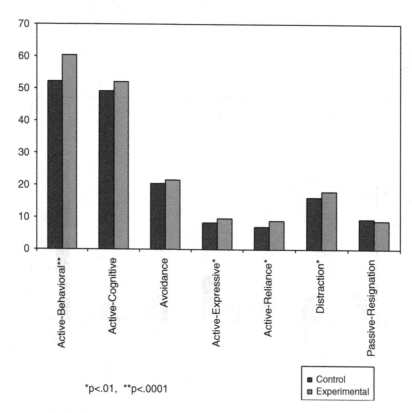

Figure 11.3 *Mean coping method and strategy scores at week six post structured psychoeducational and coping intervention for patients with early stage melanoma.*

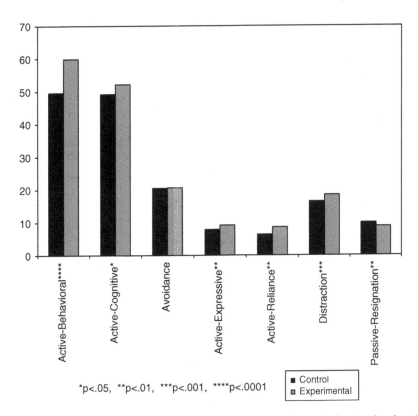

Figure 11.4 *Mean coping method and strategy scores at six months after a structured psychoeducational and coping intervention for patients with early stage melanoma.*

These studies strongly suggest that a short-term structured psychoeducational intervention may be effective for patients who are going through initial treatment and/or re-treatment in several types of cancer.

11.4 Process, Techniques and Case Example

11.4.1 Structured Psychiatric Intervention Model

Previous research on singular modes of therapies established their effectiveness but the variance accounted for by each of these modes alone was small. Therefore, based on a review of the literature and our clinical experience, we selected the specific portions of those interventions that were found to be effective and appropriate and combined them (Table 11.2). This combined intervention was first

used in a group of 50 gay men with acquired immune deficiency syndrome (AIDS) [61, 62].

The intervention model was then used for a group of newly diagnosed malignant melanoma patients, who had undergone standard surgical treatment of their tumours (consisting of wide excision of the primary site and regional lymphadenectomy when indicated) [24]. The short- and long-term effects of the intervention on psychological states were measured. Patients were assigned to either a control group receiving routine medical care or an experimental group receiving the same kind of routine medical care plus the psychoeducational group intervention below. The six week structured group intervention encompasses health education, behavioural training, coping skills and supportive therapy. Groups of 7 to 10 patients met for one and one half hours weekly for six weeks. The group meetings, which were primarily led by a qualified health care provider, were structured yet supportive.

Table 11.2   Combination of therapies effective in psychosocial interventions for cancer patients

Education	Behavioural techniques	Coping skills training	Supportive therapy
Diagnosis	*PMR*	*Stress management*	*Individual therapy*
Biopsies	Guided imagery	1. Awareness	Patient specific
Scans, X-rays	Visualisation	(a) Stress sources	*Group therapy*
Blood tests	Meditation	(b) Stress reactions	Disease specific
Symptoms	Biofeedback	2. Management Strategies	Emotional
Treatment options	Hypnosis	(a) Eliminate stress source via problem solving	support via
Side-effects	Yoga	(b) Modify stress source via problem solving	expression and peer
Dealing with effects	Tai chi, Chi gong	(c) Cognitive restructuring	validation
		(d) Change physical reaction via behavioural techniques	
Disease		*Coping*	
Prevention		1. Active behavioural coping (promote use)	
S&S of recurrence		Problem solving	
S&S of progression		Seek advice and support	
Course of disease		Partnership with doctors	
New options		Attend support groups	
Symptom manage-		Improve diet	
ment		Exercise	
Nutrition		2. Active cognitive coping (promote use)	
		Challenge	
Health enhancing		Positive opportunity	
Health inhibiting		Upward comparison	
		Sense of meaning	
		Reappraisal	
		Detoxify death	
		Grief/mourning	
		3. Avoidance coping (dissuade use)	
		Alcohol use	
		Smoking	
		Drug use	
Outcomes			
Increased knowledge	Improved physical	Decreased stress	Enhanced social support
Better compliance	symptoms	Improved coping and adjustment	

S&S, signs and symptoms; PMR, progressive muscle relaxation.

11.4.2 Health Education

The original research was done with malignant melanoma patients and the health education component of the intervention was composed of easily understood health care information specific to the diagnosis of skin cancer. They were taught about their disease, including information on risk factors that appear to be influencing the dramatic increase in skin cancer. These factors include ultraviolet radiation, skin pigmentation, genetic factors, hormonal factors and immunological factors. These risk factors are further delineated in the intervention manual. In addition to educational information, patients learn about preventive measures to avoid future sun exposure by reducing ultraviolet radiation exposure, by wearing protective clothing and by using sunscreens.

Finally, warning signs and the terms and definitions of malignant melanoma are presented. In addition, relevant booklets and informational pamphlets from the American Cancer Society and the National Cancer Institute were provided.

Subsequently, the intervention was adapted for breast cancer patients [29]. Breast cancer patients are taught about the different kinds of breast cancer (e.g. ductal carcinoma in situ (DCIS) vs. infiltrating carcinomas), the different treatment modalities (e.g. lumpectomy, mastectomy, radiation, chemotherapy and hormonal), good follow-up routines (e.g. monthly breast self-exam, annual mammograms and annual physician exams). In addition, relevant booklets and informational pamphlets from the American Cancer Society and the National Cancer Institute were provided.

11.4.3 Coping Skills Training

11.4.3.1 Behavioural Techniques and Stress Management

Stress management is divided into two main sections. Section 1 is *Awareness* which has two categories: (a) identifying the sources of stress and (b) identifying personal reactions to stress, including physiological, psychological and behavioural reactions. Section 2 involves *Management Techniques* and has four categories (a–d). The first two are: (a) totally eliminating the source of stress and (b) modifying the source of stress through the five steps of problem solving:

1. **Relaxation**. Patients are encouraged to use the relaxation techniques and collect their thoughts before launching into problem solving. This helps to bring the emotional arousal down to a level that is better for optimal performance.

2. **Identification of the problem**. Identifying the real problem may not always be clear. Patients are taught to separate out the presenting problem from the underlying problem. For example, a patient may state that he hates his job. The real problem may be related to numerous things associated with the job, including the boss, the co-workers, the type of job or even the commute necessary to get to the job. Patients learn to identify the issues that affect them and to distinguish content (the matter requiring action) from process (feelings about the problem).

3. **Brainstorming**. This step involves having patients list all possible solutions, however practical or ridiculous. This process may help to reduce tension by generating possible steps for action. After the list is complete, patients are instructed to consider the positive and negative implications of each possible solution.

4. **Selection and implementation of an appropriate strategy**. With the list developed from the brainstorming step, patients select and implement the solution that appears to be the most feasible and the most likely to succeed.

5. **Evaluation**. Patients are then encouraged to determine whether it is effective or not. If it is not effective, patients are taught to return to step 1 and proceed through the process once more.

The third category of stress management is (c) changing the attitude or perception towards the stressor by trying to look at the situation in a 'new light'. This is often referred to as cognitive restructuring. The fourth category involves (d) changing the physical reaction to the stressor through behavioural techniques. Patients are taught simple relaxation exercises (e.g. progressive muscle relaxation followed by guided imagery of a pleasant scene) that take approximately 15–20 minutes to perform. Patients are encouraged to use these techniques on a daily basis (to help them relax, to learn what a state of relaxation feels like and to learn how to achieve it) and to help them fall asleep at night or to return to sleep if they should wake up during the night. In addition, patients are taught how to use an abbreviated form of this exercise when they find themselves in an acutely stressful situation. Stress monitor questionnaires covering signs and symptoms of stress as well as sources of stress are included in the intervention manual, as are worksheets for the patients to increase awareness about their stress.

11.4.3.2 Coping Mechanisms

Patients are then introduced to the concept of coping methods and strategies. Three general theoretical methods of coping have been identified; the first two are helpful; the third is usually detrimental:

1. **Active-behavioural methods**. One tries to improve some aspect of the illness by active means such as exercise, use of relaxation techniques and frequent collaborative consultations with the physician.

2. **Active-cognitive methods**. One tries to understand the illness and accept its effect on life by focusing on positive rather than negative changes that have occurred since the onset of illness. In general, patients who use active-behavioural and active-cognitive coping methods report more positive affective states, higher levels of self-esteem and fewer physical symptoms.

3. **Avoidance methods**. One avoids being with others, hides feelings about the illness and refuses to think about the illness. Those patients who use more avoidance coping usually have higher levels of psychological distress such as anxiety, indirectly expressed anger, depression and lower quality of life.

Cognitive and behavioural responses (which have the best association with improved psychological health) may be even more specifically defined as the following strategies [61]:

1. **Active-positive strategies**, which involve increasing patients' involvement in their own care, planning action and enjoying life 'one day at a time'.

2. **Active-expressive strategies**, which include talking with others to gain information or to offer support to others with cancer.

3. **Active-reliance strategies**, which involve seeking a friend or relative for instrumental or emotional help or a physician for intervention.

4. **Cognitive-positive strategies**, which include seeking understanding of the illness, finding some meaning attached to having the illness and thinking about positive changes.

5. **Distraction strategies**, which consist of going out more socially or doing something nice for one's self.

The cognitive and behavioural strategies that generally do not result in making people feel better come under the avoidance category and include:

1. **Cognitive-passive strategies**, which involve ruminating, or daydreaming about better times and doing nothing in the hope that this would make a difference.

2. **Avoidance-solitary strategies**, which include avoiding others, taking drugs and eating, smoking or sleeping more than usual.

3. **Passive-resignation strategies**, which involve preparing for 'the worst', keeping feelings secret from others and letting the physician take all responsibility for decisions and care.

Patients are given a more complete list of strategies that people use to cope with stress. Some are identified as being more effective than others for people who are coping with serious illnesses. The patients are told that, in general, a specific strategy is not good or bad but that its effectiveness is determined by the situation. They are also told that the strategies identified as less or not effective can occasionally be used and be effective (e.g. yelling to ventilate emotions) but, if used to the exclusion of all else, can cause more problems than they solve.

11.4.3.3 Integration
The final part of the coping skills component involves integrating the stress management and problem-solving techniques with the information on coping

Table 11.3	Coping scenarios

1. Pre-diagnosis
   Worries and concerns about the possible implications of the condition
2. Diagnosis
   Accepting the diagnosis
   Informing family and friends
3. Doctor–patient relationship
   Developing a collaborative partnership
   Opening up clear lines of communication
4. Treatment issues
   Feelings of fear and isolation
   Dealing with the overwhelming technological environment
5. Body image
   Surgical scars
   Loss of body parts
   Hair and weight loss
   Sexuality
6. Depression
   Coping with varying degrees of depression
7. Interpersonal relationship issues with significant other(s)
   Communicating feelings and perceptions with significant others
8. Communication issues with friends and co-workers
   Communicating with one's extended social network
9. Returning to 'normal'
   Re-entering everyday life
   Participating in previously enjoyed activities
10. Planning for the future
   Resuming 'forward-life trajectory'

methods and strategies and applying these to specific situations.

A set of pictures illustrating 10 common problems/situations encountered by cancer patients was developed (Table 11.3) [24]. Pertinent psychosocial issues include loneliness/isolation, fear/apprehension, physician-patient relationships, change in body image, sexuality/personal contact, communication, social alienation and depression. Each situation is represented by two different pictures. The first picture generally shows the patient coping ineffectively and the second picture depicts more effective coping behaviour. The first picture is introduced and the patients are asked to identify the negative coping methods or strategies. Further discussion is encouraged that, it is hoped, will clarify why such coping is ineffective and will generate more positive options. The second picture is then introduced with the patient coping more effectively. Correct coping techniques identified by the group discussion are validated and reinforced. Any effective techniques not thought of by the group members are presented and explained by the group leader. The patients are then encouraged to apply these theoretical pictured situations to their own real-life situations. Patients are given a manual containing the coping scenarios and written descriptions of the situations and the coping techniques involved. They keep these manuals, allowing them to review the scenarios again as needed and to share them with significant others who may not have attended the meetings.

Figures 11.5a & b are an example of what one coping scenario (the physician-patient relationship) looks like in the manual. Figure 11.5a describes the patient's fear and anxiety about his diagnosis and about his relationship with his physician. Despite many questions and concerns, the patient avoids dealing with his condition and keeps his feelings locked inside. He relinquishes all decision-making power to his physician, thereby increasing the level of anxiety and loneliness. Figure 11.5b describes a positive, collaborative relationship between the patient, with his wife present to support him, and his physician. Instead of keeping his thoughts and feelings inside, the patient expresses his concerns and fears to his physician. The patient writes down his questions so that he will remember to ask his doctor.

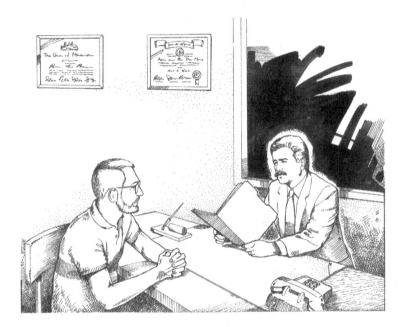

Steve has many fears and concerns about his condition. However, he has a very hard time talking with his doctor. His doctor seems distant and remote. Steve thinks he understands what the doctor tells him but when he gets home he does not remember what was said or realizes that he really did not understand. At home, Steve thinks of questions to ask his doctor but once he gets there he cannot remember what it was he was going to say. He also thinks the doctor will think he is stupid for asking about things that the doctor has already explained. As a result, Steve keeps his thoughts and feelings to himself and trusts his doctor to know what is best and to make all the decisions about his care. However, Steve is feeling more and more anxious about his condition.

What kind of coping is Steve using?

Steve is avoiding dealing with the problem directly. He is keeping his feelings to himself and giving up all decision-making powers to his doctor instead of establishing a collaborative relationship between them. He is being very solitary and passive.

AVOIDANCE

fear and concern
$\rightarrow$ (passive) $\rightarrow$ anxiety
$\rightarrow$ (solitary) $\rightarrow$ loneliness
$\rightarrow$ feel worse

Figure 11.5 *(a) Ineffective doctor-patient relationship.*

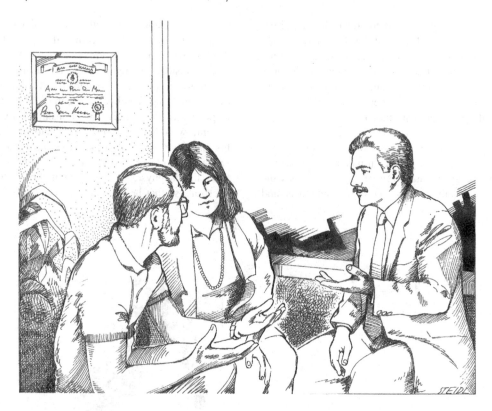

Steve finally talks to his wife, Susan, about how anxious he is and the trouble he has talking to his doctor.
Susan suggests they make a list of his questions and that they go see the doctor together. With Susan providing support, Steve is able to tell the doctor about his feelings and to ask his questions. Once the doctor realizes how Steve is
feeling, he takes extra time to reassure him and answer all the questions. The doctor also encourages Steve to ask
more questions and even the same questions again if feels he needs more explanation. The doctor says that they
would both feel better if they made decisions about Steve's treatment together. Steve feels much less anxious after
this visit. He has a sense of being more in control of his life, and he feels that a positive supportive alliance has been
established between himself and his doctor.

What kind of coping is Steve using now?

Steve is now using three forms of active-behavioral coping. He is becoming actively and positively
involved by forming a plan of action (making a list, getting wife's support, engaging the doctor). In talking to both
his wife and the doctor, he is actively expressing his feelings and actively relying on their help in dealing with the
problems.

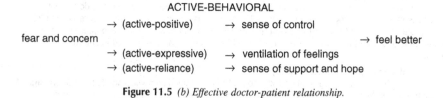

ACTIVE-BEHAVIORAL

fear and concern

→ (active-positive)   → sense of control

→ (active-expressive)   → ventilation of feelings

→ (active-reliance)   → sense of support and hope

→ feel better

Figure 11.5 *(b) Effective doctor-patient relationship.*

The patient is actively involved with his medical care, thereby increasing his sense of control and reducing his anxiety level. Having a second person (e.g. wife) present during consultations can enhance recall and review of details later.

11.4.4 Psychological Support

Psychological support is inherent throughout the intervention and is initiated with an introductory talk describing the normal assumptive world, with the forward-life trajectory of most people (Figure 11.6), and the way in which a life-threatening illness interrupts this forward-life trajectory (Figure 11.7). The underlying philosophy is that with the proper medical and psychiatric treatment, a new assumptive world can be developed and the forward-life trajectory resumed (Figure 11.8). The introductory talk ends with an analogy of how a person's support resources are similar to a building's support columns. Just as a building needs four support columns to stand, so too does a person have four sources of support. They are self, family and friends, co-workers and/or schoolmates and spirituality (Figure 11.9). Self refers to the positive facets of a person that he or she brings to an experience. These include personality, successful past experiences, coping abilities and positive attitudes towards life. Family and friends are significant sources of both instrumental and emotional social support. Recent literature has shown the importance of this type of support to an individual facing an illness. Co-workers and/or schoolmates can also be a valuable source of support. They are more likely to be supportive if they are kept informed of what is happening to the person and are given some idea of how they can be helpful (time off for medical care, temporary assistance while a person is recovering from a surgery, organising a card or letter campaign to cheer up a person in the hospital, etc.). Spirituality can be helpful in providing psychological and emotional support. Formal religious organisations are often sources of instrumental support (e.g. delivering meals to homes, transportation services, visitation and phone call networks to maintain social networks). The basic tenets of some formal religions are also helpful to some individuals in accepting and dealing with the emotional aspects of the diagnosis and treatment of cancer (e.g. 'It's God's will and He will take care of me'). Many people do not have a formal religion but rather a belief in some higher power to whom they can turn for help. Members then discuss the many topics generated by the 10 coping scenarios. The advantages of this programme are that the patients

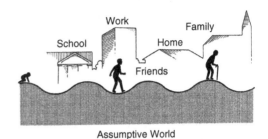

Figure 11.6 *People move forward engaging in the many domains of life.*

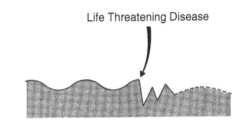

Figure 11.7 *The normal forward moving trajectory is interrupted by the illness.*

Figure 11.8 *The goal of psychological support is to help the patient establish a new assumptive world empowering resumption of the forward life trajectory.*

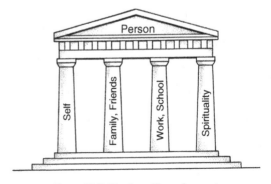

Figure 11.9 *The four pillars of support.*

are taught to collaborate with the health team and to cope actively with increased responsibility for their own health care programme. Another advantage is that the patients take away with them valuable skills that will enable them to deal more effectively with future problems.

11.5 Service Development

Our programme can be delivered by one or more competent psychosocial professionals (e.g., psychiatrists, psychologists, social workers, or nurses). Knowledge of cancer and its treatment, behavioral and cognitive techniques, group facilitation and supportive counselling is needed.

The full set of pictures used in this programme was published in General Hospital Psychiatry in 1994 [29].

Table 11.4 provides a sample outline for how the six weekly sessions might be organised for a breast cancer support group.

11.6 Summary

The psychological and medical problems encountered by cancer patients are numerous and unique. Patients are usually distressed, anxious and unable to effectively utilise their normal coping styles. Based on a review of the literature and the authors' own clinical and research experience, it appears that a short-term, structured intervention consisting of health education, behavioural training, enhancement of coping skills including stress management and problem solving and group psychosocial support offers significant benefits. The advantages of such a programme include easy implementation and replication, promotion of important illness-related, problem-solving skills and increased participation in decision making and active coping. In addition, a psychoeducational intervention offered early in the course of cancer diagnosis and treatment and offered as an integral component of their overall care may be less stigmatising and more readily accepted by both patients and staff. Such psychiatric interventions should be used as an adjunct to competent, comprehensive medical care and not as an independent treatment modality for cancer [24, 29, 63–65].

Table 11.4	Sample session outline – breast cancer support groups

Session 1

1. Health education
   (a) Surgical therapies including reconstruction
2. Stress management
   (a) Relaxation exercise taught (CD handed out)
   (b) Homework = Stress Awareness Assessment
3. Coping
   (a) Introduction – philosophy of programme
   (b) Three methods of coping
   (c) Coping scenarios 1 and 2 (pre-diagnosis and diagnosis phases)
4. Emotional support
   (a) Group members of each other
   (b) Individual member support by group leader(s) as needed

Session 2

1. Health education
   (a) Therapies (chemotherapy, hormonal, immunological, radiation)
   (b) Support drugs (e.g. anti-nausea and vomiting, colony stimulating factors)
   (c) Prognostic indicators
2. Stress management
   (a) Principles of stress management (awareness, planning for change, problem solving)
   (b) Review stress awareness assessments
3. Coping
   (a) Coping scenario 3 (doctor-patient relationships)
4. Emotional support
   (a) Group members of each other
   (b) Individual member support by group leader(s) as needed

Session 3

1. Health education
   (a) ACS booklet on sexuality
   (b) Lymphedema
   (c) Skin protection/sunscreens
2. Stress management
   (a) Review relaxation techniques
3. Coping
   (a) Coping scenario 4 (treatment issues)
   (b) Coping scenario 5 (body image changes)
4. Emotional support
   (a) Group members of each other
   (b) Individual member support by group leader(s) as needed

Session 4

1. Health education
   (a) Nutrition handouts
   (b) Efficacy of intervention (research studies)
2. Stress management
   (a) Review progress and/or problems
3. Coping
   (a) Coping scenario 6 (depression)
4. Emotional support
   (a) Group members of each other
   (b) Individual member support by group leader(s) as needed

Table 11.4	continued

Session 5
1. Health education
   (a) Bone marrow transplant
   (b) Self-exams
2. Stress management
   (a) Review progress and/or problems
3. Coping
   (a) Coping scenario 7 (relationships with significant others)
   (b) Coping scenario 8 (relationships with friends and co-workers)

Session 6
1. Health education
   (a) Answer any outstanding questions
   (b) NIH Handout – Facing Forward: A guide for Cancer Survivors
2. Stress management
   (a) Review of stress management principles
3. Coping
   (a) Review problem solving and coping
   (b) Coping scenario 9 (returning to normal)
   (c) Coping scenario 10 (planning for the future)
   (d) Closure
4. Emotional support
   (a) Group members of each other
   (b) Individual member support by group leader(s)

NIH, National Institutes of Health; ACS, American Cancer Society.

References

1. Weisman, A.D. (1979a) *Coping with Cancer*, McGraw-Hill, New York.
2. Weisman, A.D. (1979b) A model for psychosocial phasing in cancer. *General Hospital Psychiatry*, **10**, 187–195.
3. Cohen, J., Cullen, J. and Martin, L. (1982) *Psychosocial Aspects of Cancer*, Raven Press, New York.
4. McDaniel, J.S., Musselman, D.L., Porter, M.R. *et al.* (1995) Depression in patients with cancer. *Archives of General Psychiatry*, **52**, 89–99.
5. Van't Spijker, A., Trijsburg, R.W. and Duivenvoorden, H.J. (1997) Psychological sequelae of cancer diagnosis: a meta-analytic review of 58 studies after 1980. *Psychosomatic Medicine*, **59**, 280–283.
6. Zabora, J.R., Blanchard, C.G., Smith, E.D. *et al.* (1997) Prevalence of psychological distress across the disease continuum. *Journal of Psychosocial Oncology*, **15**, 73–87.
7. Grassi, L., Malacarne, P., Maestri, A. *et al.* (1997) Depression, psychosocial variables and occurrence of life events among patients with cancer. *Journal of Affective Disorders*, **44**, 21–30.
8. McDaniel, J.S., Musselman, D.L. and Nemeroff, C.B. (1997) Cancer and depression: theory and treatment. *Psychiatric Annals*, **27**, 360–364.
9. Fawzy, F.I., Fawzy, N.W., Arndt, L.A. *et al.* (1995) Critical review of psychosocial interventions in cancer care. *Archives of General Psychiatry*, **52**, 100–113.
10. Spiegel, D. and Diamond, S. (1998) Psychosocial interventions, in *American Society of Clinical Oncology Educational Book* (ed. M. Perry), American Society of Clinical Oncology, Alexandria, VA, pp. 386–395.
11. Compas, B.E., Haaga, D.A., Keefe, F.J. *et al.* (1998) Sampling of empirically supported psychological treatments from health psychology: smoking, chronic pain, cancer, and bulimia nervosa. *Journal of Consulting Clinical Psychology*, **66**, 89–112.
12. Kissane, D.W., Bloch, S., McKenzie, M. *et al.* (1998) Family grief therapy: a preliminary account of a new model to promote healthy family functioning during palliative care and bereavement. *Psychooncology*, **7**, 14–25.
13. Fawzy, F.I., Fawzy, N.W. and Canada, A.L. (1998) Psychosocial interventions programs for patients with cancer, in *American Society of Clinical Oncology Educational Book* (ed. M. Perry), American Society of Clinical Oncology, Alexandria, VA, pp. 396–411.
14. Trijsburg, R.W., van Knippenberg, F.C.E. and Rijpma, S.E. (1992) Effects of psychological treatment on cancer patients: a critical review. *Psychosomatic Medicine*, **54**, 489–517.
15. Holland, J. (1982) *The Current Concepts and Challenges in Psychosocial Oncology. Current Concepts and Challenges in Psychosocial Oncology: Syllabus of Postgraduate Course*, Sloan-Kettering Cancer Center, New York, NY.
16. Gordon, W.A., Freidenbergs, I., Diller, L. *et al.* (1980) Efficacy of psychosocial intervention with cancer patients. *Journal of Consulting and Clinical Psychology*, **48**, 743–759.
17. Pruitt, B.T., Waligora-Serafin, B., McMahon, T. *et al.* (1993) An educational intervention for newly-diagnosed cancer patients undergoing radiotherapy. *Psychooncology*, **2**, 55–62.
18. Gruber, B.L., Hersh, S.P., Hall, N.R.S. *et al.* (1993) Immunological responses of breast cancer patients to behavioral interventions. *Biofeedback and Self-Regulation*, **18** (1), 1–21.
19. Herschbach, P., Book, K., Dinkel, A. *et al.* (2010) Evaluation of two group therapies to reduce fear of progression in cancer patients. *Support Care Cancer*, **18** (4), 471–479.
20. Arakawa, S. (1997) Relaxation to reduce nausea, vomiting, and anxiety induced by chemotherapy in Japanese patients. *Cancer Nursing*, **20** (5), 342–349.
21. de Wit, R., van Dam, F., Zandbelt, L. *et al.* (1997) A pain education program for chronic cancer pain patients: follow-up results from a randomized controlled trial. *Pain*, **73** (10), 55–69.
22. Kwekkeboom, K.L., Cherwin, C.H., Lee, J.W. and Wanta, B. (2010) Mind-body treatment for the pain-fatigue-sleep disturbance symptom cluster in persons with cancer. *Journal of Pain Symptom Management*, **39** (1), 126–138.
23. Spiegel, D., Bloom, J.R. and Yalom, I.D. (1981) Group support for metastatic cancer patients: a randomized

prospective outcome study. *Archives of General Psychiatry*, **38**, 527–553.

24. Fawzy, F.I., Cousins, N., Fawzy, N.W. *et al.* (1990a) A structured psychiatric intervention for cancer patients: I. Changes over time in methods of coping and affective disturbance. *Archives of General Psychiatry*, **47**, 720–725.

25. Jacobs, C., Ross, R.D., Walker, I.M. *et al.* (1983) Behavior of cancer patients: a randomized study of the effects of education and peer support groups. *American Journal of Clinical Oncology*, **6**, 347–353.

26. Ali, N. and Khalil, H. (1989) Effects of psychoeducational intervention on anxiety among Egyptian bladder cancer patients. *Cancer Nursing*, **12** (4), 236–242.

27. Richardson, J.L., Shelton, D.R., Krailo, M. *et al.* (1990) The effect of compliance with treatment on survival among patients with hematologic malignancies. *Journal of Clinical Oncology*, **8** (2), 356–364.

28. Massie, M.J., Holland, J.C. and Straker, N. (1989) Psychotherapeutic interventions, *Handbook of Psychooncology*, (eds J.C. Holland and J.H. Rowland), Oxford University Press, New York, NY, pp. 455–469.

29. Fawzy, F.I. and Fawzy, N.W. (1994) A structured psychoeducational intervention of cancer patients. *General Hospital Psychiatry*, **16**, 149–192.

30. Burish, T.G. and Lyles, J.N. (1981) Effectiveness of relaxation training in reducing adverse reactions to cancer chemotherapy. *Journal of Behavioral Medicine*, **4**, 65–78.

31. Burish, T.G., Snyder, S.L. and Jenkins, R.A. (1991) Preparing patients for cancer chemotherapy: effect of coping preparation and relaxation interventions. *Journal of Consulting and Clinical Psychology*, **59** (4), 518–525.

32. Bridge, I.R., Benson, P., Pietroni, P.C. *et al.* (1988) Relaxation and imagery in the treatment of breast cancer. *British Medical Journal*, **4**, 65–78.

33. Decker, T., Cline-Elsen, J. and Gallagher, M. (1992) Relaxation therapy as an adjunct in radiation oncology. *Journal of Clinical Psychology*, **48**, 388–393.

34. Baider, L., Uziely, B. and De-Nour, A.K. (1994) Progressive muscle relaxation and guided imagery in cancer patients. *General Hospital Psychiatry*, **16**, 340–347.

35. Weisman, A.D., Worden, J.W. and Sobel, H.J. (1980) *Psychosocial Screening and Intervention with Cancer Patients*, Harvard Medical School, Massachusetts General Hospital, Boston, MA, Project Omega, Grant No, CA-19797.

36. Sobel, J.H. and Worden, J.W. (1982) *Helping Cancer Patients Cope: A Problem-Solving Intervention for Health Care Professionals [Audio Cassette]*, Guilford Press, New York, NY.

37. Berglund, G., Bolund, C., Gustafsson, U. *et al.* (1994) A randomized study of a rehabilitation program for cancer patients: the "starting again" group. *Psychooncology*, **3**, 109–120.

38. Hosaka, T. (1996) A pilot study of a structured psychiatric intervention for Japanese women with breast cancer. *Psychooncology*, **5**, 59–64.

39. Cocker, K., Bell, D. and Kidman, A. (1994) Cognitive behaviour therapy with advanced breast cancer patients: a brief report of a pilot study. *Psychooncology*, **3**, 233–237.

40. Dolbeault, S., Cayrou, S., Bredart, A. *et al.* (2009) The effectiveness of a psycho-educational group after early-stage breast cancer treatment: results of a randomized French Study. *Psychooncology*, **18** (6), 647–656.

41. Faul, L.A., Jim, H.S., Williams, C. *et al.* (2010) Relationship of stress management skill to psychological distress and quality of life in adults with cancer. *Psychooncology*, **19** (1), 102–109.

42. Parker, P.A., Pettaway, C.A., Babaian, R.J. *et al.* (2009) The effects of a presurgical stress management intervention for men with prostate cancer undergoing radical prostatectomy. *Journal of Clinical Oncology*, **27** (19), 3169–3176.

43. Fawzy, F.I., Wellisch, D. and Yager, J. (1977) Psychiatric liaison to the bone-marrow transplant project, in *The Family in Mourning*, (eds C.E. Hollingsworth and R.O. Pasnau), Grune & Stratton, New York, NY, pp. 181–189.

44. Fawzy, F.I., Fawzy, N.W., Hyun, C.S. *et al.* (1993) Malignant melanoma: effects of an early structured psychiatric intervention, coping, and affective state on recurrence and survival 6 years later. *Archives of General Psychiatry*, **50**, 681–689.

45. Bloom, J.R. (1982) Social support systems and cancer: a conceptual view, in *Psychosocial Aspects of Cancer* (eds J. Cohen, J. Cullen and R.L. Martin), Raven Press, New York, NY, pp. 129–149.

46. Spiegel, D. and Bloom, J.R. (1983) Pain in metastatic breast cancer. *Cancer*, **52**, 341–345.

47. Cain, E., Kohorn, E., Quinlan, D. *et al.* (1986) Psychosocial benefits of a cancer support group. *Cancer*, **57** (1), 183–189.

48. Cunningham, A.J. and Tocco, E.K. (1989) A randomized trial of group psychoeducational therapy for cancer patients. *Patient Education and Counseling*, **14**, 101–114.

49. Edgar, L., Rosberger, Z. and Nowlis, D. (1992) Coping with cancer during the first year after diagnosis: assessment and intervention. *Cancer*, **69**, 817–828.

50. Cella, D.F., Sarafian, B., Snider, P.R. *et al.* (1993) Evaluation of a community-based cancer support group. *Psychooncology*, **2**, 123–132.

51. Cunningham, A.J., Edmonds, C.V.I., Jenkins, G. *et al.* (1995) A randomized comparison of two forms of a brief, group, psychoeducational program for cancer patients: weekly sessions versus a "weekend intensive". *International Journal of Psychiatry in Medicine*, **25**, 173–189.

52. Linn, M.W., Linn, B.S. and Harris, R. (1982) Effects of counseling for late stage cancer patients. *Cancer*, **49**, 1048–1055.

53. Greer, S., Moorey, S., Baruch, J.D.R. *et al.* (1992) Adjuvant psychological therapy for patients with cancer: a prospective randomized trial. *British Medical Journal*, **304**, 675–680.

54. Moorey, S., Greer, S., Watson, M. *et al.* (1994) Adjuvant psychological therapy for patients with cancer: outcome at one year. *Psycho-Oncology*, **3**, 39–46.

55. Fawzy, N.W. (1996) A psychoeducational nursing intervention to enhance coping and affective state in newly diagnosed malignant melanoma patients. *Cancer Nursing*, **18**, 427–438.

56. Fawzy, F.I. and Fawzy, N.W. (1982) Psychosocial aspects of cancer, in *Diagnosis and Management of Cancer* (ed. D. Nixon), Addison-Wesley, Menlo Park, CA, pp. 111–123.

57. Fawzy, F.I. and Natterson, B. (1994) Psychological care of the cancer patient, in *Clinical Oncology: A Lange Clinical*

Manual (ed. R.B. Cameron), Simon & Shuster, San Mateo, CA, pp. 40–44.

58. Spiegel, D., Bloom, J.R., Kraemer, H.C. *et al.* (1989) Effect of psychosocial treatment on survival of patients with metastatic breast cancer. *Lancet*, **2** (8668), 888–891.

59. Fawzy, F.I., Fawzy, N.W., Hyun, C.S. *et al.* (1997) Brief, coping-oriented therapy for patients with malignant melanoma, in *Group Therapy for the Medically Ill* (ed. J. Spira), Guilford Press, New York, NY, pp. 133–165.

60. Boesen, E.H., Ross, L., Frederiksen K. *et al.* (2005) Psychoeducational intervention for patients with cutaneous malignant melanoma: a replication study. *Journal of Clinical Oncology*, **23** (6), 1270–1277.

61. Fawzy, F.I., Namir, S. and Wolcott, D.L. (1989) Structured group intervention model for AIDS patients. *Psychiatric Medicine*, **7** (2), 23–34.

62. Namir, S., Wolcott, D.L., Fawzy, F.I. *et al.* (1987) Coping with AIDS: psychological and health implications. *Journal of Applied and Social Psychology*, **17**, 308–328.

63. Sharp, D.M., Walker, M.B., Bateman, J.S. *et al.* (2009) Demographic characteristics of patients using a fully integrated psychosocial support service for cancer patients. *BMC Research Notes*, **2**, 253.

64. Bergelt, C., Schölermann, C., Hahn, I. *et al.* (2010) Psychooncological care for breast cancer patients in hospitals and in the outpatient sector. *Gesundheitswesen*, **72** (10), 700–706.

65. Surbone, A., Baider, L., Weitzman, T.S. *et al.*, MASCC Psychosocial Study Group (2010) Psychosocial care for patients and their families is integral to supportive care: MASCC position statement. *Support Care Cancer*, **18** (2), 255–263.

66. Fawzy, F.I., Kemeny, M.E., Fawzy, N.W. *et al.* (1990b) A structured psychiatric intervention for cancer patients: II. Changes over time in immunologic measures. *Archives of General Psychiatry*, **47**, 729–735.

12 Meaning-Centered Group Psychotherapy

William Breitbart[1,2] and Allison Applebaum[1]

[1]Department of Psychiatry and Behavioral Sciences, Memorial Sloan-Kettering Cancer Center, New York, NY, USA
[2]Weill Medical College of Cornell University, New York, NY, USA

12.1 Introduction

A famous Talmudic question asks: 'What is truer than the truth?' The answer: 'The story.' This, dear reader, is the story of Meaning-Centered Group Psychotherapy (MCGP), at least in abbreviated form.

Like many clinical interventions in our field of psycho-oncology, Meaning-Centred Psychotherapy (MCP) arose from a need to deal with a challenging clinical problem, that of despair, hopelessness and desire for hastened death in advanced cancer patients who were, in fact, not suffering from a clinical depression [1], but rather confronting an existential crisis of loss of meaning, value and purpose in the face of a terminal prognosis. While our group ultimately demonstrated that desire for hastened death in the presence of a clinical depression could be reversed with adequate antidepressant therapy [2], no effective intervention appeared available for loss of meaning and hopelessness in the absence of clinical depression.

Inspired primarily by the works of Viktor Frankl [3–6] and further informed by the contributions of Irvin Yalom [7], our research group adapted Frankl's concepts of the importance of meaning in human existence (and his 'logotherapy'), and initially created MCGP, intended primarily for advanced cancer patients. The goal of the intervention was to diminish despair, demoralisation, hopelessness and desire for hastened death by sustaining or enhancing a sense of meaning, even in the face of death. While MCP relies heavily on Frankl's concepts of meaning, its sources

and related resources to re-connect with meaning in the midst of suffering, MCP also incorporates fundamental existential concepts and concerns that do not directly focus on meaning, but are clearly related to the search for, connection with and creation of meaning. MCGP is an eight-week intervention, composed of didactics and experiential exercises, designed to help patients understand the importance of meaning to diminish despair near the end of life.

12.2 Background

As we deepen our understanding of the psychosocial needs of palliative care patients, it is apparent that our present concepts of adequate care must be expanded beyond simple pain and physical symptom control to include psychiatric, psychosocial, existential and spiritual domains of care [8–12]. While physical symptoms are indeed distressing, those relating to psychological distress and existential concerns are even more prevalent than pain and other physical symptoms [13]. Acknowledging the psychological and spiritual domains of end-of-life care are clear priorities for both medical professionals and patients themselves.

12.2.1 Defining Spirituality as a Construct of Meaning and/or Faith

The Consensus Conference on Improving Spiritual Care as a Dimension of Palliative Care defined

Handbook of Psychotherapy in Cancer Care, First Edition. Edited by Maggie Watson and David W. Kissane.
© 2011 John Wiley & Sons, Inc. Published 2011 by John Wiley & Sons, Inc.

spirituality as 'the aspect of humanity that refers to the way individuals seek and express meaning and purpose and the way they experience their connectedness to the moment, to self, to others, to nature and to the significant or sacred' [14]. Others have defined spirituality as a construct that combines concepts of meaning and religious faith [15, 16]. Meaning, or having a sense that one's life has meaning, involves the conviction that one is fulfiling a unique role and purpose in a life that is a gift. This comes with a responsibility to live to one's full potential as a human being; in so doing, one gains a sense of peace, contentment or even transcendence, through connectedness with something greater than one's self [4]. Faith is a belief in a higher transcendent power, not necessarily, but typically, identified as God, and usually, but not necessarily, through participation in the rituals or beliefs of a specific organised religion. The faith component of spirituality is most often associated with religious belief, while the meaning component appears to be a more secular and potentially universal concept that can exist in religious or non-religiously identified individuals.

12.2.2 Spiritual Well-Being/Meaning and Its Impact on Psychosocial Outcomes in Advanced Cancer

There has been great interest in the impact of faith and religious beliefs on health outcomes [17–21]. Religion and spirituality generally play a positive role in patients' coping with illnesses such as cancer or HIV [17, 22, 23]. However, the link between religion and health is weaker than that between spirituality/meaning and health outcomes [24, 25]. Importantly, researchers theorise that religious beliefs may help patients construct meaning in suffering inherent to illness, which may in turn facilitate acceptance of their situation [19].

There is extensive evidence for the significance of spiritual well-being at the end-of-life. For example, Singer and colleagues found that 'achieving a sense of spiritual peace' was a domain that was most important from the patients' perspective [26]. Moadel and colleagues reported that 51% of patients wanted help overcoming fears, while 41% needed help finding hope, 40% the meaning in life, 43% peace of mind and 39% spiritual resources [27]. Among Japanese hospice inpatients, psychological distress was related to meaninglessness in 37%, hopelessness in 37% and loss of social role and feeling irrelevant in 28% [28]. Finally, Meier and colleagues noted that 'loss of meaning in life' accounted for 47% of the requests

for assisted suicide [29]. Clearly, spirituality is an essential element of quality end-of-life care.

Several studies expand on the importance of these concepts. A high degree of meaning corresponds with higher satisfaction with quality of life and better tolerance of severe physical symptoms [30]. Our research group [1, 23] demonstrated the central role for spiritual well-being (i.e. meaning) as a buffering agent, protecting against depression, hopelessness and desire for hastened death. We also found that spiritual well-being was significantly associated with end-of-life despair, even after controlling for the influence of depression [31]. Similarly, Yanez and colleagues found that increases in meaning/peace significantly predicted better mental health and lower distress, whereas increases in faith did not [32].

Depression, hopelessness and loss of meaning are associated with poorer survival [33] and higher rates of suicide, suicidal ideation and desire for hastened death [1, 34–37]. Additionally, hopelessness and loss of meaning predict desire for death, independently of depression [1]. There is a critical need for psychosocial interventions that address loss of meaning as a mechanism for improving psychosocial outcomes (e.g. quality of life, depression, anxiety, hopelessness, desire for death and end-of-life despair).

12.3 Theoretical Conceptual Framework Underlying Meaning-Centred Psychotherapy

12.3.1 Frankl's Concepts of Meaning

Frankl's logotherapy was not designed for the treatment of cancer patients or those with life threatening illness. His main contribution to human psychology was to raise awareness of the spiritual component of human experience, and the central importance of meaning (or the will to meaning) as a driving force or human instinct. Basic concepts related to meaning, proposed by Frankl and adapted for MCP in the cancer setting include:

1. **Meaning of life** – life has and never ceases to have meaning, from the first moment through to the very last. Meaning may change through the years, but it never ceases to exist. When we feel our lives have no meaning, it is because we have become disconnected from such meaning, rather than because it no longer exists.

2. **Will to meaning** – the desire to find meaning in existence is a primary motivating force in

Table 12.1	Frankl's sources of meaning
Creativity	*Engaging in life* through work, deeds, causes, artistic endeavours, hobbies, and so on. Examples include our careers/job, volunteer work, involvement with church/synagogue, political and social causes.
Experience	*Connecting with life* through love, relationships, nature, art and humour. Examples include our family, children, loved ones, the sunset, gardening, beaches, museums, playing with pets, and so on.
Attitude	*Encountering life's limitations* by turning personal tragedy into triumph, things we have achieved despite adversity, rising above or transcending difficult circumstances. Examples include achieving an education despite personal/financial challenges, overcoming grief/loss, persevering through cancer treatment, and so on.
History	*Legacy given (past), lived (present) and left (future).* Examples include our story, our family history, the history of our name, our accomplishments and whatever we hope to leave behind.

our behaviour. Human beings are creatures who innately search for and create meaning in their lives.

3. **Freedom of will** – we have the freedom to find meaning in life and to choose our attitude towards suffering. We have the responsibility to discover meaning, direction and identity. We must respond to the fact of our existence and create the 'essence' of what makes us human.

4. **Sources of meaning.** Meaning in life has specific and available sources (Table 12.1). The four main sources of meaning are derived from creativity (work, deeds, dedication to causes), experience (art, nature, humour, love, relationships, roles), attitude (the stance one takes towards suffering and existential problems) and legacy (meaning exists in a historical context, thus legacy – past, present and future – is a critical element in sustaining or enhancing meaning).

Drawing from these principles, MCGP enhances patients' sense of meaning by helping them to capitalise on the various sources of meaning in their lives. Enhanced meaning is conceptualised as the catalyst for improved quality of life, reduced psychological distress and despair. Specifically, meaning is viewed as both an intermediary outcome, as well as a mediator of change.

12.3.2 Meaning-Focused Coping

More recently, Park and Folkman [38] described helpful conceptual models for meaning in relation to traumatic events and coping, which seem relevant to the theoretical framework of MCP and MCGP. They describe meaning as a general life orientation, as personal significance, as causality, as a coping mechanism and as an outcome. Critically important is their concept of meaning-based coping, assessed in terms of reevaluating an event as positive, answering the question of why or 'Why me?', enumerating ways in which life changed (sometimes for the positive) because of an event, and appreciating that

one has 'made sense of' or 'found meaning' in these circumstances [3–6, 39–42]. Park and Folkman [38] also describe two levels of meaning: global meaning and situational meaning. Unlike this conceptualisation of global or situational, Frankl viewed meaning as a state; individuals can move from feeling demoralised and as if their lives hold no value (see Kissane [37]), to recognising personal meaning and purpose, which allows them to value even more intensely the time remaining. Conceptualising meaning as a state subject to change suggests its potential responsiveness to intervention. Frankl also viewed suffering as a potential springboard, both for having a need for explanation and for finding meaning [3, 4]. Hence, the diagnosis of a terminal illness may be seen as a crisis in the fullest sense of the word – an experience of distress or even despair that may in itself offer an opportunity for growth and meaning.

12.3.3 Concepts Central to Existential Philosophy and Psychology

Underlying the development of MCP and MCGP are concepts central to existential philosophy, psychology and psychiatry, developed by such pioneers as Kierkegaard, Nietzsche, Heidegger, Sartre and Yalom [7, 43–46]. Much of the psychotherapeutic work is richer when the therapists are well grounded in the basic theories of existential philosophy and psychotherapy. Important concepts include: freedom, responsibility, choice, creativity, identity, authenticity, engagement, existential guilt, care, transcendence, transformation, direction, being unto death, being and temporality and existential isolation. These existential concepts richly inform the intervention and are utilised primarily to reinforce the goals of MCP related to the search for, connection with and creation of meaning.

12.4 Target Groups of Patients

MCGP, as it has been developed and shown to be effective in clinical trial to date, has been targeted towards advanced cancer patients with poor prognosis. Patients with physical limitations sufficient to preclude participation in outpatient group psychotherapy (as indicated by a Karnofsky Performance Rating below 50 [47]) are not suited for this intervention. The efficacy of MCGP in improving patients' spiritual well-being and sense of meaning, and decreasing anxiety and desire for death, makes it particularly appropriate for patients who are experiencing at least moderate distress, (as indicated by a score of 4 or higher on the *Distress Thermometer*, NCCN Clinical Practice Guidelines in Oncology [48]), predominantly in the areas of emotional problems and spiritual/religious concerns.

12.5 Main Themes and Format of the Therapy

MCGP is an eight-week (1 1/2 hour weekly sessions) group intervention, which uses a mix of didactics, discussions and experiential exercises that are centred around particular themes related to meaning and advanced cancer (Table 12.2). The intention is to sustain or enhance a sense of meaning and purpose by teaching patients how to use the breadth of possible sources of meaning as coping resources through a combination of: (i) instructed teaching on the concepts of meaning; (ii) group experiential exercises to enhance learning, followed by homework for practice; and (iii) group leader-facilitated discussion aimed at reinforcing the importance of re-connecting to sources of meaning and using these as resources. Other existential concepts, such as freedom, responsibility, authenticity, existential guilt, transcendence and choice

are incorporated into session content as these themes arise. Elements of support and expression of emotion are inevitable in each session (but are limited by the psycho-educational focus of MCGP).

The following is an overview of each session, including the experiential exercises used to facilitate discussion and deepen understanding.

12.5.1 Session 1: Concepts and Sources of Meaning

The first session involves introductions of each group member and an overall explanation of the group's goals. Patient introductions include biographical/demographic information, as well as their expectations, hopes and questions relating to the group. The session concludes with a discussion of what *meaning* means to each participant, stimulated by an experiential exercise which helps patients discover how they find a sense of meaning and purpose in general, as well as specifically in relation to having been diagnosed with cancer. As an adjunctive to the group, all patients are given a copy of Frankl's 'Man's Search for Meaning' [4] as a means of facilitating each patient's understanding of the main themes of the intervention.

12.5.1.1 Session 1: Experiential Exercise
List one or two experiences or moments when life has felt particularly meaningful to you – whether it sounds powerful or mundane. For example, it could be something that helped get you through a difficult day, or a time when you felt most alive. And say something about it.

Session	MCGP	Content
	Table 12.2 Topics of meaning-centered group psychotherapy weekly sessions	
1	Concepts and sources of meaning	Introductions of group members; introduction of concept of meaning and sources of meaning; experiential exercise; homework
2	Cancer and meaning	Identity – before and after cancer diagnosis; experiential exercise; homework
3	Historical sources of meaning (legacy: past)	Life as a legacy that has been given (past); experiential exercise; homework
4	Historical sources of meaning (legacy: present and future)	Life as a legacy that one lives (present) and gives (future); experiential exercise; homework
5	Attitudinal sources of meaning: encountering life's limitations	Confronting limitations imposed by cancer, prognosis and death; experiential exercise; introduction to legacy project; homework
6	Creative sources of meaning: engaging in life fully	Creativity, courage and responsibility; experiential exercises, homework
7	Experiential sources of meaning: connecting with life	Love, nature, art and humour
8	Transitions: reflections and hopes for the future	Review of sources of meaning, as resources, reflections on lessons learned in the group, experiential exercise on hopes for the future

12.5.2 Session 2: Cancer and Meaning

The emphasis of session 2 is the linking of identity as a central element of meaning. The session begins as a continuation of sharing meaningful experiences, as well as a detailed explanation of what, or who, made these experiences meaningful. Identity, as a component of meaning, is addressed through the experiential exercise in which patients are asked to respond to the question 'who am I?' This exercise provides the opportunity to discuss pre-cancer identity and roles, and then how cancer has affected their identity and what they consider to be meaningful in their lives.

12.5.2.1 Session 2: Experiential Exercise
'Identity and Cancer'

1. *Write down four answers to the question, 'Who am I?' These can be positive or negative, and include personality characteristics, body image, beliefs, things you do, people you know, and so on ... For example, answers might start with, 'I am someone who _____', or 'I am a _____'.*

2. *How has cancer affected your answers? How has it affected the things that are most meaningful to you?*

The following MCGP excerpt exemplifies the type of interaction that occurs between group members and leaders during the Session 2 Experiential Exercise:

PATIENT 1: *I am a daughter, a mother, a grandmother, a sister, a friend and a neighbour. I attempt to respect all people in their views, which sometimes can be difficult. I represent myself honestly and frankly without being offensive, or at least I try. And my philosophy is to do unto others as they would have done unto you. I'm somebody who can be very private and not always share all my needs and concerns. I also have been working on accepting love and affection and other gifts from other people. I'm more of a caregiver than someone who gets care from others, I don't like to receive care, but I'm beginning to, ... actually ... this may be the one thing that my illness has caused me to mull over. That I'm more accepting of people wanting to do things.*

GROUP LEADER: *Thank you. That's really interesting. I want to make some comments, but first let's hear from someone else. Patient 2, would you like to go?*

PATIENT 2: *Well in terms of pre-cancer, I'm my niece's loving aunty whom she currently adores ... she's seven, I'm not sure how long that will last, but right now, that's really important to me, and it's brought*

my brother and me closer. I'm active and am always ready for an adventure. All my friends knew I was a 'yes, let's do it, person', enthusiastic, open. I'm a young adult librarian, with a real connection to the teens. I really loved working with them, especially on the advisory council; I really just loved it, and oftentimes would stay very late with them, into the night. I was just, really ... connected.... I ran around a lot and I was rarely home before 11 p.m. ... My friends always asked why I wasn't home more. It wasn't that I didn't like home, it's just that I wanted to be out, experiencing life. I also love concerts, and I danced. And I dated; I was the essence of positive, a very good friend, I'm really proud of that.*

(Several other patients discussed their responses to this exercise)

GROUP LEADER: *Thanks. Do you have any questions for each other about the things that you said? Were there any commonalities that you noticed?*

PATIENT 1: *I guess the commonality that most of us spoke about, is being a member of a unique group, a family and for most of us, that was in the top position. That was most important.*

PATIENT 2: *I have a comment but I don't know if it's what you're asking for. Patient 1 was talking about being a giver, but that it's basically hard for her to receive. I've had friends who are like that and it's frustrating to want to give to a person like you, but you also don't want to take people's wishes lightly ... I know I'm probably speaking out of turn for all of your friends, who want to be generous back to you.*

PATIENT 1: *Most of them have been, because they, you know, sit me down and do what they want to do. I guess most of my good friends are very strong willed people like me and they listen and do for the most part what they want. And I don't get offended for the most part.*

GROUP LEADER: *It was actually quite striking ... that there were many similarities in what you all shared about your identities pre-cancer. For many people, the first, the most important source of your identity, had to do with your love relationships, family relationships, your role in a family, being a daughter, father, an aunt, being a member of immediate family. So it's from these connections that we derive meaning in life, through our connectedness with people we love. And often they are members of our family. And, often, these are our sources of identity, as a member of a family, as a father, an aunt...*

PATIENT 1: *These roles are also a source of pain.*

GROUP LEADER: *Yes, that can be true, but they are also clearly a source of meaning. Do you remember* which source of meaning? It's the 'experiential' source of meaning. Through love, through connectedness with people. ... Someone made a comment that Patient 3 didn't mention this source of meaning. Patient 3, you said something interesting. You said you've been alone too long. But you also said that you're a loyal friend, loyal as a puppy and a good lover. So for you, love is very relevant too. You derive a sense of meaning through friendship and romantic love. Those are all similar, all love, right? Let me ask you something, Patient 3, did you leave out being a son, or a family member, for a specific reason?

PATIENT 3: Well, I never knew my dad. I didn't really know my mother until I was older. And I have a brother and a sister, but I'm not close to either of them. So, in a way, my job became more of my family, the people I worked with, people in recovery, they were my family. Because I became more connected to them. But outside of that, no ... no real family. So in a sense, family has been a disappointment, pain. So everyone talks about family reunions, I don't have that. That's not a part of my life.

GROUP LEADER: So again this idea comes up that the things that give us meaning, like love and relationships and family, are also potential sources of pain. We have to be aware of that, don't we! The other thing I heard that was common in the responses, besides love and connectedness to other people, is connectedness to other kinds of experiences in life, like dancing, and Patient 4, you were talking about baking, cooking ... so it's not just relationships with people, it's relationships to the world, and being in nature, and engaging in pleasurable things, like dancing and eating. And in addition to that, several people talked about their identity coming from what they did for work, being a nurse, a lawyer, a librarian ... your work, these are creative sources of meaning, because we derive meaning through things we create, the work we do in our lives. And you added something interesting, Patient 1, that had to do with ... I think I would used the word compassion ... It had to do with caring for other people?

PATIENT 1: Well, you know, you talked about our professions, but I didn't actually talk today about my professional life, I didn't say anything about being a nurse or a health care provider, but I talked about being caretaker. A caretaker, in general, to the people in my life.

GROUP LEADER: Exactly. So this creative source of meaning doesn't just come from a job you get paid to do, but from the person you create in the world. You've created a person who is loving, giving and caring. You've created a virtue, a value, compassion is important, caring for others is important. So it's not just the job you do, but the kind of person you become and create in the world, and what values that represents, that is meaningful to you. That's all part of 'creative' sources of meaning.

12.5.3 Sessions 3 and 4: Historical Sources of Meaning

Sessions 3 and 4 focus on giving each patient a chance to share their life story with the group, which helps them to better appreciate their inherited legacy and past accomplishments while still elucidating current and future goals. The theme of Session 3 is 'Life as a legacy that has been given' via the past, such as legacy given through one's family of origin. The facts of our lives that have been created by our genetics and the circumstances of our past are discussed in terms of how they have shaped us and perhaps motivated us to transcend limitations. Session 4 focuses on 'Life as a legacy that one lives and will give', in terms of patients' living legacy, and the legacy they hope to leave for others. The Session 3 experiential exercise helps patients to understand the ways in which their pasts have shaped what they find meaningful, and the Session 4 exercise fosters a discussion of future goals, no matter how small. As a homework assignment after Session 4, patients are asked to tell their life story to a loved one(s), highlighting experiences that have been a source of meaning and pride for them, and things they wished they might have accomplished but have yet to do.

12.5.3.1 Session 3: Experiential Exercise
'Life as a Legacy That Has Been Given'

When you look back on your life and upbringing, what are the most significant memories, relationships, traditions, and so on, that have made the greatest impact on who you are today?

For example: Identify specific memories of how you were raised that have made a lasting impression on your life (e.g. your relationship with parents, siblings, friends, teachers, etc.) What is the origin of your name? What are some past events that have touched your life?

12.5.3.2 Session 4: Experiential Exercise
'Life as a Legacy That You Live and Will Give'

1. As you reflect upon who you are today, what are the meaningful activities, roles or accomplishments that you are most proud of?

2. *As you look towards the future, what are some of the life-lessons you have learned along the way that you would want to pass on to others? What is the legacy you hope to live and give?*

12.5.4 Session 5: Attitudinal Sources of Meaning

This session examines each patient's confrontation with limitations in life and the ultimate limitation – our mortality and the finiteness of life. The focus is on our freedom to choose our attitudes towards such limitations and find meaning in life, even in the face of death. In discussing the experiential exercise, group leaders emphasise one of Frankl's core theoretical beliefs, that by choosing our attitude towards circumstances that are beyond our control, (e.g. cancer and death), we may find meaning in life and suffering, which will then help us to rise above or overcome such limitations. One of the more critical elements of this session involves the experiential exercise in which patients are asked to discuss their thoughts, feelings and concepts of what constitutes a 'good' or meaningful death. Common issues that have arisen include where patients prefer to die (e.g. at home in their own bed), how they want to die (e.g. without pain, surrounded by family), and what patients expect takes place after death, funeral fantasies, family issues and the afterlife. This exercise is designed to detoxify the discussion of death and to allow for a safe examination of the life they have lived and how they may be able to accept that life. Inherent in these discussion are issues of tasks of life completion, forgiveness and redemption. At the end of session 5, patients are presented with the 'Legacy Project', which integrates ideas presented in treatment (e.g. meaning, identity, creativity and responsibility), in order to facilitate the generation of a sense of meaning in light of cancer. Some examples of Legacy Projects include creating a legacy photo album or video, mending a broken relationship or undertaking something the patient has always wanted to do but has not yet done.

12.5.4.1 Session 5: Experiential Exercise
'Encountering Life's Limitations'

1. *Since your diagnosis, are you still able to find meaning in your daily life despite your awareness of the finiteness of life? (If yes, how? If no, what are the obstacles?)*

2. *During this time, have you ever lost a sense of meaning in life – that life was not worth living? (If yes, please briefly describe.)*

3. *What would you consider a 'good' or 'meaningful' death? How can you imagine being remembered by your loved ones? (e.g. what are some of your personal characteristics, the shared memories or meaningful life events that have made a lasting impression on them?)*

12.5.5 Session 6: Creative Sources of Meaning

Session 6 focuses on 'Creativity' as a source and resource of meaning in life. One important element of the experiential exercises deals with the issue of 'Responsibility' (our ability to respond to the fact of our existence, to answer the question, 'what life have we created for ourselves?'). Each patient is asked to discuss what their responsibilities are, as well as for whom they are responsible. Any unfinished business or tasks patients may have is also examined. This discussion invites group members to focus on the task at hand, as opposed to focusing only on their suffering. Additionally, by attending to their responsibility to others, meaning may be enhanced by the realisation that their lives transcend themselves and extend to others.

12.5.5.1 Session 6: Experiential Exercise
'Engaging in Life Fully'

1. *Living life and being creative requires courage and commitment. Can you think of time(s) in your life when you've been courageous, taken ownership of your life or made a meaningful commitment to something of value to you?*

2. *Do you feel you've expressed what is most meaningful to you through your life's work and creative activities (e.g. job, parenting, hobbies, causes)? – If so, how?*

3. *What are your responsibilities? Who are you responsible to and for?*

4. *Do you have unfinished business? What tasks have you always wanted to do, but have yet to undertake? What's holding you back from responding to this creative call?*

12.5.6 Session 7: Experiential Sources of Meaning

Session 7 focuses on discussing experiential sources of meaning, such as love, beauty and humour. While creative and attitudinal sources of meaning require more of an *active involvement with life*, experiential sources embody more of a *passive or even sensory engagement with life*. Patients explore moments and experiences when they have felt connected with life through love, beauty and humour. Often, the discussions highlight how these sources of meaning become particularly important for patients since their cancer diagnosis. Feelings concerning the group's upcoming termination are discussed in preparation for the final session.

12.5.6.1 Session 7: Experiential Exercise
'Connecting with Life'

List three ways in which you 'connect with life' and feel most alive through the experiential sources of: LOVE: BEAUTY: HUMOUR:

12.5.7 Session 8: Transitions

The final session provides an opportunity to review patients' Legacy Projects, as well as to review individual and group themes. Additionally, the group is asked to discuss topics such as: (i) How has the group been experienced? (ii) Have there been changes in attitudes towards your illness or suffering? (iii) How do you envision continuing what has been started in the group? The experiential exercise that ends this session focuses on answering the question, 'What are your hopes for the future?'

12.5.7.1 Session 8: Experiential Exercise
'Group Reflections and Hopes for the future'

1. *What has it been like for you to go through this learning experience over these last eight sessions? Have there been any changes in the way you view your life and cancer experience having been through this process?*

2. *Do you feel like you have a better understanding of the sources of meaning in life and are you able to use them in your daily life? If so, how?*

3. *What are your hopes for the future?*

12.6 Key Therapist Techniques in the Application of MCGP

12.6.1 Group Process Skills and Techniques

MCGP is essentially a group intervention, and as such, attention to basic tenets of group process and dynamics remains important. Co-facilitators must be cognizant of group etiquette, especially in terms of working together as co-facilitators, attending to and promoting group cohesion and facilitating an atmosphere that is conducive to productive exchanges between patients. While MCGP is not intended to be primarily a supportive group intervention, elements of support are in fact quite inevitable, but are not intentionally promoted or specifically fostered.

12.6.2 Psycho-Educational Approach: Didactics and Experiential Exercises to Enhance Learning

MCGP is also essentially an educational intervention. The goal of MCGP is to have patients understand the concept of meaning, and its importance, particularly as one faces a terminal illness, and the ultimate limitation of death. Additionally, MCGP strives to have patients learn about sources of meaning in order for these to become resources in coping with advanced cancer. This educational process is achieved primarily through a set of brief didactics which introduce each session, followed by an experiential exercise designed to link learning of these abstract concepts with patients' own emotional experiences. Patients each share the content of their experiential exercises, and the process of experiential learning is reinforced through the comments of co-facilitators and patients, as well as through the identification of commonalities among patients' responses.

12.6.3 A Focus on Meaning and Sources of Meaning as Resources

MCGP is designed to have patients learn Frankl's concepts of meaning and to incorporate these sources of meaning as resources in their coping with advanced cancer. In each session, the co-facilitators listen carefully for and highlight content shared by patients that reflect sources of meaning. Co-facilitators identify 'meaningful moments' described by patients, and also draw attention to 'meaning shifts' when patients begin to incorporate the vocabulary and conceptual framework of meaning into the material they share. An emphasis is also placed on the importance of the patient's ability to shift from one source of meaning to another, as selected sources of meaning become unavailable due to disease progression. A specific technique used to facilitate this process is called 'Moving from ways of doing to ways of being'. This refers to helping patients to become aware that meaning can be derived in more passive ways. For example, patients can still be good fathers even if they cannot go out to the backyard and play ball with their sons, by being fathers in less action-oriented ways, such as sitting and talking about their son's life goals and fears, and through expressing affection. In MCGP, it is also important for co-facilitators to be aware of the 'co-creation of meaning' between group members. All present are 'witnesses' or repositories of meaning for each other, and are thus part of a meaningful legacy created by the group-as-a-whole.

12.6.4 Incorporating Basic Existential Concepts and Themes

A central concept in MCGP is that human beings are creatures. We create key values and, most importantly, we create our lives. In order to live fully, we must create a life of meaning, identity and direction. 'Detoxifying death' through the therapeutic stance and attitude of the co-facilitators is an important technique utilised throughout MCGP. Co-facilitators speak openly about death as the ultimate limitation that causes suffering and for which meaning can still be derived through the attitude that one takes towards suffering (e.g. transcendence, choice). Another technique, the 'existential nudge', occurs when co-facilitators gently challenge the resistance of patients to explore difficult existential realities, such as the ultimate limitation of death or existential guilt.

12.7 Case Example

Allen is a 56 year old gay man who has worked in the advertising field for 30 years. His work is fast paced, taxing and consuming. While he enjoyed his work, he had begun to think of doing other things in recent years that may be more fulfilling. However, such feelings were usually overtaken by fears of what he would do with his life and what identity he would subsequently have. He has had a long and satisfying relationship with his partner of many years, a relationship in which Allen finds great solace and comfort.

His initial battle with cancer began 16 years ago, when he was diagnosed with thyroid cancer. The subsequent surgeries left him with significant scarring of his neck, which impacted his self-image and sense of self. He stated, 'I felt like a fish that had been filleted.' Despite this, he felt he had overcome cancer and that the 'battle was won'. However, a routine examination three years ago revealed advanced prostate cancer. Allen stated that this 'completely overwhelmed me. I felt crushed'. He began to experience anxiety and depression, and to question the value of fighting

this battle once again. His current life felt empty and meaningless in the face of his new cancer; he felt alone and 'singled out' by having to face this challenge again. Allen began seeing a psychiatrist for help with his mood symptoms, and hence his referral to MCGP.

After the first session, Allen reported that he felt 'overwhelmed by all these other people with cancer'. He considered ending the group, but discussed this with his psychiatrist and decided to stick it out. He was relieved when other group members shared similar feelings, and he felt more connected to them. He no longer felt as alone and now, in addition to the support of his psychiatrist, he had people who understood his experience of facing cancer and possible death.

As the group progressed, Allen began to alter his world view significantly. He began to view the pressures of work, which had seemed so compelling and all-consuming, as being secondary to his own needs and quality of life. His long-standing desire to leave his work began to take on a new intensity. Session 6, which focuses on patients' feelings of responsibility to themselves and others, as well as any unfinished business, was an important turning point for Allen. 'I used to be so afraid of what I would do and who I would be. But I've battled cancer twice! If I can fight these kinds of fights, those fears really seem to pale. My work was important for me. But it's the "me" that counts here. Me and my partner count so much more.' Such a change is a good example of the type of cognitive re-structuring in the face of illness that often occurs. Allen's shift of taking into account not only himself, but his partner as well, illustrates this session's goal of enhancing patients' sense of meaning through the realisation that their lives transcend themselves and extend to others as well.

For his 'Legacy Project', Allen resolved to accomplish two goals. The first was to finish his employment and put his available resources into his relationship. The second was to begin the process of renovating his home, something he and his partner had wanted to do, but his illness had up until now prevented from occurring. Allen related that he used to think, 'I'm dying. Why bother?' His new outlook on life and his illness allowed him to view his remaining time as precious and worthy of investment. In addition, he came to the realisation that despite the anxieties and pain his illness caused, he still lived and therefore he should carry on living to the end. 'Until I go, I'm still here. Why should I stop experiencing the simple joy of still existing? I won't let it rob me of that.'

At the conclusion of the group, Allen reported that he felt it to have been of great value to him. 'I would not have seen the purpose or even the possibility of making these changes without this group and all of you.' At the two-month follow-up we conduct with patients, Allen had indeed carried out the twin goals of his 'Legacy Project'. He felt an enhanced sense of meaning in his life, and was finding it easier to cope with his illness.

12.8 Key Challenges in Application of MCGP

The key challenge in applying MCGP in an advanced cancer population is related to inflexibility, which is innate to a weekly group intervention that requires regular attendance at a specified day and time. MCGP also has specific themes that are covered weekly, with a logical progression of content as the sessions unfold. Therefore, attending all sessions is desirable. Research with palliative care populations suffers from attrition due to illness, death, conflicts with scheduling chemotherapy, diagnostic tests, other doctor appointments and brief hospitalisations. Our trials of MCGP have had attrition rates as high as 50% (interestingly, the rate is the same for Supportive Psychotherapy).

12.9 Overview of Evidence on Efficacy

Early research by Yalom, Spiegel and colleagues demonstrated that a one-year supportive-expressive group psychotherapy, which included a focus on existential issues, decreased psychological distress and improved quality of life [49–51]. More recent studies have described short-term interventions that included a spiritual or existential component, including individually-based approaches [36, 52–54]. However, results are inconsistent in their effects on depression, anxiety and desire for death. More importantly, specific aspects of spiritual well-being and meaning were not consistently targeted as outcomes. Thus, despite the seeming importance of enhancing one's sense of meaning and purpose, few clinical interventions have been developed that attempt to address this critical issue.

A randomised controlled trial of MCGP [55] demonstrated its efficacy in improving spiritual well-being and a sense of meaning, as well as in decreasing anxiety, hopelessness and desire for death. Ninety patients were randomised to either eight sessions of MCGP or Supportive Group Psychotherapy (SGP). Of the 55 patients who completed the eight-week intervention, 38 completed a follow-up assessment two months later (attrition was largely due to death or physical deterioration). Outcome assessments included measures of spiritual well-being, meaning, hopelessness, desire for death, optimism/pessimism, anxiety, depression and overall quality of life.

Results demonstrated significantly greater benefits from MCGP compared to SGP, particularly in enhancing spiritual well-being and a sense of meaning. Treatment effects for MCGP appeared even stronger two months after treatment ended, suggesting that benefits not only persist, but may grow over time. Patients who participated in SGP failed to demonstrate any such improvements, either post-treatment or at the two month follow-up assessment.

12.10 Service Development and Future Directions

While MCGP is effective for patients with advanced cancer, it is demanding, inflexible and associated with significant attrition. We therefore developed the more flexible individual format, Individual Meaning-Centred Psychotherapy (IMCP). IMCP has proved to be equally effective, but allows for flexibility in time and place (e.g. office, bedside or chemo suite) for scheduling sessions, and has significantly reduced attrition and enhanced rates of intervention completers [56]. We are currently adapting and testing MCP for other cancer populations, (e.g. early stage cancer, cancer survivors) as well as for oncology care providers [57]. Additionally, we are developing briefer forms of IMCP that can be applied to hospice populations.

12.10.1 Training

Clinicians can be readily trained to deliver MCP through one-day workshops and supervision sessions. Its psycho-educational format as a structured intervention makes mastery more straightforward, although the experience that well trained therapists bring is invaluable.

12.10.2 Manuals

Both formats of MCP – MCGP and IMCP – have been manualised, with manuals developed both for therapists and patient participants. By the end of 2011, these manuals, along with a textbook on MCP, will be available and published through Oxford University Press.

12.11 Summary

MCGP and IMCP have been developed by W. Breitbart and colleagues in the Department of Psychiatry and Behavioral Sciences, Memorial Sloan-Kettering Cancer Center. MCGP is a novel and unique intervention demonstrated to be effective in enhancing meaning and diminishing despair in advanced cancer patients.

Acknowledgement

All research, particularly intervention development, is collaborative. MCGP benefitted significantly by the contribution of Mindy Greenstein PhD, and IMCP similarly benefitted from the contribution of Shannon Poppito PhD (both of whom worked with Dr. W. Breitbart as post-doctoral research fellows). Drs Rosenfeld, Pessin and so many other research collaborators must be duly recognised as well. This work was funded by Grant # **1RO1 CA128187** from the National Cancer Institute, Grant # **1R21AT/CA0103** from the National Institute of Health-Center for Complementary and Alternative Medicine, and grants from The Fetzer Institute and The Kohlberg Foundation, all to William Breitbart, M.D. as PI.

Recommended Reading

Breitbart, W. and Heller, K.S. (2003) Reframing hope: Meaning-centered care for patients near the end-of-life. *Journal of Palliative Medicine*, **6** (6), 979–88.

Breitbart, W., Gibson, C., Poppito, S. and Berg, A. (2004) Psychotherapeutic interventions at the end-of-life: a focus on meaning and spirituality. *Canadian Journal of Psychiatry*, **49**, 366–372.

Breitbart, W., Rosenfeld, B., Gibson, C. *et al.* (2010) Meaning-centered group psychotherapy for patients with advanced cancer: a pilot randomized controlled trial. *Psycho-oncology*, **19** (1), 21–28.

Fillion, L., Duval, S., Dumont, S. *et al.* (2009) Impact of a meaning-centered intervention on job satisfaction and on quality of life among palliative care nurses. *Psycho-Oncology*, **12**, 1300–1301.

Frankl, V.F. (1959/1992) *Man's Search for Meaning*, 4th edn, Beacon Press.

References

1. Breitbart, W., Rosenfeld, B., Pessin, H. *et al.* (2000) Depression, hopelessness, and desire for hastened death in terminally ill cancer patients. *Journal of the American Medical Association*, **284**, 2907–2911.

2. Breitbart, W., Rosenfeld, B., Gibson, C. *et al.* (2010) Impact of treatment for depression on desire for hastened death in patients with advanced AIDS. *Psychosomatics*, **51**, 98–105.

3. Frankl, V.F. (1955/1986) *The Doctor and the Soul*, Random House, New York.

4. Frankl, V.F. (1959/1992) *Man's Search for Meaning*, 4th edn, Beacon Press.

5. Frankl, V.F. (1969/1988) *The Will to Meaning: Foundations and Applications of Logotherapy, Expanded Edition*, Penguin Books, New York.

6. Frankl, V.F. (1975/1997) *Man's Search for Ultimate Meaning*, Plenum Press, New York.

7. Yalom, I.D. (1980) *Existential Psychotherapy*, Baisc Books, New York.

8. Breitbart, W., Bruera, E., Chochinov, H. *et al.* (1995) Neuropsychiatric syndromes and psychiatric symptoms in patients with advanced cancer. *Journal of Pain and Symptom Management*, **10**, 131–141.

9. Breitbart, W., Chochinov, H.M. and Passik, S.D. (1998) Psychiatric aspects of palliative care, in *Oxford Textbook of Palliative Medicine*, 2nd edn (eds D. Doyle, G.W. Hanks and N. MacDonald), Oxford University Press, New York, pp. 216–246.

10. Chochinov, H.M. and Breitbart, W. (2000) *The Handbook of Psychiatry in Palliative Medicine*, Oxford University Press, New York.

11. Rousseau, P. (2000) Spirituality and the dying patient. *Journal of Clinical Oncology*, **18**, 2000–2002.

12. Puchalski, C. and Romer, A.L. (2000) Taking a spiritual history allows clinicians to understand patients more fully. *Journal of Palliative Medicine*, **3**, 129–137.

13. Portenoy, R., Thaler, H.T., Kornblith, A.B. *et al.* (1994) The Memorial Symptom Assessment Scale: an instrument for evaluation of symptom prevalence, characteristics and distress. *European Journal of Cancer*, **30A**, 1326–1336.

14. Pulchalski, C., Ferrell, B., Virani, R. *et al.* (2009) Improving the quality of spiritual care as a dimension of palliative care: the report of the consensus conference. *Journal of Palliative Medicine*, **12**, 885–904.

15. Brady, M.J., Peterman, A.H., Fitchett, G. *et al.* (1999) A case of including spirituality in quality of life measurement in oncology. *Psycho-Oncology*, **8**, 417–428.

16. Karasu, B.T. (1999) Spiritual psychotherapy. *American Journal of Psychotherapy*, **53**, 143–162.

17. Baider, L., Russak, S.M., Perry, S. *et al.* (1999) The role of religious and spiritual beliefs in coping with malignant melanoma: an Israeli sample. *Psycho-Oncology*, **8**, 27–35.

18. Koenig, H.G., Cohen, H.J., Blazer, D.G. *et al.* (1992) Religious coping and depression among elderly, hospitalized medically ill men. *American Journal of Psychiatry*, **149**, 1693–1700.

19. Koenig, H.G., George, L.K. and Peterson, B.L. (1998) Religiosity and remission of depression in medically ill older patients. *American Journal of Psychiatry*, **155**, 536–542.

20. McCullough, M.E. and Larson, D.B. (1999) Religion and depression: a review of the literature. *Twin Research*, **2**, 126–136.

21. Sloan, R.P., Bagiella, E. and Powell, T. (1999) Religion, spirituality, and medicine. *Lancet*, **353**, 664–667.

22. Brady, M.J., Peterman, A.H., Fitchett, G. *et al.* (1999) A case of including spirituality in quality of life measurement in oncology. *Psycho-Oncology*, **8**, 417–428.

23. Nelson, C., Rosenfeld, B., Breitbart, W. *et al.* (2002) Spirituality, depression and religion in the terminally ill. *Psychosomatics*, **43**, 213–220.

24. McCullough, M.E. and Larson, D.B. (1999) Religion and depression: a review of the literature. *Twin Research*, **2**, 126–136.

25. Sloan, R.P., Bagiella, E. and Powell, T. (1999) Religion, spirituality, and medicine. *Lancet*, **353**, 664–667.

26. Singer, P.A., Martin, D.K. and Kelner, M. (1999) Quality end-of-life care: patients' perspective. *Journal of the American Medical Association*, **281**, 163–168.

27. Moadel, A., Morgan, C., Fatone, A. *et al.* (1999) Seeking meaning and hope: self-reported spiritual and existential needs among an ethnically diverse cancer patient population. *Psycho-Oncology*, **8**, 1428–1431.

28. Morita, T., Tsunoda, J., Inoue, S. *et al.* (2000) An exploratory factor analysis of existential suffering in Japanese terminally ill cancer patients. *Psycho-Oncology*, **9**, 164–168.

29. Meier, D.E., Emmons, C.A., Wallerstein, S. *et al.* (1998) A National survey of physician-assisted suicide and euthanasia in the United States. *New England Journal of Medicine*, **338**, 1193–1201.

30. Brady, M.J., Peterman, A.H., Fitchett, G. *et al.* (1999) A case of including spirituality in quality of life measurement in oncology. *Psycho-Oncology*, **8**, 417–428.

31. McClain, C., Rosenfeld, B. and Breitbart, W. (2003) The influence of spirituality on end-of-life despair among terminally ill cancer patients. *Lancet*, **361**, 1603–1607.

32. Yanez, B., Edmondson, D., Stanton, A.L. *et al.* (2009) Facets of spirituality as predictors of adjustment to cancer: relative contributions of having faith and finding meaning. *Journal of Consulting and Clinical Psychology*, **77**, 730–741.

33. Watson, M., Haviland, J.J., Greer, S. *et al.* (1999) Influence of psychological response on survival in breast cancer population-based cohort study. *Lancet*, **354**, 1331–1336.

34. Breitbart, W. and Rosenfeld, B. (1999) Physician-assisted suicide: the influence of psychosocial issues. *Cancer Control*, **6**, 146–161.

35. Chochinov, H.M., Wilson, K., Enns, M. *et al.* (1994) Prevalence of depression in the terminally ill: effects of diagnostic criteria and symptom threshold judgments. *American Journal of Psychiatry*, **51**, 537–540.

36. Chochinov, H.M., Wilson, K.G., Enns, M. *et al.* (1995) Desire for death in the terminally ill. *American Journal of Psychiatry*, **152**, 1185–1191.

37. Kissane, D., Block, S., Miach, P. *et al.* (1997) Cognitive-existential group therapy for patients with primary breast cancer – techniques and themes. *Psycho-Oncology*, **6**, 25–33.

38. Park, C. and Folkman, S. (1997) Meaning in the context of stress and coping. *Review of General Psychology*, **1**, 115–144.

39. Andrykowski, M.A., Brady, M.J. and Hunt, J.W. (1993) Positive psychosocial adjustment in potential bone marrow transplant recipients: cancer as a psychosocial transition. *Psycho-Oncology*, **2**, 261–276.

40. Folkman, S. (1997) Positive psychological states and coping with severe stress. *Social Science and Medicine*, **45**, 1207–1221.

41. Taylor, S.E. (1983) Adjustment to threatening events: a theory of cognitive adaptation. *American Psychologist*, **38**, 1161–1173.

42. Taylor, E.J. (1993) Factors associated with meaning in life among people with recurrent cancer. *Oncology Nursing Forum*, **20**, 1399–1405.

43. Kierkegaard, S., Hong, H. and Hong, E. (1983) *Fear and Trembling/Repetition*, Princeton University Press, Princeton.

44. Heidegger, M. (1996) Translated by Stambaugh, J., *Being and Time*, State University of New York Press, Albany.

45. Nietzsche, F. (1986) *Human, All Too Human: A Book for Free Spirits*, Cambridge University Press, Cambridge.

46. Sartre, J.P. (1984) *Being and Nothingness*, Citadel Press, New York.

47. Schag, C.C., Heinrich, R.L. and Ganz, P.A. (1984) Karnofsky performance status revisited: reliability, validity, and guidelines. *Journal of Clinical Oncology*, **2**, 187–193.

48. National Comprehensive Cancer Network (2003) NCCN distress management clinical practice guidelines. *Journal of National Comprehensive Cancer Network*, **1**, 344–374.

49. Spiegel, D. and Yalom, I. (1978) A support group for dying patients. *International Journal of Group Psychotherapy*, **28**, 233–245.

50. Spiegel, D., Bloom, J. and Yalom, I.D. (1981) Group support for patients with metastatic breast cancer. *Archives of General Psychiatry*, **38**, 527–533.

51. Yalom, I. and Greaves, C. (1977) Group therapy with the terminally ill. *American Journal of Psychiatry*, **134**, 396–400.

52. Lee, V., Cohen, S.R., Edgar, L. *et al.* (2006) Meaning-making and psychological adjustment to cancer: development of an intervention and pilot results. *Oncology Nursing Forum*, **33**, 291–302.

53. Kissane, D.W., Bloch, S., Smith, G.C. *et al.* (2003) Cognitive-existential group psychotherapy for women with primary breast cancer: a randomised controlled trial. *Psycho-Oncology*, **12**, 532–546.

54. Coward, D.D. (2003) Facilitation of self-transcendence in a breast cancer support group: II. *Oncology Nursing Forum*, **30**, 291–300.

55. Breitbart, W., Rosenfeld, B., Gibson, C. *et al.* (2010) Meaning-centered group psychotherapy for patients with advanced cancer: a pilot randomized controlled trial. *Psycho-Oncology*, **19**, 21–28.

56. Breitbart, W., Poppito, S., Rosenfeld, B. *et al.* A randomized comparison of meaning-centered psychotherapy and massage therapy for patients with advanced cancer. *Journal of Clinical Oncology* (Under Review).

57. Fillion, L., Duval, S., Dumont, S. *et al.* (2009) Impact of a meaning-centered intervention on job satisfaction and on quality of life among palliative care nurses. *Psycho-Oncology*, **12**, 1300–1301.

13 Couple-Focused Group Intervention for Women with Early Breast Cancer and Their Partners

Sharon Manne[1] and Jamie Ostroff[2]

[1]Fox Chase Cancer Center, Cheltenham, PA, USA
[2]Department of Psychiatry and Behavioral Sciences, Memorial Sloan Kettering Cancer Center, New York, NY, USA

13.1 Background

The diagnosis and treatment of early stage breast cancer can be stressful and upsetting. Patients deal with the emotional consequences of being diagnosed with a life-threatening illness, cope with surgery, chemotherapy and radiation which can result in difficult side effects such as surgical and radiation scarring and worries about attractiveness, nausea, weight gain and fatigue. In addition to these emotional concerns, breast cancer diagnosis and treatment can result in a number of day-to-day practical stressors that patients deal with, particularly after surgery and when they undergo chemotherapy and/or radiation. These stressors include changes in family and marital roles, interference with social plans and managing household responsibilities. Even after treatment is completed, patients must negotiate the transition back to 'normal' life, deal with life long concerns about recurrence and alter their life plans and goals upon the realisation that life may be foreshortened. These experiences can take an emotional toll on some patients, both in the short- and long-term. Between 7 and 46% of women with early stage breast cancer report clinically significant levels of depressive symptoms within the first six months of diagnosis and between 32 and 45% of women report clinically significant levels of anxiety [1, 2].

A diagnosis of early stage cancer in one partner can adversely affect the other partner in similar ways. Indeed, research suggests that partners report elevated levels of depressive symptoms after diagnosis as compared with the general population [3] with between 25 and 30% of spouses reporting clinically significant levels of depression or distress [3, 4]. When comparisons with the patient diagnosed with breast cancer are conducted, some studies report similar levels of psychological distress [5], whereas other studies suggest that spousal distress exceeds that of the patient [6–8]. Distress appears to decline over time [6]. It is unclear whether such comparisons of patient and partner distress reflect gender differences in the reporting of psychological distress [9]. Nevertheless, a large body of research suggests that spouses struggle with similar worries and issues as patients – concerns about the patient's treatment side effects, worry about how she is managing her illness, worries about possible loss of their life partner, concerns about the children, worries about how to provide the best support and assistance and managing practical disruptions to day-to-day marital and family roles and responsibilities [10–18]. Recent evidence suggests that job functioning may also be detrimentally impacted in the year after diagnosis [19].

In order to deal with the many challenges and stresses of breast cancer, couples are likely to depend on one another as a key resource for both emotional and practical support. Indeed, both patients and partners typically nominate their spouse as their primary confidante [20, 21]. Unfortunately, while breast cancer

Handbook of Psychotherapy in Cancer Care, First Edition. Edited by Maggie Watson and David W. Kissane.
© 2011 John Wiley & Sons, Inc. Published 2011 by John Wiley & Sons, Inc.

can both serve as an opportunity to enhance the closeness of the marital relationship [22], it can also strain the marital relationship and reduce relationship quality [8]. To address these challenges and value the importance of the marital relationship in maintaining and enhancing psychosocial adaptation, we developed and evaluated a couple-focused group (CFG) intervention for women diagnosed with early stage breast cancer and their partners. Before describing the intervention, we describe the theoretical and empirical data guiding its development. We used two social and clinical psychology theoretical models to guide our intervention strategies: the cognitive-social-affective processing model and the interpersonal process model of intimacy. Cognitive-social-affective processing theory suggests that successful adaptation to a difficult life experience involves actively assimilating or accommodating the event into one's 'world view' which typically involves finding some meaning or purpose in the event [23, 24]. While some processing is done on an individual level, the social network can aid or interfere with effective processing [25]. As discussed by Tait and Silver [26], talking with others may facilitate successful processing through allowing the expression of emotions, by helping the person learn to tolerate aversive feelings, by provision of support and encouragement of effective coping and by direct assistance in finding meaning and benefit in the experience. In sum, significant others can also be a source of 'coping assistance', helping one to deal successfully with a difficult life event. Work by Stanton and colleagues [27] suggests that expression of emotions to a receptive social network may be particularly important for women with breast cancer. Conversely, not being able to talk about a difficult experience with one's network of family and friends because one perceives one's family or friends as overtly critical, unreceptive or uncomfortable with the topic, may place individuals at higher risk for adverse psychological reactions. Barriers to sharing the cancer experience with one's spouse may be particularly problematic because of the level of importance the spouse has as both a confidante and primary source of support [28]. Fewer opportunities to share thoughts and feelings and receive spouse feedback may result in less assistance in finding benefits and meaning, less assistance in tolerating aversive thoughts and feelings and less assistance in identifying and utilising effective coping strategies. In short, criticism and other unsupportive behaviour on the part of significant others affords individuals fewer opportunities to successfully cognitively process the event. Indeed, our studies are consistent with these explanations. We have found that the association between partner unsupportive behaviour and distress is mediated by greater utilisation of maladaptive coping mechanisms such as avoidance [29] and lower appraisals of coping efficacy [30].

Our couples' work has also been guided by relationship intimacy theories from the social psychology literature which highlights the critical role of communication and support among couples dealing with a serious life event. The Interpersonal Process Model of Intimacy [31] emphasises two fundamental components of relationship intimacy: self-disclosure and partner responsiveness [31, 32]. According to this theory, more intimate interactions occur when the person (the speaker) communicates personal information to another person (the listener) and the listener is responsive. In order to be characterised as responsive, the listener must convey that he or she understands the content of the speaker's disclosure, accepts or validates the speaker and expresses that he or she feels positively towards the speaker [31, 32]. Intimacy may also develop from personal disclosures between partners [33]. We were also guided by an older literature on the value of equity in affective self-disclosure in marriage [34–37]. These theories propose that relationship satisfaction increases with increasing levels of mutual affective self-disclosure and that equity in level of affective disclosure is an important determinant of closeness and relationship satisfaction. These theories also suggest that emotional inexpressiveness is a deterrent to the development of an intimate relationship [37, 38] because sharing feelings promotes trust and respect and willingness to make oneself vulnerable. According to all relationship intimacy theories, criticism and avoidance by either partner towards the other is damaging because it erodes perceived understanding, caring and closeness. Our findings are consistent with the Interpersonal Process Model of Intimacy and suggest that patients, who have partners who reciprocate self-disclosure [39] and who are perceived as being responsive during discussions of cancer-related concerns [40], are less distressed and perceive greater closeness with their spouses. These findings suggest that perceived responsiveness, degree of self- and perceived partner disclosure, as well as perceived empathy and caring, are important to target in a couple-focused intervention.

A number of studies bolster our focus on enhancing the quality of marital communication and relationship intimacy. Cross-sectional studies have indicated that spouse emotional support is an important correlate of patient adaptation to breast cancer [28, 41, 42]. Higher quality spousal support, particularly emotional support, is associated with lower distress (e.g. [20]). In our work, we have examined couples' support-related communication in a number of different ways, using observational and survey methods. Our results have identified three consistent aspects of couple communication about breast cancer that are linked with patient outcomes: open communication, partner responsiveness/mutual self-disclosure and partner spouse unsupportive behaviours. We have several findings suggesting that open and constructive communication is important. Mutual constructive communication, which is defined as mutual discussion of problems, expression of feelings about the problem, understanding of one another's views and feeling the issue was resolved, has also been shown to predict less distress and higher marital satisfaction in longitudinal studies [43]. In addition, we have found that patient emotional expression predicts greater posttraumatic growth among early stage breast cancer patients and patients whose husbands engage in more emotional expression report more posttraumatic growth [44]. As noted above, reciprocal disclosure is associated with lower distress on the part of patients [40], and perceived partner disclosure is associated with greater intimacy. Conversely, protective buffering, a dynamic where couples hesitate to share their concerns and fears because they do not want to upset one another [45], has been shown to be associated with increased distress among patients with early stage breast cancer and their partners [46]. Mutual avoidance, defined as the couple avoiding discussing cancer-related problems and stressors, is associated with later distress for both patients and partners [43], and demand-withdraw communication, which is defined as one partner pressuring the other to talk while the other partner withdraws from the conversation, is associated with greater distress and lower relationship satisfaction for both patients and partners [43]. Taken together, these results support the notion that open communication is beneficial to patients' short- and long-term adjustment to breast cancer and guided the development of the CFG intervention. As described more fully below, CFG incorporates strategies to assist couples in improving their cognitive, affective

and social processing of the cancer experience and enhance their ability to communicate openly and effectively with their spouse.

13.2 Intervention Strategies and Main Themes of the Couple-Focused Group (CFG)

Based on the theory and empirical data described above, CFG targets both individual-level cognitive processing of the cancer experience and couple-level communication and affective processing of the cancer experience. The intervention is conducted in a multiple couples' group format to facilitate the goal of affective and social processing, because couples can model good communication for one another, as well as provide opportunities to listen and provide support regarding concerns and issues raised by other patients and partners. The primary goals of this intervention are: (i) to facilitate psychological adaptation of both partners by improving their cognitive, affective and social processing and (ii) to improve relationship intimacy.

To achieve these aims, we use both *cognitive-behavioural* and traditional *behavioural marital enhancement* intervention strategies (e.g. [47, 48]). On an individual level, intervention content focuses on cognitive-behavioural techniques such as effective stress management (e.g. relaxation), appraising the stressor and then matching the coping strategy to the controllability of the stressful situation, choosing an effective coping strategy that fits the situation, soliciting support effectively and achieving an understanding of ways that the cancer experience has affected one's priorities and goals. On a couple-level, intervention content focuses on learning effective communication skills with a particular emphasis on constructive expression of feelings and needs and empathic listening to one's partner, enhancing communication and understanding of physical intimacy needs and maintaining a sense of normalcy in the relationship by engaging in non-cancer related relationship strengthening activities.

Psycho-educational content also included reviewing the sexual side effects of breast cancer treatments and educating the participants regarding common survivorship concerns. The group leaders use common behavioural marital therapy approaches such as in-session practice of skills with therapist observation and feedback and couple-focused home assignments. All content is specifically directed towards stressful life experiences associated with the diagnosis and treatment of breast cancer.

13.2.1 Target Groups of Patients and Partners

This treatment has been offered to women diagnosed with stage 0 (Ductal Carcinoma In Situ) to IIIA breast cancer who are in active treatment for this disease, who are married or in a committed relationship, have a partner of either gender, are English speaking, and do not have a serious psychiatric illness or active substance abuse condition. Because of its short-term nature, this is not a therapy, that is appropriate for seriously distressed relationships, and therefore the group has not been offered to couples who are separated or seriously considering divorce. We have included couples where the patient or partner is clinically distressed and we have included couples who are experiencing marital conflict or strain. We have included same-sex couples. In terms of group process, we have found that a diversity of ages, relationship durations, clinical medical experiences and ethnicities works well. Group size ranges between three and five couples. The ideal size for groups is about four couples. Sessions are 90 minutes in duration and the recommended number of sessions is six.

13.3 Evidence on Efficacy

We have initial evidence of treatment efficacy in a randomised clinical trial comparing the CFG intervention to Usual Care (UC) [49]. We approached 710 women diagnosed with early stage breast cancer for this study and 238 agreed (33.5%). Couples were randomly assigned to receive either six sessions of CFG or UC. Patients completed measures of global psychological distress, cancer-specific distress, partner unsupportive behaviours, physical impairment and a treatment evaluation pre-intervention, one week post-intervention and six months post intervention. Measures were collected from all patients, even if they did not attend sessions. No measures from partners were included in the original analyses. One hundred twenty couples were assigned to the CFG intervention arm of the study and 118 couples were assigned to the UC arm of the study. Seventy-eight couples attended between one and six group sessions (65%). Seventy-one of the 78 patients (91%) in the CFG arm who attended between one and six sessions completed the Time 2 assessment and 66 of the 78 patients (85%) in the CFG arm who attended sessions completed

the Time 3 assessment. Completion rates for Time 2 and 3 assessments among those patients not attending any group sessions was much lower (52 and 42%, respectively, for Time 2 and 3). Ninety-four patients (79.7%) in the UC arm completed the Time 2 assessment and 79 (84%) completed the Time 3 assessment. The groups were rated for treatment fidelity and achieved a high degree of fidelity (97–100%). Data were analysed using growth curve models approach [50] and an intent-to-treat approach which includes all participants who signed consents and agreed to be randomised, regardless of whether they attended sessions. We also conducted subgroup analyses comparing participants who were assigned to CFG but did not attend any group sessions. Intent-to-treat analyses evaluating depression, anxiety, loss of behavioural and emotional control, Impact of Event Scale (IES) and general well being indicated a significant group effect for reducing depressive symptoms in favour of CFG compared with UC. There were no main effects for CFG on the other outcomes. However, when possible moderating effects for partner unsupportive behaviour and physical impairment were evaluated, several moderating influences were noted. Among women who rated their partners as more unsupportive pre-intervention, women assigned to CFG reported less loss of behavioural and emotional control than women in the UC group and greater psychological well-being at follow-up. In addition, women assigned to the CFG who rated their partners as more unsupportive reported marginally lower depressive symptoms at follow-up as compared with women in UC. There was also marginally significant cancer-specific distress among women reporting more physical impairment pre-intervention in CFG as compared with UC.

Our second analyses compared those women who did and did not attend the CFG and women assigned to UC. Results indicated that women in CFG reported lower depressive symptoms, anxiety, loss of behavioural and emotional control than women assigned to CFG who did not attend sessions (CFG-Attrition, i.e. CFG-A group) and women in UC. A similar moderating effect was found for partner unsupportive behaviour on depressive symptoms, such that women who had higher than average ratings of partner unsupportive behaviour at baseline reported significantly lower depressive symptoms at follow up in the CFG group as compared with UC and CFG-A. A similar moderating effect was found for physical impairment on loss of behavioural and emotional control in that, for women participating in CFG whose impairment increased over time, there was a lower level of loss of behavioural and emotional control as compared to women in UC and CFG-A.

Overall, our results indicated that the treatment impacted women's depressive symptoms but not other indicators of distress and well-being. The group was more beneficial for women rating their partners as more unsupportive and women reporting more physical impairment. Treatment evaluation ratings were very high for patients (item $M = 3.7$ on a 5-point scale) and partners ($M = 3.7$). Patients reported that they learned something new from the group ($M = 4.2$), that they will use the skills they learned in the group in the future ($M = 3.9$), felt the topics covered were important ($M = 4.1$), and that they would recommend the group to other patients and their partners ($M = 4.8$). Similarly, partners reported that they learned something new from the group ($M = 4.7$), felt the group improved their relationship with their partner ($M = 3.5$), felt that they would use the skills that they learned in the future ($M = 3.7$) and felt the topics covered were important ($M = 4.9$).

In a second publication [51], we evaluated additional potential individual and relationship level social-cognitive factors which may alter treatment effects: emotional expression, emotional processing (e.g. trying to understand one's feelings), acceptance coping and protective buffering. Results indicated that women who began CFG reporting higher levels of emotional processing and emotional expression evidenced lower depressive symptoms compared with women who did not use either type of emotional approach coping. We did not find that pre-intervention levels of protective buffering and acceptance coping, moderated treatment effects for CFG. Overall, our results suggest that CFG is an effective group psychological intervention approach for women with breast cancer that has stronger effects on distress among women who perceive that their partners are unsupportive before the group begins and among women who begin the group with more emotionally expressive coping style. To date, we do not know whether the treatment is effective for spouses or whether non-specific treatment effects such as group cohesion or group support account for treatment effects. We also do not know what the mechanisms for treatment effects are. These questions are currently being addressed in a second randomised clinical trial.

13.4 Processes and Techniques

CFG is a highly structured and manualised treatment stipulating session content, time allowances, format,

co-facilitator roles and home assignments. A complete description of the content of each session is contained in our therapy manual [52]. The goals and highlighted summary for each group session are presented below.

During *session 1*, the group leaders introduce themselves and describe the goals, objectives, rationale and format for the groups, including home assignments. This is followed by an icebreaker exercise where couples break up and interview one another to learn about the relationship, family and important facts about the cancer. The group members then introduce another couple. The next activity is a group 'fishbowl' exercise where the patients meet in the middle of the room, while the partners observe from the outside of that circle [53]. Patients discuss the impact of cancer on themselves and their relationship. Next, partners meet in the middle of the room and discuss the impact of cancer on themselves and their relationship. Following the group discussion, the leaders ask the patients to summarise and reflect back what they heard the partners say and the partner summarise and reflect what they heard the patients say. The leaders summarise common themes and then end the group by asking members how they felt about the group, what the members' goals are for the sessions, and asking if the group participants have questions.

The theme of the *second session* is learning about signs of stress, recognising and respecting differences in how couples deal with stress and learning relaxation skills. The leaders begin the group by asking group members about any reactions they had to the first group. The primary goal of session 2 is to discuss coping with stress. The couples are asked to discuss the most challenging aspects of the cancer experience, and the leader supplements this discussion with a list of commonly experienced stressors. Next, the leader asks members to generate observable signs of heightened stress (mental, emotional, physical and relationship signs). Next, the leader discusses the importance of being able to recognise signs of stress in oneself and one's partner. The group engages in the 'Signs of Stress Activity'. During this activity, participants list both their own signs of stress and their partner's signs of stress. Next, each couple tallies how many signs of stress they correctly recognised in their partner and the couple who recognises the most signs of stress in one another wins the 'not-so-newlywed' couple of the week. The group leader asks the couples to take home the signs of stress lists that they have created and discuss together how stress affects them both individually and as a couple. They are given a list of questions to guide this discussion. In closing this session, the leader engages the group in a Focused Breathing relaxation exercise. Afterwards, the leader assigns the homework which entails the discussion of the impact of stress personally and on the relationship and practicing relaxation exercises.

The theme of the *third session* is stress and intimacy. After a review of the home assignments, the leader presents material on coping with the stress of illness and its treatment. The group discusses non-productive and productive forms of coping with cancer, reviews effective ways of coping with cancer and its treatment and the importance of respecting differences between partners in ways of coping with cancer-related stressors, as well as how to handle differences in coping styles. Next the leader brings up the topic of sexuality and cancer. A videotape is shown of a woman with breast cancer and her partner discussing how cancer has affected their sexual relationship and the patient's body image. The clip also includes discussion by health care professionals about sexuality concerns commonly raised by patients and partners. Afterwards, the group discusses their reactions to the tape as well as any personal issues raised in the video. This discussion, which is typically very brief, is followed by a presentation by the leader on the effects of the diagnosis and treatment of breast cancer on the physical intimacy aspects of the relationship. Couples are encouraged to engage one another in a discussion at home about how cancer has changed their sexual relationship and what accommodations or changes they would like to make to their sexual relationship. Next, the couples are asked to create an Intimacy Deck, which is a list of brief, inexpensive, fun activities that the couples can engage in together to enhance their closeness and enjoyment of time spent together. The couples are asked to do one activity together as a home assignment. The leaders add one activity to the intimacy deck, which is non-genital sensate focus exercise. Finally, the leader engages the group in a progressive relaxation exercise. The homework is relaxation practice, intimacy deck and sensate focus.

The *fourth session* focuses on relationship communication. After reviewing the home assignment, the leader introduces the topic of good communication, and asks group members for their thoughts about what good communication is. Afterwards the leader defines good communication, explains the two levels of communication (verbal and non-verbal) and reasons communications are less effective (communication filters). The group then discusses poor communication and the leaders review examples of unhelpful communication (e.g. cross-complaining), and ask

group members whether they can relate to any of the patterns. Specific strategies for constructive communication are discussed next, followed by an illustration of a method of conveying negative feedback, the 'X–Y–Z' statement. Several videotapes illustrating couples using both poor and constructive communication are shown, and group members are asked to identify the communication patterns they see in each video clip. Finally, the group leader reviews the Speaker–Listener skill, which is a way for couples to communicate effectively about a difficult issue or concern. Group members are given handouts containing guidelines, and an in-session exercise was to use speaker–listener to discuss a relationship concern. Leaders provide feedback to each couple during the time they break up and engage in the speaker–listener exercise. Next, the leaders conduct a guided imagery relaxation exercise. The home assignment is for the couples to use speaker–listener exercise at home to discuss a cancer-related stressor in the next week and to practice guided imagery relaxation.

The goal of *session 5* is relationship communication and support needs. After reviewing the homework, the leaders engage the couples in a discussion of reasons people may not share feelings, why it is important to share feelings, what people generally hope for when they disclose feelings and what people generally do not want when they disclose feelings. Ways of openly communicating support needs effectively are then reviewed. The leader reviewed different types of support needs that individuals diagnosed with cancer and their partners may have (e.g. needs for emotional support), and then asks each couple to privately discuss what their support needs are during the cancer experience with one another and use good communication skills during the in-session exercise. Next, the couples return to the group and discuss what it was like to listen to their partner's needs, and what might prevent them from fulfiling their partner's needs. The Caring Days exercise is introduced. Each partner is asked to create a wish list of ten small activities that they wish their partner would do for them that would bring them enjoyment. Afterwards, partners are asked to exchange wish lists and discuss the lists. The home assignment is for couples to fulfil some of the wishes during the week.

Session 6, the final session, focuses on survivorship. After reviewing the home assignment, the group leader reviews common emotional reactions that women and their partners may have to the end of active medical treatment, as well as the importance of re-evaluating life goals and priorities. Next, group members are asked to complete a priority Pie Chart together (separately from the group). This is a graphic way for the couples to illustrate their priorities as a couple before the cancer diagnosis and after the cancer diagnosis. Next, couples are asked to consider new priorities and goals they may have for the future and to discuss a 'Living with Cancer' motto together (separately from the group). After this exercise, couples are asked to share their pies and mottos and the leader interviews each couple about them.

Finally, the group leaders will wrap up the group by asking couples what their thoughts and feelings are about the final group, what they learned from the group, what the most memorable session and most useful skill learned was, what was least helpful about the group, and any additional suggestions. The leader emphasises the importance of using good communication and relaxation to manage the stresses of cancer. Couples are provided with a list of resources for cancer survivors and their loved ones and the leaders say goodbye.

13.5 Case Example

Because this intervention is delivered in a group format, we have several options for illustrating cases. We can either describe individual participant couples or describe an illustrative group. The former may best illustrate how couples work within the CFG context to acquire coping and communication skills. We will utilise a couple enrolled in the CFG intervention to illustrate several themes related to how the CFG helps couples.

Kim and Kate[1] were a same-sex couple who participated in a group consisting of three other couples. Kate, recently diagnosed with Stage 2 breast cancer, had a recent mastectomy and was undergoing radiation treatments during the group sessions. Kim was about 20 years younger than Kate. Although commitment to the relationship was very high, the level of pre-intervention relationship satisfaction was average (e.g. the patient's pre-intervention score on the Dyadic Adjustment Scale was 109 and the partner's score was 111). Both reported elevated general distress and the partner reported elevated levels of cancer-specific distress. The couple had two adopted teenage children. Both Kate and Kim were very active participants in the group. They were typically the first to provide examples and disclose relationship concerns

[1] Actual names have been changed to protect the privacy of the couple.

and issues during the group discussions and both readily engaged with the material and practiced skills during the in-session exercises and home assignments. Kate and Kim easily identified some of the relationship stresses brought about by the cancer diagnosis which included Kim's realisation that the significant age difference may result in her dealing with a disabled partner much sooner than she thought, age differences in interest in sexual activity that were exacerbated by the cancer treatment, ongoing difficulties with spending sufficient quality time together due to fatigue related to the treatment, and difficulties using constructive communication strategies when dealing with cancer-related problems. They both reported having difficulties focusing on specific problems during discussions, because both partners tended to discuss issues not related to the problem being addressed (kitchen sinking), and because both had difficulty listening and reflecting what they heard the other partner say. Both partners tended to come to negative conclusions about the other partner's intentions. During the course of the group, they were able to begin to use constructive communication skills such as listening and reflection more readily, were able to slow down their communication, and were able to listen more attentively to one another during difficult conversations. They were also able to plan time to spend more time together and to assist one another with behavioural change goals (e.g. exercising more). At the end of the group, the couple reported feeling more comfortable discussing difficult topics related to the breast cancer experience.

Like other group interventions, group dynamics can both hinder and facilitate the effectiveness of the CFG intervention. For instance, we have observed the disruptive impact of enrolling a highly conflictual couple who presents challenges to the group members and leaders in staying focused on the session format and content. Similarly, couples who present an 'overly rosy' view of the impact of cancer on their relationship often seem to alienate other group members who are overtly acknowledging the struggles of dealing with cancer and its treatment. On the other hand, it can be highly therapeutic to witness other couples who are coping with shared challenges and losses and we routinely see the powerful therapeutic effect of behavioural modelling, cathartic self-expression, mutual problem-solving and interpersonal learning.

13.6 Service Development

Each group is co-led by a therapist team. Traditionally, leaders have been social workers, psychologists or advanced psychology graduate students enrolled in clinical or counselling psychology programmes. The majority of leaders have had some group therapy experience and all have had individual therapy experience. Most therapists have some experience with cognitive behavioural therapy techniques. Few therapists have had experience working with cancer populations. Previous training in behavioural marital therapy is helpful, because this facilitates effective feedback during couples' in session communication exercises. Group leaders receive 6 hours of in-person training that consists of review of the manual and all study materials and role play exercises. Group leaders are supervised weekly after videotapes of the group have been coded for treatment fidelity. Fidelity to the CFG treatment model has been good but leaders typically have required ongoing supervision to ensure that all session topics are covered. Because this group intervention has been evaluated only in the research setting, we have paid careful attention to the degree to which the leaders adhere to the treatment manual. In a purely clinical setting, where the level of adherence to the treatment would not be as closely monitored, it is not clear whether the treatment would remain efficacious. This conclusion would await an effectiveness trial, which has not been conducted.

Group sessions are co-facilitated with co-therapists rotating the leadership of a specific session and the co-leader keeping the time and facilitating the in-session exercises. The co-leader closely observes treatment session goals and tracks process so as to attend to any session material, that is overlooked by the main leader. Group leaders typically debrief after sessions and check in with one another between groups.

Attendance for each group has been confirmed by the study staff. In addition, the group schedule is set by research staff in advance, and, in most cases, groups are held weekly. If one partner cannot make the group, then the other partner is told they can attend alone. We have rescheduled groups when one or more partners or couples cannot attend. In our experience, it is difficult to conduct in-session dyadic communication exercises when one partner in a couple does not attend. CFG is run as a closed group. That is, new couples cannot join after the initial group session.

In terms of difficult situations, there are several common situations that are challenging for the group leaders. The first, and most common, issue is low group participation secondary to disrupted or curtailed attendance. Unfortunately, this situation leads to a group, that is too 'didactic', less engaged and not well-bonded. To address this, leaders can use a more conversational style to engage couples in the material. Typically, leaders ask group members for their thoughts and personal examples. Thorough pre-group evaluation and orientation with interested couples is essential for establishing realistic expectations and securing firm commitment for group participation.

The second situation that arises is when the group goes off topic and it is difficult to re-engage them in the group material. While the non-relevant topics can be interesting for the group members, it is important to try to find some relevance of the topic being discussed as a way of leading members back to the topic. The third difficult situation is the couple who has an overt relationship conflict in the group. In over five years of conducting groups, we have not found this to be a common event as these couples typically opt out of participation. However, if it does occur we typically normalise this in the group and attempt to address the conflict during an in-session exercise where the group leader can utilise the time to facilitate good communication about the topic causing conflict. We have referred couples to marital therapy after the group session.

The final challenge is when couples do not complete home assignments. Because this is a skill-based therapy, it is important for couples to complete home assignments and we recommend emphasising this point during group orientation. As is the case in any behavioural therapy, our strategy is to review the home assignments with the entire group present, reinforce completion, trouble shoot barriers to completion and then emphasise importance of completion of home assignments.

13.7 Summary

We have developed and evaluated the efficacy of a CFG intervention for women diagnosed with early stage breast cancer and their partners. In the research context, we have found that the CFG group intervention results in lower levels of distress among patients, particularly among those patients reporting that their partners were unsupportive prior to the onset of the group. Couples report enjoying the groups and benefiting from the communication and stress management skills they learn. In a research context, we have been able to maintain relatively high levels of group attendance and high levels of treatment fidelity.

There are a number of challenges to transferring this CFG therapy model to the clinical setting. These issues include the fact that our uptake was not exceptionally high (33.5% of couples accepted). We do not know what the level of interest would be in such a group in the community oncology setting. We also do not know whether therapists working solely in a clinical context would maintain fidelity to treatment, and, if fidelity was low, whether the treatment would remain effective. These questions will require an effectiveness trial, which has not been conducted to date.

13.8 Supporting Materials

Each session has handouts for participants. All handouts are contained in our participant manual [53].

Acknowledgements

This work was supported by R01 CA 78084 from the National Cancer Institute and an Established Investigator in Cancer Prevention and Control Award (K05 CA109008) awarded to Sharon Manne.

References

1. Gallagher, J., Parle, M. and Cairns, D. (2002) Appraisal and psychological distress six months after diagnosis of breast cancer. *British Journal of Health Psychology*, **7**, 365–376.

2. Omne-Ponten, M., Holmberg, L., Burns, T. *et al.* (1992) Determinants of the psycho-social outcome after operation for breast cancer. Results of a prospective comparative interview study following mastectomy and breast conservation. *European Journal of Cancer*, **28A** (6-7), 1062–1067.

3. Bigatti, S.M., Wagner, C.D., Lydon-Lam, J.R. *et al.* (2010) Depression in husbands of breast cancer patients: relationships to coping and social support. *Support Care Cancer*.

4. Segrin, C., Badger, T., Sieger, A. *et al.* (2006) Interpersonal well-being and mental health among male partners of women with breast cancer. *Issues Mental Health Nursing*, **27** (4), 371–389, http://www.springerlink.com/content/e24uh40x1t673028.

5. Northouse, L.L. and Swain, M.A. (1987) Adjustment of patients and husbands to the initial impact of breast cancer. *Nursing Research*, **36** (4), 221–225.

6. Baider, L., Ever-Hadani, P., Goldzweig, G. *et al.* (2003) Is perceived family support a relevant variable in psychological distress? A sample of prostate and breast cancer couples. *Journal of Psychosomatic Research*, **55**, 453–460.

7. Foy, S. and Rose, K. (2001) Men's experiences of their partner's primary and recurrent breast cancer. *European Journal of Oncology Nursing*, **5** (1), 42–48.

8. Langer, S., Abrams, J. and Syrjala, K. (2003) Caregiver and patient marital satisfaction and affect following hematopoietic stem cell transplantation: a prospective, longitudinal investigation. *Psycho-Oncology*, **12** (3), 239–253.

9. Hagedoorn, M., Sanderman, R., Bolks, H.N. *et al.* (2008) Distress in couples coping with cancer: a meta-analysis and critical review of role and gender effects. *Psychological Bulletin*, **134** (1), 1–30.

10. Ben-Zur, H., Gilbur, O. and Lev, S. (2001) Coping with breast cancer: patient, spouse, and dyad models. *Psychosomatic Medicine*, **63**, 32–39.

11. Fletcher, K.A., Lewis, F.M. and Haberman, M.R. (2009) Cancer-related concerns of spouses of women with breast cancer. *Psycho-Oncology*, **19** (10), 1094–101. [E-pub ahead of print].

12. Hilton, B.A., Crawford, J.A. and Tarko, M.A. (2000) Men's perspectives on individual and family coping with their wives' breast cancer and chemotherapy. *Western Journal of Nursing Research*, **22** (4), 438–459.

13. Hoskins, C.N. (1995) Adjustment to breast cancer in couples. *Psychological Reports*, **77** (2), 435–454.

14. Lethborg, C.E., Kissane, D.W. and Burns, W.I. (2003) 'It's Not the Easy Part': the experience of significant others of women with early stage breast cancer, at treatment completion. *Social Work in Health Care*, **37** (1), 63–85.

15. Longman, A.J., Braden, C.J. and Mishel, M.H. (1996) Side effects burden in women with breast cancer. *Cancer Practice*, **4** (5), 274–280.

16. Northouse, L.L. (1992) Psychological impact of the diagnosis of breast cancer on the patient and her family. *Journal of the American Medical Women's Association*, **47** (5), 161–164.

17. Northouse, L.L., Dorris, G. and Charron-Moore, C. (1995) Factors affecting couples' adjustment to recurrent breast cancer. *Social Science and Medicine*, **41** (1), 69–76.

18. Wellisch, D.K., Jamison, K.R. and Pasnau, R.O. (1978) Psychosocial aspects of mastectomy: II. the man's perspective. *American Journal of Psychiatry*, **135** (5), 543–546.

19. Sjovall, K., Attner, B., Lithman, T. *et al.* (2010) Sick leave of spouses to cancer patients before and after diagnosis. *Acta Oncologica*, **49** (4), 467–473.

20. Pistrang, N. and Barker, C. (1995) The partner relationship in psychological response to breast cancer. *Social Science and Medicine*, **40**, 789–797.

21. Maunsell, E., Guay, S., Yandoma, E. *et al.* (2009) Patterns of confidant use among patients and spouses in the year after breast cancer. *Journal of Cancer Survivorship*, **3** (4), 202–211.

22. Dorval, M., Guay, S., Mondor, M. *et al.* (2005) Couples who get closer after breast cancer: frequency and predictors in a prospective investigation. *Journal of Clinical Oncology*, **15**, 3588–3596.

23. Horowitz M.J. (1986) *Stress Response Syndromes*, 2nd edn, Jason Aronson Press, Northvale, NJ.

24. Janoff-Bulman, R. (1992) *Shattered Assumptions: Towards a New Psychology of Trauma*, Free Press, New York.

25. Clark, L.F. (1993) Stress and the cognitive-conversational benefits of social interaction. *Journal of Social and Clinical Psychology*, **12**, 25–55.

26. Tait, R. and Silver, R.C. (1989) Coming to terms with major negative life events, in *Unintended Thought* (eds J.S. Uleman and J.A. Bargh), Guilford, New York, pp. 351–382.

27. Stanton, A., Danoff-Burg, S., Cameron, C. *et al.* (2000) Emotionally expressive coping predicts psychological and physical adjustment to breast cancer. *Journal of Consulting and Clinical Psychology*, **68** (5), 875–882.

28. Pistrang, N. and Barker, C. (1992) Disclosure of concerns in breast cancer. *Psycho-Oncology*, **1**, 183–192.

29. Manne, S.L., Alfieri, T., Taylor, K. and Dougherty, J. (1999) Spousal negative responses to cancer patients: the role of social restriction, spouse mood and relationship satisfaction. *Journal of Consulting and Clinical Psychology*, **67** (3), 352–361.

30. Manne, S.L. and Glassman, M. (2000) Perceived control, coping efficacy and avoidant coping as mediators between spouses' unsupportive behaviors and cancer patients' psychological distress. *Health Psychology*, **19** (2), 155–164.

31. Reis, H. and Shaver, P.R. (1988) Intimacy as an interpersonal process, in *Handbook of Personal Relationships: Theory, Research and Interventions* (ed. S. Duck), John Wiley & Sons, Inc., New York, pp. 367–389.

32. Reis, R. and Patrick, B. (1996) Attachment and intimacy: component processes, in *Social Psychology: Handbook of Basic Principles* (eds E. Higgins and A. Kruglanski), John Wiley & Sons, Ltd, England, pp. 523–563.

33. Perlman, D. and Fehr, B. (1987) The development of intimate relationships, in *Intimate Relationships: Development, Dynamics and Deterioration* (eds D. Pearlman and S.W. Duck), Sage, Beverly Hills, CA, pp. 219–230.

34. Worthy, M., Gary, A.L. and Kahn, G.M. (1969) Self-disclosure as an exchange process. *Journal of Personality and Social Psychology*, **3**, 59–63.

35. Davidson, B., Balswick, J. and Halverson, C. (1983) Affective self-disclosure and marital adjustment: a test of equity theory. *Journal of Marriage and the Family*, **45**, 93–102.

36. Jorgensen, S.R. and Gaudy, J.C. (1980) Self-disclosure and satisfaction in marriage: the relation examined. *Family Relations*, **29**, 281–287.

37. Balswick, J. and Peek, C. (1970) The inexpressive male and family relationships during early adulthood. *Sociological Symposium*, **1** (4), 1–12.

38. Balswick, J. (1981) Inexpressiveness as a role behavior for men, in *Men in Difficult Times* (ed. R. Lewis), Random House, New York, pp. 105–125.

39. Manne, S.L., Ostroff, J., Rini, C. *et al.* (2004) The interpersonal process model of intimacy: the role of self-disclosure, partner disclosure and partner responsiveness in interactions between breast cancer patients and their partners. *Journal of Family Psychology*, **18**, 589–599.

40. Manne, S.L., Ostroff, J., Winkel, G. *et al.* (2005) Partner unsupportive responses, avoidant coping, and distress among women with early stage breast cancer: patient and partner perspectives. *Health Psychology*, **24** (6), 635–641.

41. Giese-Davis, J., Hermanson, K. and Koopman, C. (2000) Quality of couples' relationship and adjustment to metastatic breast cancer. *Journal of Family Psychology*, **14** (2), 251–266.

42. Zemore, R. and Shepel, L.F. (1989) Effects of breast cancer and mastectomy on emotional support and adjustment. *Social Science Medicine*, **28**, 19–27.

43. Manne, S.L., Ostroff, J., Norton, T. *et al.* (2006) Cancer-related relationship communication in couples coping with early stage breast cancer. *Psycho-Oncology*, **15** (3), 234–247.

44. Manne, S.L., Ostroff, J., Winkel, G. *et al.* (2004) Posttraumatic growth after breast cancer: patient, partner, and couple perspectives. *Psychosomatic Medicine*, **66**, 442–454.

45. Coyne, J.C. and Smith, D.A. (1991) Couples coping with a myocardial infarction: a contextual perspective on wives' distress. *Journal of Personal and Social Psychology*, **61** (3), 404–412.

46. Manne, S.L., Norton, T.R., Ostroff, J.S. *et al.* (2007) Protective buffering and psychological distress among couples coping with breast cancer: the moderating role of relationship satisfaction. *Journal of Family Psychology*, **21** (3), 380–388.

47. Floyd, F.J. and Markman, H. (1995) Preventive intervention and relationship enhancement, in *Clinical Handbook of Couple Therapy* (eds N.S. Jacobson and A.S. Gurman), The Guilford Press, New York.

48. Gottman, J. and Notarius, C. (1976) *Couples Guide to Communication*, Research Press.

49. Manne, S., Ostroff, J., Winkel, G. *et al.* (2005) Couple-focused group intervention for women with early stage breast cancer. *Journal of Consulting and Clinical Psychology*, **73** (4), 634–646.

50. Moskowitz, D.S. and Hershberger, S.L. (2002) *Modeling Intraindividual Variability with Repeated Measures Data*, Lawrence Erlbaum Associates, Mahwah, NJ.

51. Manne, S.L., Ostroff, J. and Winkel, G. (2007) Social-cognitive processes as moderators of a couple-focused group intervention for women with early stage breast cancer. *Health Psychology*, **26** (6), 735–744.

52. Manne, S.L. and Ostroff, J. (2008) *Coping with Breast Cancer: A Couples-Focused Group Intervention: Therapy Guide*, Oxford University Press, New York.

53. Manne, S.L. and Ostroff, J. (2008) *Coping with Breast Cancer: Workbook for Couples*, Oxford University Press, New York.

Section C

Couple and Family Therapies

14 Couples Therapy in Advanced Cancer: Using Intimacy and Meaning to Reduce Existential Distress

Talia I. Zaider and David W. Kissane

Department of Psychiatry and Behavioral Sciences, Memorial Sloan-Kettering Cancer Center, New York, NY, USA

14.1 Introduction

There are things that I feel we don't talk about and ... I understand why ... but I feel like I – it's something I'd like to – I would like to use some of our time ... [pause] We don't talk about me dying ... and I'd like to (Patient, Case 009)

We don't talk about the essence of it ... that this person that perhaps you love is not going to be here anymore. I hit the surface with you [turns to husband] but I can't really talk about it with you because you talk me out of it (Patient, Case 019)

In each excerpt above, a family member with advanced cancer makes a courageous bid for open and direct conversation about their death. Yet the grief and existential threat associated with such conversations can easily overwhelm the most well functioning couple, giving rise to a host of dilemmas: How will we sustain and deepen intimacy while preparing for loss? How will we savour and enrich our lives while we face an uncertain future? How will we accommodate the demands of illness while preserving our identity and honouring our history together? How will we continue to give and receive mutually when our roles have been severely skewed?

In this chapter, we present a brief model of couples therapy, called Intimacy and Meaning-Making Couples Therapy (IMMCT), that strives to optimise communication about these concerns, while helping the couple identify, affirm and 'keep in circulation' [1] sources of relational meaning that counter the distress which these dilemmas bring.

14.1.1 Why Work with the Couple?

When asked what constitutes a 'good death', family caregivers, cancer patients and health care professionals alike have described a common set of needs that include good symptom management, collaborative decision-making, preparation for death, sense of life completion, support and affirmation of the whole person [2, 3]. A closer look reveals that relational concerns predominate across these domains. Valued experiences include saying goodbye, being able to spend time with and confide in intimate others, resolving longstanding conflicts and feeling that one is of value to others.

The psychosocial impact of cancer can be construed in relational terms [4, 5]. Indeed, couples affected by cancer often function as an interdependent emotional unit, such that their needs, goals and emotional responses are correlated and mutually influencing [6]. Furthermore, the quality of the relationship is strongly associated with the psychological adaptation of each individual, both in the period close to death and well into bereavement [4, 7, 8]. When it

Handbook of Psychotherapy in Cancer Care, First Edition. Edited by Maggie Watson and David W. Kissane.
© 2011 John Wiley & Sons, Inc. Published 2011 by John Wiley & Sons, Inc.

is mutually supportive and communicative, the intimate relationship can be a crucial, distress-buffering resource for both parties [9].

For this reason, there has been increased interest in approaching the psychosocial care of the cancer patient with a relational lens. Yet, in the oncology setting, advanced cancer patients and their significant others are typically offered support separately, with services delivered in an individualised or support group format. Conjoint, couple-based interventions in end-of-life care have been largely underutilised and understudied [10]. This stands in contrast to the proliferation of supportive interventions tested for couples coping with early stage cancers [11]. The lack of couples-based support at the end-of-life leaves a potential resource untapped, as the close relationship shared by patient and partner is often the primary context in which distress is regulated, end-of-life wishes and priorities are defined and meaning-making is nurtured or constrained. The emphasis on themes of caregiving, anticipated loss and existential concerns differentiates the support of advanced-stage couples from early-stage interventions [7].

14.1.2 Whom Do We Target?

The model of couples therapy presented here targets the distress carrying dyad. This follows a growing trend in psycho-oncology to limit delivery of supportive interventions to individuals and families with the greatest need, while respecting the inherent resilience of those who are able to cope independently. For example, following an initial trial of Family Focused Grief Therapy (FFGT), a relationally-based intervention delivered to families of cancer patients in palliative care, effect sizes were strongest for the most distressed families and significant improvements were noted for individuals with the top 10% of scores on the Brief Symptom Inventory (BSI) or Beck Depression Inventory (BDI) at baseline [12]. Similarly, an intervention to promote problem solving skills in caregivers was found to be effective only for the distressed sub-sample [13]. In their review of interventions for caregivers in palliative care, Harding and Higginson [14] concluded that broad delivery of supportive interventions lacks evidence to support benefit, and that greater promise lies with targeted interventions that identify a significantly distressed or depressed sub-group.

Distress can include elevated symptoms of anxiety or depression, but does not necessarily imply the presence of a DSM-IV diagnosis. Couples are thus identified for couples therapy either by referral from the oncologist, nurse or social worker, or through a preventive screening process whereby scores on surveys such as the BSI [15] are used to determine clinical 'caseness'. Distress may be present to a large degree in one partner (the so-called 'symptom bearer'), which is sometimes suggestive of complementary relationship processes. Regardless of the source of distress, intervening at the relational level serves to strengthen the couples' capacity to 'metabolise' distress by empowering each partner to draw comfort from the relationship. Advanced illness and loss present distinct challenges for all couples, but can be particularly challenging for couples who have had limited capacity to comfort each other to begin with. As noted by McWilliams, 'It is very painful to say goodbye when you are vaguely aware of not having said a satisfactory 'hello' to the other person' [16].

Documented rates of clinically significant distress reported by cancer patients and their partners range from 15 to 50%, with increased rates and worsened quality-of-life noted as the illness progresses [17, 18]. In a longitudinal study of couples affected by prostate cancer, the majority of which had advanced disease, approximately 23% had at least one partner who scored above threshold on the BSI and partners appeared to be particularly vulnerable, with 22% meeting DSM-IV criteria for major depression or an anxiety disorder [19]. Furthermore, across a six month period, partners reported a decline in significant marital quality, with 25% perceiving reduced teamwork, 18% reporting poor communication and 17% perceiving excessive conflict [19].

14.2 Integrating Meaning-Making and Intimacy: Working Models

As notions of meaning-making and intimacy underpin the intervention model presented here, we elaborate below on theoretical models that help define these constructs.

14.2.1 Meaning-Making

Susan Folkman's [20] seminal study of caregiving partners of men with AIDS yielded the important insight that alongside the intense grief and emotional pain associated with illness and loss, it is possible, even common, for loved ones caring for a dying partner to experience positive emotional states. This capacity for positive emotional experiences in the face of adversity has been understood as the outcome of meaning-based coping, a term that describes a range of coping strategies such as reordering one's life priorities, infusing ordinary events with positive meaning, and drawing on one's beliefs, values and existential goals (e.g. purpose in life) to sustain well-being during a difficult life event. Park and Folkman [21] developed a model of meaning-making, wherein people engage in meaning-making efforts when their appraisal of a stressful event is discrepant with their global beliefs, goals, priorities and sense of purpose in life. Most research and theoretical work on meaning-making in the face of adversity has emphasised intrapsychic processes [22]. An exception to this is the work of Lepore [23], who demonstrated the important role of social relationships in hindering or facilitating a person's capacity for growth, benefit finding and cognitive processing in the setting of a severe stressor.

How do we understand the process of meaning-making in a relational context? Patterson and Garwick [24] developed the notion of *family meanings*, which they define as the 'interpretations, images and views that have been collectively constructed by family members as they interact with each other, as they share time, space and life experience and as they talk with each other and dialogue about these experiences' (p. 2). Theirs is a systemic and social constructivist definition, according to which meaning-making *requires* interaction, and is the emergent property of the family-as-a-whole, rather than belonging to any one member. They describe three levels of family meaning, which move from most concrete and observable, to most abstract and implicit:

1. Meanings pertaining to the situation at hand (i.e. immediate, subjective appraisals of the stressful event, why it happened, who is responsible for managing it, what demands will be faced and whether resources exist to meet these demands);

2. Meanings pertaining to family identity (i.e. the family's view of itself, including implicit relationship rules, routines, rituals and role assignments);

3. Meanings pertaining to the family's world view (i.e. how the family views the outside world and their purpose in it, including their shared ideology, shared control, trust in others, sense of coherence and meaningfulness).

Whether viewed as an individual effort or an interpersonal process, there is increased recognition that a person's efforts to find meaning during a serious life event occur in a social context, and are shaped by social transactions that can restrict or enable this process. In IMMCT, the couple is invited to find meaning at the end-of-life together, through a shared, deeply relational process.

14.2.2 Intimacy

Our work is guided by two conceptualisations of intimacy. One is the widely cited Interpersonal Process Model of Intimacy [25], according to which intimacy is something we *feel* when we engage in mutual disclosure (sharing of thoughts or feelings with one another), and experience mutual responsiveness (feeling cared for, accepted and understood). The premise that these two components (disclosure and responsiveness) culminate in feelings of intimacy during couples' interactions has garnered considerable empirical support [26], and has been shown to take effect in couples affected by breast cancer [27]. The implication for our model of therapy is that to build or sustain intimacy, we must help couples become curious about and accepting of one another's thoughts, concerns and fears. We thus use circular questioning ([28]; also see Chapter 16 on FFGT) to encourage each partner to consider the other's experience and facilitate open expression of feelings. Intimacy has secondly been construed as something we *do*, a relational act (not necessarily verbal), that is performed in a particular context and moment [29]. Thus, couples may broadly describe their relationship as close, having enjoyed many years of companionship, yet still struggle to 'do' intimacy in the context of advanced illness. Common constraints to intimacy in this setting would include protectiveness (e.g. desire to avoid distressing topics), a wish to remain hopeful (e.g. desire to avoid consideration of future outlook) or pre-emptive distancing as a way to manage anticipatory grief. In his behavioural model of intimacy, James Cordova [30] emphasised that an intimate interaction is one in which behaviour that is interpersonally 'vulnerable' (i.e. acting or speaking in ways that risks disapproval), is reinforced in the relationship. When vulnerable behaviour (e.g. expressing 'soft' feelings, such as sadness, shame, anxiety) is validated and encouraged more often than it is punished, partners experience greater intimacy. An accumulation of such experiences produces an affective climate in which partners feel comfortable expressing a broad range of thoughts and feelings. In the model of couple therapy described here, intimate interactions are 'performed' during sessions when we facilitate the expression of vulnerable feelings about illness and empower the couple to take the risk of drawing comfort from one another, even when the likelihood of separation through loss is acknowledged.

Weingarten [29] proposed a definition of intimacy that incorporates meaning-making as a central feature, without privileging verbal disclosure over nonverbal interactions. Weingarten suggests that an intimate interaction cannot be judged by the degree or content of disclosure per se, but rather the extent to which the interaction carries a meaning, that is shared, understood and constructed by *both partners*:

'Intimate interaction occurs when people share meaning or co-create meaning and are able to coordinate their actions to reflect their mutual meaning-making. Meaning can be shared through writing, speech, gesture or symbol. In the process of co-creating meaning, individuals have the experience of knowing and being known by the other' [29, p. 7].

14.3 Processes: Structure and Overview of Therapy

IMMCT is a brief intervention targeting couples in which one partner is facing advanced illness and one or both partners are experiencing high levels of psychological distress. The *goals* of IMMCT are to (i) improve psychological adjustment of the distressed partner(s) and (ii) reduce existential distress. We work towards these goals by strengthening intimacy (e.g. facilitating shared disclosure of concerns about the future, building effective support processes, facilitating sharing of grief) and promoting meaning-making, especially at the relational level (e.g. reviewing relational priorities and wishes, building a relational legacy). We work with couples across four 'core' sessions, the first two held one week apart, and the second two held two to three weeks apart. This spacing between sessions is designed to give couples time to integrate and reinforce what is learned in therapy. An additional two 'maintenance' sessions may be offered at one to two month intervals to affirm the couples' progress and review set-backs or unresolved areas of concerns.

14.3.1 Session Content

Session content is distributed as follows:

- Session 1: Eliciting the story of cancer, understanding its impact on individual and couple adaptation, identifying relevant domains for future focus.
- Session 2: Conducting a genogram assessment and relational life review, with a goal of identifying values and patterns of relating inherited from prior

generations, as well as models of resilience and adaptation to loss that are evident in the couples' history.

- Session 3: Identifying sources of meaning, improving communication about difficult topics and discussing the legacy project.
- Session 4: Consolidation, reviewing support processes, anticipating future concerns and set backs.

14.3.2 The Therapist's Style

The following points highlight the key ways in which the therapist facilitates this model of therapy:

- The therapist uses his or her warmth to forge a trusting relationship with the couple that becomes increasingly open to exploration and deepens understanding of their relational world.

- The therapist strives to remain neutral in relationship to the couple, consciously avoiding an unequal alliance with either party. Should this stance of neutrality be put aside temporarily for therapeutic intent, it will be redressed with a reciprocal movement that re-establishes the neutral position for the greater benefit of the couple-as-a-whole.

- The therapist facilitates rather than teaches, so that what is incorporated from any session's material is chosen by the couple rather than imposed by the therapist.

- Open ended questions from the therapist will be linear, circular and strategic in style as commonly used in systemic therapies (see Chapter 16 on FFGT).

- Summaries are balanced and inclusive of both sides, reflecting strengths alongside issues or concerns. The couple is typically invited to extend, confirm or amend any summary until consensus is reached about the understanding of any lived experience.

- The therapist takes responsibility for the process of the therapy, explains steps along the way and moderates the pace of therapy in response to the needs and understanding of each individual couple. In this way, the therapist outlines the goals of the therapy, its structure, arranges appointments and monitors the time spent on different sections of the model.

- As the therapy is with distressed couples, the therapist liaises actively with the treating oncologist about symptom management issues, the need for medication, including psychotropic treatment of clinical depression or anxiety.

14.3.3 Main Themes

Three content areas relevant to couples facing advanced disease are addressed: (i) loss and grief; (ii) existential distress and meaning-making and (iii) relationship skew. These domains are described below, followed by case examples to illustrate the therapeutic processes and couple exercises used.

14.3.3.1 Loss and Grief

Loss is experienced universally in advanced cancer and is derived from several sources. The illness brings loss of wellness, with the usual expectations for a long life being cast aside with its many dreams. Body integrity may be lost with disfigurement exemplified by mastectomy, colostomy or amputation of a limb. Alteration of the face from surgery for head and neck cancers can profoundly change body image, inducing deep shame at one's appearance. Weight loss from cancer cachexia syndrome can be accompanied by a growing sense of frailty, fatigue and ability to pursue one's career and interests. Several social losses follow as physical weakness restricts capacity to mix with friends and travel.

Anti-cancer treatments add further to this cumulative experience of loss as side-effects are generated, illustrated by neuropathic pain from chemotherapy, xerostomia from radiation, hot flushes from hormonal ablation, fistulae and wound breakdown from surgeries... the list could go on. Many of the simple pleasures of life found in tasting food, swallowing a drink, enjoying sex, reading a book, listening to music and walking freely can be forfeited or impaired.

Accompanying progressive illness is the loss of any perceived sense of certainty, loss of control over life's taken-for-granted choices, loss of mastery of many skills and talents developed through the years – losses that stack up to deepen the sadness brought by such change and create the potential for anguish and despair about what lies ahead. Several fears may follow, including the fear of being dependent, a burden to one's family, of suffering and of a painful death. A sense of futility about continued living can lead to a desire for hastened death.

14.3.3.2 Dealing with Loss and Grief

A sound principle for therapists working with advanced cancer patients and their partners is to acknowledge the grief first. It is always there, albeit sometimes concealed by a brave smile or merry disposition. Naming the grief is helpful to many who feel the sadness, but have not made the intellectual connection to the process of mourning. When couples recognise the normality of their grief and begin to share it, they deepen their intimacy through efforts to mutually support one another. Such trusting communication of what hurts and what they fear tends to unite the couple as long as well-intentioned avoidance (the common protective motivation) can be overcome.

Couples express grief differently, and hence consideration of who expresses these feelings easily, who with difficulty, the role of sharing and the benefit of reciprocal support become important patterns to explore. Therapists used to individual psychotherapy will naturally move towards offering their own empathic support for any distressed individual. While there is no harm in such compassionate care, a therapist is potentially more effective when they succeed in fostering mutual support within the couple's relationship. Questions help here:

'What helps Sue when you see her crying?' 'How do you know when to comfort and when to withdraw?' 'What helps and what hinders your conversation about grief?' 'Who tends to ask the other for a hug?'

A therapeutic goal for a couple struggling with grief is to have them adopt the observer's meta-position, from which they can identify respective needs for comfort, patterns of avoidance or withdrawal, tendency to problem-solving instead of emotional support or any cultural or family style of coping. Choice is empowered by helping them to better understand each other's need for support and preferred coping style.

In such work, therapists need skill at differentiating grief from depression, recognising coping styles, tracking expressions of ambivalence (e.g. suicidal thought), acknowledging and helping refocus maladaptive anger, and pacing the session to address mutual needs. When differential coping patterns are evident, these are named to promote acceptance. Use of reflexive and strategic questions foster adaptive coping responses (see Chapter 16 on FFGT).

14.3.3.3 Existential Distress

Challenges that arise from the very givens of our human existence are known as existential issues,

Table 14.1	Existential challenges met by couples in the setting of advanced cancer	
Existential challenge	**Nature of distress**	**Features of adaptation**
Death	Death anxiety	Courage and focus on living life out to fullest
Loss	Complicated grief	Adaptive mourning, with openness to creativity
Freedom	Loss of control	Acceptance of frailty and loss of independence
Self/dignity	Threat to self worth	Maintain self worth despite disfigurement
Aloneness	Isolation and alienation	Accompaniment by partner, family and friends
Meaning	Demoralisation	Sense of fulfilment with celebration
Unknowable/mystery	Spiritual despair	Reverence for the sacred

and serve as a common source of distress [31, 32]. Table 14.1 lists these, with the form of related distress that comes from each existential challenge and the usual pathway through which couples cope and adapt. While conceptually these can be experienced individually, they are commonly shared, with the couple better able to grapple with each issue through mutual support and discussion.

Therapists do well to put names to these existential challenges as they hear couples give voice to them, so that there is acknowledgement of the normality and universality of each theme, with subsequent exploration of the coping approach that the couple feels will best help them to move forward.

Death Anxiety

Fear of the process of dying or the state of being dead is readily exacerbated by pessimism, selective attention to the negative, magnification and catastrophisation. In most couples, one party will tend to the more negative style, and the help of the other can be enlisted as a co-therapist to reframe negative cognitions as realistically as one can. Thus, 'Yes, one day we will all die. Should we spoil the living with constant worry about that prospect? Or can we use the truth of our mortality to harness energy into living well in the present moment?'

Uncertainty

In truth, we live every day with considerable amounts of uncertainty. Therapists can use this reality to invite couples to consider hypothetical scenarios that clarify their priorities and wishes. 'What would you do if you had one full year to live?' 'If it was only six months, how might this change?' 'If you only had three months, what becomes your first priority?' In this so-called 'Hypothetical Timeline Exercise', the couple is asked to reflect on three such hypothetical scenarios and to discuss how they would fill their time accordingly: what events, people, relationships or pastimes would be most important to them? Take time to explore

how well each party understands the other's priorities and help them to mutually consider each other's needs. A case example is described below (see Section 14.4).

Obsessional Control

When threatened by the experience of loss of control, expectations about what should and ought to be come to the fore. How has the couple negotiated differing expectations in the past? Can 'all-or-nothing' thinking be seen in their comments? How do they help each other exercise control over what remains within their mastery and let go of things they can no longer influence?

Unfairness

Assumptive beliefs about the need for a just world are common, including a just god, and deep frustration can be felt by couples who perceive the illness and its treatment as unfair. Regrettably, illness has never respected person, age or timing in the life cycle. It never has been fair! Hopefully one party will hold less rigid expectations about the functioning of nature, enabling their views to be held in balance with those sensing deep unfairness. Thus the competency of one partner is used to help achieve a shift in the cognitions of the other.

Fear of Being a Burden

Here, for every couple, there is a natural balance between giving and receiving, together with the reality of aging. Can care-giving be talked about openly, so that any strain is acknowledged, the support of adult children and friends welcomed and the necessity of respite understood? Loving reassurance by a supportive family can be responded to with expressions of gratitude.

Disfigurement and Dignity

Use of cognitive distortions that include negative labelling and stereotyping can induce embarrassment and deep shame. Drawing out the narrative of who the ill person is, naming the strengths of their character, affirming their accomplishments and highlighting the commitment evident in the relationship help to shore up resilience as a counter to any sense of loss of worth. For couples, the perception of the onlooker can be worse than the experience of the patient. Nevertheless, horror and disdain occur; ugliness can be named; realistic truth warrants acknowledgement. Black humour can help deal with the smelly, the revolting parts of a body that becomes abject. There is also a place for professional nursing to take responsibility for wound care and dressings, such that two people who have been lovers can focus on tender ways to maintain the dignity of their relationship. Direct guidance from therapists can bring maturity and commonsense to bear here.

Spiritual Anguish

Spirituality has been variously described as the cohesive relationship with the inner self, the deepest and most genuine aspect of a person or the inner life force that emerges as the soul of each individual. Whatever its form, couples understand this best in each other. As such, the expression of spirituality is typically relational and meaning-based. And while it is a universal concept reflected in all religions, these usually focus more on external forms of expression, while true spirituality is most importantly reflected in the inner self. Spiritual peace is then gained through transcendence over everyday living, with its ordinary condiments, and with a focus on connectedness with some sense of ultimacy, whether this is understood as a cosmic force, God or the deep beauty of one's most precious relationships. Symptomatic distress emerges when this is not attained, when religious doubt sets in, bewilderment over the chaos of life prevails, anguish emerges over perceived futility or when indeed the mystery of life is lost.

One response to the unknowable dimensions of life, to the abyss of existential mystery, is found through the old virtue of reverence. This is the 'awe phenomenon' that wonders at the beauty of nature or the romanticised aspects of a spouse. For reverence is found in healthy relationships, where deep regard, respect and tolerance is the basis of civility and love for others. Reverence is also found through humility, which is open to personal shame and vulnerability, while affirming the talents, success and contribution of others with deep gratitude. As a result, acceptance of self develops, of one's true rather than false self (as described

by object relations theory). Therapists can help couples to recognise where they direct reverence in their lives, to share practices and rituals that foster this in each other, and to understand the religious dimension in their partner.

Among the existential philosophers, Paul Tillich [33] saw faith and mysticism as pathways towards union (or relationship) with the ultimate reality. However, he was clear that faith is not about believing in the unbelievable! Rather he saw faith as 'the state of being grasped by the power of being which transcends everything, that is' [33, p.106]. In his tome, *The Courage to Be*, he went on to say, 'The courage of the modern period (is) not a simple optimism. It (has) to take into itself the deep anxiety of nonbeing in a universe without limits and without a humanly understandable meaning.' [33, p.106]. This construct of the unknowable is found in human relationships, as well as those with a higher power. And through reverence, couples can search to more deeply understand each other, their spiritual selves, their inner lives, the richness and wonderment that strengthens every relationship, transcending the ordinary and appreciating the deep dignity of the other.

Couples then can be helped to understand the spiritual other, support any rituals or customs that assist this and converse openly about spiritual doubt, alongside accessing any additional help that a chaplaincy or pastoral care service might offer.

Let us turn now to meaning and purpose in life, a key existential domain, and one that we prioritise in a major way in this model of therapy because of its prime importance to most patients towards the end of their lives.

14.3.4 Meaning and Purpose of Life

Relational meaning is of prime importance to each couple. This is understood through the story of the relationship, its early beginnings, any struggles, the forces of attraction that brought them together, what is shared in common and where their differences lie. It is often a story of family as well. The narrative includes the families-of-origin, with patterns of relationship seen in parents and grandparents and passed so often from one generation to the next. Many nuances will unfold, but the therapist must understand and bring out the story of roles, goals and intentions, accomplishments, shared creativity, occupations and leisure pursuits (see Section 14.4). Ultimately, the therapist must be able to offer a summary of the couple's story, one that highlights their strengths and accomplishments alongside any challenges and vulnerabilities, balancing the good and the hard aspects of their shared life.

A well understood story will engender a coherence that is discernable to the astute listener. This sense of coherence needs to be wisely balanced, temporal in its logical development, comprehensive in spanning what occupies each partner's days and historical in containing necessary features like medical and sexual history, events, tragedies, losses and stresses that have been borne, whether individually or together.

Commonly, a major portion of established relational life will be directed towards procreation, whether successful or not in their raising of children. This helps to define roles within their nuclear family, points to respective capacity as care-givers/parents and helps understand their teamwork and complementarity, in short, it tells a lot about their relational style as these phases of life are negotiated.

14.3.5 Relational Skew

Relational skew or the loss of reciprocity in a close relationship is inevitable in the setting of advanced illness, as the healthy partner increasingly assumes a caregiving role and the ill partner becomes less functional across various domains of shared life. Strong ambivalence may be felt by the caregiver, who is both striving to protect and care for the ill partner, while managing his or her own emotional response. Naming and normalising ambivalence about the burden of care is a key task of the therapist, particularly as the couple may not fully appreciate the extent to which their roles have changed over time. John Rolland [34] usefully refers to a problem of 'emotional currency' [34, p. 176], whereby concern about the patient's disability or death can sometimes eclipse and therefore can seem to devalue the burden experienced by the other. Concerns about the burden can become silenced. Complicating matters further is the common belief that competence in caregiving connotes a practical and stoic coping style. Spouses may unwittingly follow the culturally sanctioned imperative to 'stay strong' or 'think positively', making it difficult to tolerate the complexity of emotional reactions experienced.

Inequity in the caregiving relationship has been associated with greater distress, relationship dissatisfaction and perceived burden [35]. By exploring with *both partners* how they support one another (e.g. *'What gestures of support does your partner appreciate most?'*, *'How will you know when your partner needs respite?'*), we aim to restore a realistic balance

of supportive exchange so that caregivers perceive more benefit relative to their investment and patients also perceive themselves as having some – albeit limited – contributory role. Equally important here is for the therapist to draw insights from each partner's family-of-origin genogram (see Section 14.4), looking for clues about the implicit rules and expectations that may have been inherited or reinforced regarding caregiving (e.g. *'How was caregiving valued in the family-of-origin?'*, *'From where did family caregivers draw strength?'*, *'Were caregivers isolated or cheered on by supportive others?'*, *'How did caregivers find respite or ways to care for themselves?'*).

The therapist is well reminded to appreciate the occasional need for distance in the couples' relationship, as a necessary and at times restorative counterpoint to the promotion of intimacy. Caregivers may indeed need permission to allow themselves respite from the intensity of their role. Couples are also encouraged to find 'islands of couplehood' untouched by illness. Across sessions of IMMCT, the therapist offers the couple opportunities to articulate and reinforce their relational identity, their shared values and priorities and their unique history together. In so doing, the couple is encouraged to honour and re-experience dimensions of their relationship that will ultimately transcend illness and loss. Rolland [34] and McDaniel [36] similarly discuss the importance of drawing a boundary around illness so that it does not fully dominate the couples' identity.

Relational skew often pertains to inequity in the distribution of instrumental tasks (e.g. household chores). However, couples commonly present with a kind of emotional skew, that is, a perception that one partner consistently carries greater distress or worry than the other. The 'worried' or 'depressed' partner may become locked into this role, generating frustration for the other and creating mounting tension as efforts to mitigate one partner's distress prove ineffective. When there is flexibility in a marital system, partners' roles can be complimentary, as each partner takes turns harbouring distress. Similarly, one partner may 'specialise' in focusing on the grim realities of illness, so that the other can occupy a more hopeful and removed stance. Reframing what may seem like one partner's psychological problem into a relational style can help the couple appreciate the common source of distress (advanced illness) and develop ways to share recognition of its impact. Often, one partner's distress derives from fears or worries about loss and/or the future that have been difficult to voice before the other. Facilitating the safe expression of these thoughts while normalising them can foster intimate interactions and provide relief to the distressed partner.

14.4 Couple Exercises and Case Examples

As noted above, IMMCT leans more heavily on exploratory than didactic methods of intervention. Nevertheless, there are specific couple exercises that are used to facilitate exploration of the content areas described above, and to stimulate direct conversation between partners. These exercises are reviewed below, with case examples to illustrate their use.

14.4.1 Genogram Exercise

During the second couple's session, the therapist sets aside time to learn about each partner's family-of-origin through a focused genogram, or 'family tree' exercise (for more information about this common family therapy tool, see McGoldrick and colleagues [37]). The goal is to identify aspects of each partner's family history that shape their response to illness, and/or contribute to their relational style at present. The therapist uses a pad or whiteboard to construct a genogram that depicts at least three generations of family (e.g. the parental generation, the couples' own generation with siblings and their children's generation, if relevant). Using circular questioning, the therapist asks each partner to comment on relationship patterns in his or her spouse's family-of-origin. (e.g. *'How openly did the parents communicate?', 'How was affection shown?', 'What coping styles were most dominant at times of stress or illness?', 'How did the parents manage differences of opinion or conflict?', 'What styles of relating does your partner bring from his family?', 'Who is he/she most like?', 'Are there any styles you/your partner has been determined to leave behind?'*). A key objective of conducting this historical review is to honour the strengths and values that are evident in each partner's family history. A summary that synthesises key themes of family life that have influenced each partner can reinforce the insights gained from this exercise, making it more therapeutic than information-gathering.

14.4.1.1 Case 1

Mr. C was a 66 year old retired electrician with metastatic pancreatic cancer seen with his wife, *Mrs. C. Mr. C had discontinued chemotherapy and recognised that he was growing weaker, but agreed to attend sessions at the suggestion of his wife, who worried that he was showing signs of depression. The couple had raised four children, three of whom lived at considerable geographical distance, a source of sadness and bewilderment. In the second session, a genogram revealed that Mr. C had been estranged from his younger sister for seven years. The decision to stop talking to his sister had been enforced by Mrs. C, following a financial dispute related to the family business. Mrs. C, angered by her sister-in-law's 'self-ishness', had refused to invite her to family events and insisted on distance. When reviewing these incidents, the therapist asked Mrs. C, 'How much do you think your husband misses his sister?' Mr. C proceeded to describe his double bind: on the one hand, he wished to speak with his sister 'before it's too late'; on the other hand, he wished to remain loyal to his wife. At the next session, Mr. C announced that with his wife's blessing, he had reconnected with his sister, updated her on his condition and they arranged a family gathering. Mr. C said, 'it felt good to hear my sister's voice again, and I'm proud of (my wife) for encouraging me to do that'. Cut-offs were identified as a common occurrence in Mrs. C's family history, with distance seen as a way to resolve differences. The couple recognised the difference in their styles, and worried that their own children may adopt a distant style of relating as well. Opportunities to encourage greater cohesiveness in their family relationships were explored.*

14.4.2 Communication Exercise

At the end of the first session, the therapist asks the couple to set aside a mutually agreed upon day and time to plan a shared activity that will allow for conversation (e.g. a mealtime, a walk). Couples are asked to use this time to discuss the impact of illness on their relationship. The therapist provides a list of questions to guide discussion about sources of shared meaning. These questions invite the couple to reflect on valued roles (e.g. *'Think about the roles you play in your life – wife/husband/mother/father/friend – which of these roles has been most meaningful to you? Which have been most impacted by cancer? Which do you think have been most meaningful to your partner? What role have you had in your marriage and how has that changed during your illness?'*). This exercise, deliberately assigned early in the intervention, aims to stimulate discussion and shared reflection outside of the therapy setting. The couple is asked to review what was discussed at the following session.

14.4.2.1 Case 2

Mr. L was a 48 year old architect with advanced stage prostate cancer who was seen with his wife. The couple had been married for 23 years and raised two children, now teenagers. Mrs. L complained that she thinks about her husband's illness 'constantly', while Mr. L says, 'it doesn't always bother me the same way'. While the couple recognised the importance of communicating openly and 'putting things on the table', they acknowledged that they are often protective of one another and do not easily share their grief. Mr. L explained that they 'talk about the cancer in terms of symptoms', but not address its emotional impact. Mrs. L added that they sit in front of the television at night to avoid discussion. The therapist highlighted the protectiveness that avoidance brings, while acknowledging the comfort and intimacy felt in sitting together without talking. Following the first session, the couple was asked to complete the communication exercise. When they returned to the following session, they told the therapist that they had gone out to a cafe, where they had an emotional conversation about the impact of illness on their lives. Mrs. L shared her worries about being left alone in the future and they shared their grief more openly than they had done before.

14.4.3 Hypothetical Timeline Exercise

The couple is presented with three *hypothetical* scenarios in which their future together is limited by different degrees (e.g. one year, six months, two months; or not make a christening, not be there for graduation, not be around for a wedding). The couple is asked to reflect on how they would fill their time in each of these 'best case' to 'worst case' scenarios: what events, people, relationships, accomplishments or pastimes would be important to them? This exercise was developed in order to help the couple clarify shared priorities and reflect on the experiences that they value most given the likelihood of a limited and uncertain future. Although the emphasis could easily be on the ill partner's wishes and priorities at the end-of-life, the therapist deliberately asks each partner to provide their perspective, thus ensuring the couple determines collaboratively what is most meaningful at present. This exercise may be done in session or can be assigned as a home exercise, and the therapist is encouraged to select hypothetical time periods that suit the patient's disease status.

14.4.3.1 Case 3

Mrs. S is a 69 year old former dancer with stage IV breast cancer, who was seen in couples therapy with her husband of 42 years, a musician. The couple has one child, a son who lives in California, and had been pleading with his parents to move to California, where he could support them financially, keep them comfortable and make arrangements for their care. Several years ago, the couple had sold their home for a smaller apartment that afforded better access to the hospital. The move into a more urban area also enabled the couple to visit museums and concerts without travelling any considerable distance. Mr. S had been in favour of moving to California, and when pressed, shared in session that he preferred to be near his son so that he was not left alone should his wife pass away. Mrs. S, however, was indecisive, in part feeling tied to her treatment team, even though her oncologist assured her that he would facilitate her referral to a new treatment centre. Completing the timeline exercise encouraged the couple to clarify their priorities within the constraints of hypothetical time limits. The exercise evoked feelings of sadness and disappointment at the loss of future plans, but empowered the couple to make choices about their future. Mrs. S realised how important it was that she feel rooted in an area that felt like 'home', and that moving would deny her this comfort. Mr. S acknowledged that their return to city life recalled their early years together, and noted that it felt a more fitting setting for them to share their remaining time. The couple decided to stay where they were, surrounded by close artist friends and shared interests.

14.4.4 Relational Legacy Exercise

During the last one to two sessions, the therapist invites the couple to honour their shared life by working on an activity that would help to define and celebrate their love for one another. This can take any form, either verbal or symbolic, and has typically included activities such as writing together, collecting photos and creating an album of memories or collecting meaningful music that celebrates their couple-hood. Unlike individual legacy work, this exercise gives couples an opportunity to concretise what they have built together. In doing this activity, the couple is asked to consider and discuss the following questions: *"If you were to look back on your married life, what accomplishments as a couple would please you most? What are you most proud of in your marriage? What would you say your life goals and priorities have been? If you had a 'motto' as a couple that described your history together, what would it be?"*

14.4.4.1 Case 4

Mr. R was a 55 year old man with advanced prostate cancer, who came to couples therapy with his wife of 28 years. Mr. R's diagnosis occurred shortly after their retirement. The therapist used future oriented questions to anticipate concerns or worries about how the future will look for Mrs. R (to Mr. R: 'If we consider a future time when you are no longer with us, how will your wife fare? What will give her strength? Where will she turn for support?'). This led to a discussion about building a shared legacy. Mr. and Mrs. R had received a video camera as a gift from their daughter. They decided to use it to film themselves sitting together and looking through early photo albums. With each album page, they told stories about the courting period of their relationship, their travels and memorable family events.

14.5 Evidence on Efficacy

A growing evidence base supports the utility of couple-based interventions in the setting of advanced illness. The emphasis on themes of caregiving, anticipated loss and existential concerns differentiates the support of advanced-stage couples from early-stage couple interventions [7]. These range from psychoeducational interventions that primarily promote adaptive coping in the caregiving spouse [38], to attachment-based interventions that aim to strengthen the couples' emotional bond [39]. Kuijer and colleagues [35] demonstrated improved relationship quality and reduction in perceived relationship skew following a five-session couple-based intervention that strengthened mutual support. Sessions aimed to restore a realistic balance in the relationship by addressing instrumental needs and psychological processes (revising the patient and partner's own standards about how much investment is possible). McLean and Nissim [39] found preliminary support for an empirically supported intervention called emotion-focused couples therapy (EFT-C) to address disruptions in emotional engagement that occur for some facing advanced cancer. The goal of EFT-C is to strengthen a couple's capacity to shore up safety and connectedness, particularly during periods of vulnerability. Rather than instructing couples to use communication or problem solving skills per se, the EFT-C therapist assumes that these skills already exist and will emerge spontaneously in a context of safe connection. McLean and her colleagues [39] showed improved marital functioning, decreased depression and subjective reports of benefit and satisfaction.

14.6 Service Development

The therapeutic approach presented here relies heavily on the identification and enlistment of couples who may benefit from this modality of care. As discussed above, this therapy is well suited to couples who feature distress (e.g. symptoms of anxiety and/or depression) in one or the other partner. Routine distress screening for both the patient *and his or her spouse* is therefore an important mechanism for identifying couples who would benefit from these sessions. This process may require a paradigm shift in some medical settings, where the patient's individual care is prioritised and less attention is given to the psychosocial adjustment of the spouse. The family-centred approach promoted here recognises loved ones as both a crucial resource to the patient, and as harbouring considerable worry and distress themselves that easily remains unmanaged. In offering support to the couple as a unit, we call attention to the value of protecting and strengthening their relationship as a 'third patient', that is more than the sum of its parts. Thus, caregiving spouses who may be reluctant to prioritise their own psychosocial needs if offered individual support may more easily join the patient in pursuing goals of improved teamwork, mutual support, increased closeness and enhanced meaning.

Couples are best approached when the patient's prognosis is approximately one to two years or less. While the brief nature of this intervention eases any practical concerns about attending sessions, couples who suffer from longstanding discord (e.g. history of unresolved infidelity, high conflict or periods of separation) will likely benefit from more than four to six sessions and may require some initial effort to de-escalate conflict before embarking on intimacy or meaning-enhancing work.

As with any systemically oriented therapy, it is assumed that therapists working with couples have a skill base that enables them to maintain neutrality with respect to each partners' perspective, and to appreciate relational strengths. There is evidence that brief training in conducting conjoint family or couple meetings in the palliative care setting can effectively empower multi-specialty health care professionals to deliver systemic care (Gueguen *et al.*, 2009).

At the authors' institution, a bi-weekly couple and family therapy peer supervision group creates a mechanism for the involved psychologists, psychiatrists and social workers to discuss challenging cases, consider goals of care, review co-therapy options and support the development and application of systemic therapies. Bringing the male-female dyad together as co-therapists when caring for challenging couples can assist balancing the unconscious dynamics influencing alliances, sustain neutrality and foster greater hypothesising about beneficial outcome options.

14.7 Summary

Couples facing advanced illness face the formidable task of sustaining intimacy and preserving their identity as a couple, while simultaneously weathering the cascade of losses that accompany serious illness [16]. A portion of couples carry clinically significant distress, whether in the patient or partner, or both [17, 18]. Conjoint therapy can be an effective way to reinforce the couples' capacity to draw comfort from one another, and to ease communication about existential fears, grief and the burden of illness. There is substantial evidence that a supportive, communicative and close relationship can buffer distress for patients and their partners and ensure optimal adaptation to severe stress [9]. A model of couples therapy was presented here that aims not only to strengthen the buffering capacity of the relationship, but also to empower couples to notice and honour relational sources of meaning, and co-create a legacy founded on their shared history. Thus, meaning-making as a *shared* process becomes a pathway to greater intimacy in the face of advanced disease.

Recommended Reading

Greenberg, L.S. and Goldman, R.N. (2008) *Emotion-Focused Couples Therapy*, American Psychological Association, Washington, DC.
Moderation of affect regulation is the key method of enhancing the relationship.

References

1. White, M. and White, M. (1989) Saying hello again: the incorporation of the lost relationship in the resolution of grief, in *Selected Papers* (ed. M. White), Dulwich Centre Publications, Adlalide, pp. 29–35.
2. Steinhauser, K.E., Christakis, N.A., Clipp, E.C. *et al.* (2000) Factors considered important at the end of life by patients, family, physicians, and other care providers. *Journal of the American Medical Association*, **284** (19), 2476–2482.
3. Steinhauser, K.E., Clipp, E.C., McNeilly, M. *et al.* (2000) In search of a good death: observations of patients, families, and providers. *Annals of Internal Medicine*, **132** (10), 825–832.
4. Kissane, D.W., Bloch, S., Burns, W. *et al.* (1994) Psychological morbidity in the families of patients with cancer. *Psychooncology*, **3**, 47–56.

5. Zaider, T. and Kissane, D.W. (2007) Resilient families, in *Resilience in Palliative Care* (eds B. Monroe and D. Oliviere), Oxford University Press, Oxford, pp. 67–81.
6. Hagedoorn, M., Sanderman, R., Bolks, H.N. *et al.* (2008) Distress in couples coping with cancer: a meta-analysis and critical review of role and gender effects. *Psychology Bulletin*, **134** (1), 1–30.
7. McLean, L.M. and Jones, J.M. (2007) A review of distress and its management in couples facing end-of-life cancer. *Psycho-Oncology*, **16** (7), 603–616.
8. Kissane, D.W. and Bloch, S. (2002) *Family Focused Grief Therapy: A Model of Family-Centred Care during Palliative Care and Bereavement*, Open University Press, Buckingham and Philadelphia.
9. Roberts, K.J., Lepore, S.J. and Helgeson, V. (2006) Social-cognitive correlates of adjustment to prostate cancer. *Psycho-Oncology*, **15**, 183–192.
10. Lantz, J. and Gregoire, T. (2000) Existential psychotherapy with couples facing breast cancer: a twenty year report. *Contemporary Family Therapy*, **22** (3), 315–327.
11. Manne, S.L., Ostroff, J.S., Winkel, G. *et al.* (2005) Couple-focused group intervention for women with early stage breast cancer. *Journals of Consulting and Clinical Psychology*, **73** (4), 634–646.
12. Kissane, D.W., Bloch, S., McKenzie, M. *et al.* (2006) Family focused grief therapy: a randomized controlled trial in palliative care and bereavement. *American Journal of Psychiatry*, **163**, 1208–1218.
13. Toseland, R.W., Blanchard, C.G. and McCallion, P. (1995) A problem solving intervention for caregivers of cancer patients. *Social Science and Medicine*, **40** (4), 517–528.
14. Harding, R., Higginson, I.J. and Donaldson, N. (2003) The relationship between patient characteristics and carer psychological status in home palliative cancer care. *Support Care Cancer*, **11** (10), 638–643.
15. Derogatis, L.R. and Melisaratos, N. (1983) The brief symptom inventory: an introductory report. *Psychological Medicine*, **13**, 595–605.
16. McWilliams, A.E. (2004) Couple psychotherapy from an attachment theory perspective: a case study approach to challenging the dual nihilism of being an older person and someone with a terminal illness. *European Journal of Cancer Care (English)*, **13** (5), 464–472.
17. Northouse, L., Templin, T., Mood, D. and Oberst, M. (1998) Couples' adjustment to breast cancer and benign breast disease: a longitudinal analysis. *Psycho-Oncology*, **7**, 37–48.
18. Kaufman, B., Peretz, T., Baider, L. *et al.* (1996) Mutuality of fate: adaptation and psychological distress in cancer patients and their partners, in *Cancer and the Family* (eds L. Baider, C.L. Cooper and A. Kaplan De-Nour), John Wiley & Sons, Ltd, Chichester, pp. 173–186.
19. Couper, J.W., Bloch, S., Love, A. *et al.* (2006) Psychosocial adjustment of female partners of men with prostate cancer: a review of the literature. *Psycho-Oncology*, **15** (11), 937–953.
20. Folkman, S. (1997) Positive psychological states and coping with severe stress. *Social Science and Medicine*, **45**, 1207–1221.

21. Park, C.L. and Folkman, S. (1997) Meaning in the context of stress and coping. *Review of General Psychology*, **2**, 115–144.

22. Park, C. (2010) Making sense of the meaning literature: an integrative review of meaning making and its effects on adjustment to stressful life events. *Psychological Bulletin*, **136** (2), 257–301.

23. Lepore, S.J. and Helgeson, V.S. (1998) Social constraints, intrusive thoughts, and mental health after prostate cancer. *Journal of Social and Clinical Psychology*, **17** (1), 89–106.

24. Patterson, J.M. and Garwick, A.W. (1994) Levels of meaning in family stress theory. *Family Process*, **33**, 287–304.

25. Reis, H.T., Shaver, P. and Duck, S. (1998) Intimacy as an interpersonal process, in *Handbook of Personal Relationships* (ed. S. Duck), John Wiley & Sons, Ltd, Chichester, pp. 367–389.

26. Laurenceau, J.P., Barrett, L.F. and Rovine, M.J. (2005) The interpersonal process model of intimacy in marriage: a daily diary and multilevel modeling approach. *Journal of Family Psychology*, **19**, 314–323.

27. Manne, S., Ostroff, J., Rini, C. *et al.* (2004) The interpersonal process model of intimacy: the role of self-disclosure, partner disclosure, and partner responsiveness in interactions between breast cancer patients and their partners. *Journal of Family Psychology*, **18** (4), 589–599.

28. Tomm, K., Campbell, D. and Draper, R. (1985) Circular interviewing: A multifaceted clinical tool, in *Applications of Systemic Family Therapy: The Milan Approach* (eds D. Campbell and R. Draper), Grune & Station, London, pp. 33–45.

29. Weingarten, K. (1991) The discourses of intimacy: adding a social constructivist and feminist view. *Family Process*, **30**, 285–305.

30. Cordova, J.V. and Scott, R. (2001) Intimacy: a behavioral interpretation. *The Behavior Analyst*, **24**, 75–86.

31. Yalom, I. (1980) *Existential Psychotherapy*, Basic Books.

32. Kissane, D. (2000) Psychospiritual and existential distress. The challenge for palliative care. *Australian Family Physician*, **29** (11), 1022–1025.

33. Tillich, P. (2000) *The Courage to Be*, Yale University Press.

34. Rolland, J. (1994) *Families, Illness, and Disability: An Integrative Treatment Model*, Basic Books.

35. Kuijer, R.G., Buunk, B.P., De Jong, G.M. *et al.* (2004) Effects of a brief intervention program for patients with cancer and their partners on feelings of inequity, relationship quality and psychological distress. *Psycho-Oncology*, **13** (5), 321–334.

36. McDaniel, S., Hepworth, J. and Doherty, W. (1992) *Medical Family Therapy: A Biopsychosocial Approach to Families with Health Problems*, Basic Books.

37. McGoldrick, M., Gerson, R. and Shellenberger, S. (1999) *Genograms: Assessment and Intervention*, 2nd edn, WW Norton & Company.

38. Northouse, L., Kershaw, T., Mood, D. and Schafenacker, A. (2005) Effects of a family intervention on the quality of life of women with recurrent breast cancer and their family caregivers. *Psycho-Oncology*, **14** (6), 478–491.

39. McLean, L.M. and Nissim, R. (2007) Marital therapy for couples facing advanced cancer: case review. *Palliative and Supportive Care*, **5** (3), 303–313.

40. Gueguen, J., Bylund, C.L., Brown, R. *et al.* (2009) Conducting Family Meetings in Palliative Care: Themes, Techniques and Preliminary Evaluation of a Communication Skills Module. *Palliative & Supportive Care*, **7** (2), 171–179.

15 Therapies for Sexual Dysfunction

Mary K. Hughes

The University of Texas M.D. Anderson Cancer Center, Houston, TX, USA

15.1 Background

According to Thaler-DeMers, all cancers can impact sexuality and intimacy [1]. Schover reports sexuality to be one of the first elements of daily living disrupted by a cancer diagnosis and in 2008 found that unlike other side effects of cancer and its treatments, these problems do not tend to resolve after several years of disease-free survival [2, 3]. According to Leiblum, all patients regardless of age, sexual orientation, marital status or life circumstances should have the opportunity to discuss sexual matters with their health care professional [4]. But it is not easy to talk about despite living in a culture, that is saturated with overtly sexual images, graphic lyrics and explicit advertising [5]. Bruner and Boyd assert that the promotion of sexual health is vital for preserving quality of life and is an integral part of total or holistic cancer management [6].

According to Tomlinson, the main difference between taking a history about a sexual problem and an ordinary medical history is the level of embarrassment and discomfort of the patient and the health care provider [7]. A discussion of sexual changes can begin by acknowledging the sexual changes brought about by the cancer or the treatment of the cancer [1]. Sexual changes after treatment is not routinely addressed or only barely touched on despite patients having significant needs for education, support and practical help with managing them.

Maslow described sexual activity to be a basic need on his hierarchy of needs while love and connection to others was at a higher level [8]. Everyone has a lifelong need for touch and emotional connection to others regardless of current relationship status [9]. Sexual intercourse is not the defining characteristic of a person's sexuality; a sexual relationship includes the need to be touched and held along with closeness and tenderness [10, 11].

In a study of sexual problems and distress in United States women, Shifren et al. found that although 44% report a sexual problem, only 21% felt this caused personal distress [12]. Sexual concerns must be associated with distress to be considered a medical problem. Malcarne et al. report that because of the emotional and physical changes in the person with cancer the quality of a couple's relationship can be altered even by successful treatment [13].

15.1.1 Review of Sexuality

Masters and Johnson described the human sexual response cycle that begins with libido or the desire for sexual activity [14]. Gregorie reports that men are more attracted to visual sexual stimuli, whereas women are more attracted to auditory and written material, particularly stimuli associated within the context of a loving and positive relationship [15]. Women aren't linear in their sexual response, but more circular and may experience sexual excitement before they have a desire for sexual activity [16]. Sexual excitement is the phase where the penis becomes rigid enough to use and in the female, the vagina lubricates and enlarges in depth and width, and the clitoris enlarges [17–19]. Erection is the male counterpart to vaginal secretions from the sexual physiology perspective [20]. Orgasm is the height of sexual pleasure and the release of sexual tension. The penis emits semen through muscular spasms and there are rhythmic contractions of the vagina and the cervix lifts up out of the vaginal vault. The last phase of the cycle is the resolution phase where the genitals

Handbook of Psychotherapy in Cancer Care, First Edition. Edited by Maggie Watson and David W. Kissane.
© 2011 John Wiley & Sons, Inc. Published 2011 by John Wiley & Sons, Inc.

return to their normal, non-excited state. During this phase, there is an evaluation of the sexual experience as well as relaxation and contentment [21, 22]. The refractory period, where the genitals are resistant to sexual stimulation happens during this stage. In males, this period can be a matter of minutes in youth, but take days in older men or with certain medications or medical conditions like cancer.

15.1.2 Sexual Dysfunction

Sexual dysfunction is failure of any aspect of the sexual response cycle to function properly [23]. Goldstein reports that sexual dysfunction is 90% psychological and 75% physiological which overlap [24]. However, when a person with cancer has sexual dysfunction, it is mostly physiological.

What constitutes a sexual problem?

- physiological dysfunction;
- altered experiences;
- own perceptions and beliefs;
- partner's perceptions and expectations;
- altered circumstances;
- past experiences [15].

Thaler-DeMers report that treatment decisions made at the time of diagnosis impact interpersonal relationships, sexuality and reproductive capacity of all cancer survivors [1]. Most often sexual dysfunction is treatment related due to the changes in physiologic, psychological and social dimensions of sexuality and disruption in one or more phases of the sexual response cycle [9, 25]. As early as 1981, Derogatis and Kourlesis reported that the majority of patients have sexual problems after cancer treatment [26].

Besides chemotherapy, biologic agents and hormones, there are numerous medications that can have sexual side effects that range from decreased desire to difficulty reaching orgasm. It should be remembered that sexual dysfunctions are not all or nothing phenomena, but occur on a continuum in terms of frequency and severity. Co-morbidity of sexual dysfunctions is common. Gregorie reports that almost half the men with low libido also have another sexual dysfunction, and 20% of men with Erectile Dysfunction (ED) have low libido [15]. The patient's partner and their relationship probably have a more profound effect on sexual health than on any other aspect of health.

15.1.3 Fertility

Schover reports one of the greatest concerns of cancer survivors of childbearing age is the effect of treatment on fertility [27]. Wenzel et al. report reproductive concerns that emerge within the cancer experience are negatively associated with quality of life [28]. Studies show that most young survivors are interested in having children, especially if they were childless at the time of their cancer diagnosis [29, 30]. Difficulties with fertility increase with age and are much more common for women greater than 40 years [31, 32]. Pregnancy does not appear to increase the risk of cancer recurrence [33].

The ability to preserve fertility depends on:

- age;
- type of cancer;
- combination of treatments;
- type of treatment [34–37].

The American Society of Clinical Oncologists recommends that:

- Oncologists address the possibility of infertility with patients in their reproductive years.
- Fertility preservation should be considered as early as possible during treatment.
- Standard fertility preservation practice is:
  - sperm cryopreservation for men;
  - embryo cryopreservation for women;
  - other methods considered investigational [38, 39].

Carter et al. found significant depression, grief and sexual difficulties in women whose cancer treatment caused infertility [40]. A study by Katz found that homophobia does not affect current cancer care experiences of gay and lesbian patients, and health care providers accepted the support of the patient's same-sexed partners [41]. Often the health care practitioner does not know the sexual orientation or gender identity of their patients [42]. Dibble et al. further state that because of heterosexism, those who do not share a heterosexual orientation may have difficult lives especially when they are ill [42]. Heterosexism is the belief that heterosexuality is the only 'normal' option for relationships [42]. Most of the research on the effects of cancer and its treatment on sexuality has been limited to heterosexual women or women assumed to be heterosexual [43].

Many people have adopted a pattern of sexual behaviour before their diagnosis and attempt to return to it after treatment. If they experience discomfort or failure to function as before, they will stop trying and feel they cannot enjoy sexual activity [44]. Couples who are cancer survivors and are in a stressful relationship with an unsupportive partner tend to have more distress that can lead to avoidant coping behaviours and avoid talking about difficult issues including sexuality [45]. During the time of treatment, the cancer experience encourages a more intimate and intense interpersonal relationship, but there are few studies that have attempted any type of psychosocial intervention to assist survivors in integrating the cancer experience into their personal life [1].

15.1.4 Sexual Assessment

Regardless of our role in providing care to the patient, most of us do not have experience talking about sexuality and intimacy in a frank, direct and authentic manner [5]. Annon's PLISSIT model can provide a framework for doing a sexual assessment.

It has four components:

- **P** Permission to be sexual while ill or undergoing treatment.

- **LI** Limited Information of possible sexuality side effects of treatments.

- **SS** Specific Suggestions to help with intimacy.

- **IT** Intensive Therapy where there are complex underlying problems [46].

The practitioner gives the patient permission (**P**) to think about cancer and sexuality at the same time by asking,

'*What sexuality changes have you noticed since your cancer?*' which lets them know that they aren't the only ones to experience sexuality changes. By asking open-ended questions, the health care provider is better able to get a thoughtful response from the patient [47]. Giving them time to answer is important. Try to remain relaxed with good eye contact to let them know that you are interested in this area of their lives. Addressing sexuality issues early on in the assessment and treatment of the patient allows the practitioner to open up a line of communication with the patient so that these issues can be addressed as they come up in the future [47].

15.1.5 Sexual Assessment Models

PLEASURE Model

P – Partner

L – Lovemaking

E – Emotions

A – Attitude

S – Symptoms

U – Understanding

R – Reproduction

E – Energy

Schain, W.S. (1988) The sexual and intimate consequences of breast cancer treatment. *CA Cancer J. Clin.*, **38** (3), 154–161.

ALARM Model

A – Activity

L – Libido (desire)

A – Arousal and orgasm

R – Resolution

M – Medical history

Andersen, B.L. (1990) How cancer affects sexual functioning. *Oncology*, **4** (6), 81–88.

PLISSIT Model

P – Permission

LI – Limited information

SS – Specific suggestions

IT – Intensive therapy

Annon, J.S. (1976) A proposed conceptual scheme for the behavioral treatment of sexual problems. *The Behavioral Treatment of Sexual Problems: Brief Therapy*, Harper and Row, Hagarstown, MD, pp. 43–47.

BETTER Model

B – Bring

E – Explain

T – Tell

T – Timing

E – Educate

R – Record

Mick, J.A., Hughes, M. and Cohen, M.Z. (2004) Using the BETTER Model to assess sexuality. *Clin. J. Oncol. Nurs.*, **8** (1), 84–86.

15.2 Processes and Techniques

Giving them **LI** about side effects from treatments by saying, '*Sometimes people notice sexuality changes when they get this treatment*', lets them know that you are comfortable talking about sexuality issues. One of the first steps towards sexual rehabilitation is sex education [48].

Describing **SS** such as books to read, positions to use, can offer them help with the problem.

Table 15.1 lists other suggestions.

Some patients are in difficult relationships, which only get worse with cancer treatment and need **IT** from a marital or a sex therapist. Having a list of those resources in the community can be helpful to the patient. However, Schover reports that patients often prefer to receive information from a member of the health care team instead of being sent to a sex specialist [53].

Giving referrals depends on the patients who may benefit from specialised assistance if they need it.

Table 15.2 describes some of these referrals.

Interventions for sexual dysfunction resulting from cancer treatment can be limited because of the hormone status of the tumour. Women with oestrogen receptive positive breast cancer are often unable to use any oestrogen products, while some oncologists give them the go-ahead to use an oestrogen vaginal ring, vaginal creams or tablets. A study reported that use of vaginal oestradiol tablet was associated with a rise in systemic oestradiol levels which reverses oestrogen suppression achieved by aromatase inhibitors and should be avoided [58].

Greenwald reported that women with cervical cancer had their sexual desire and enjoyment rebound six years after treatment, but they struggled with sexuality issues until then [59]. Furthermore, there are some oncologists that will agree to the use of off-label androgen gel for those women to improve libido. Studies have shown that testosterone has positive effects on women's sexuality and that higher doses show greater effects [60]. It is controversial and should be left up to the discretion of the medical oncologist. Women with other types of cancer can use oral oestrogen replacement if they are comfortable with that and their oncologist gives them agreement.

15.3 Case Examples

15.3.1 Case 1

Mrs. Annie Alpha is a 46 year-old-married white female currently being treated for oestrogen-positive, progestin-positive and her-2neu negative left breast cancer. Three years ago, she had a segmental mastectomy, taxane chemotherapy, and 5-fu, adriamycin and cytoxan chemotherapy, which threw her into premature menopause. Currently, she is on tamoxifen and is complaining of sexuality dysfunction. She has

Table 15.1	Suggestions for treating sexual dysfunction
Suggestion	**Example**
Vaginal dilator	Different sizes to find comfortable fit with partner or to be able to tolerate gynaecological examination
Using erotica	Videos, magazines
Vaginal lubricants and moisturisers	K-Y® or Astroglide® lubricants for sexual activity, Replens® moisturiser for vaginal health and comfort
Videos	Better Sex Videos®, an inexpensive, tastefully done option
Contraceptive options	Oral contraceptives may not be option, use barrier protection
Planning for sexual activity	Take medications to control symptoms 30 minutes before encounter Schedule encounters when energy is highest
Communicating more openly about sexual needs	Tell partner what feels good; when sexual desire is highest
Exploring one's own body	Finding out new erogenous zones, pleasuring self
Safer sexual practices	If not in committed relationship, use barrier protection (condoms)
Different means of sexual expression	Oral–genital activity, different sexual positions
Better symptom control	Take medications for pain, nausea, diarrhoea as needed
Using erotic devices	Vibrators can enhance sexual activity
Sensate focus	Focuses on receiver's pleasure, no genital activity, uses all of the senses

Refs. [49–52].

Table 15.2	Types of referrals for sexual dysfunction
Treatment	**Example**
PDE5inhibitors	Tadafil, vardenafil, sildenafil
Penile implants	Genito-urinary specialist referral
Penile injections	Alprostadil
Penile suppositories	Alprostadil
Vacuum erection device	Need prescription
Fertility specialists	Both male and female
EROS-CT for women	Vacuum device for female (need prescription)
Physical therapist for pelvic floor exercises	P.T. must have specialised training
Reconstructive surgery	Plastic surgeon, dentists, wound ostomy nurses
Breast implants	Plastic surgeon
Hormone therapy	Endocrinology
Psychosexual therapy	Sexual therapist
Lymphoedema	P.T. who specialises in treating this

Refs. [2, 18, 54–57].

been married 15 years and has two children, ages 6 and 12 and works as an architect.

Upon further questioning, she reveals that her relationship with her husband, Alex, is stable and that he understands her sexual changes. She doesn't like the way her body looks with the scars and weight gain, but Alex is just glad that she is alive. She complains that she has no libido, vaginal dryness, dyspareunia and unpredictable orgasms and they have sexual intercourse less than once a month. Before her cancer experience, they would make love three to four times a week and she would always orgasm at least once. She misses their sexual activities and is hoping you can help.

After interviewing Mrs. Alpha, you find out that her breasts are erogenous zones, but Alex has not touched them since the surgery. They have attempted sexual intercourse several times, but it has mainly been unsatisfying to her. She misses the intimacy with Alex, but is just not interested in engaging in sexual activities with him, nor do they talk about this. She has not much experience with masturbation, nor has she used a vibrator, so she doesn't know how sensitive her erogenous zones are now. They have engaged mainly in penile/vaginal sexual activities, but have some experience with oral–genital sexual activity that she reports as satisfying.

She is aware that she cannot take oestrogen replacement hormones, but is interested in trying anything to improve her sexual life. She describes Alex as a very patient and understanding man, but she knows how

important sexual activity had been to him in the past. After interviewing Alex, you find that he is very concerned about Annie's health and wants to make sure she continues to remain cancer-free. He does admit that he would like to engage in sexual activity more frequently than they have, but he wants his wife to enjoy it, too.

You describe **sensate focus exercises** to them in an attempt to get them to begin touching each other in a sexual, but non-threatening way. You tell them to focus on the receiver's pleasure and that there is to be no genital activity or sexual intercourse during this exercise. They are to use all of their senses: taste, touch, smell, sight and hearing. You suggest sensuous foods, music and aromatherapy.

They are given **written information** about this and agree to try it. They were also given information about sexual vibrators which could be another way to increase her sexual arousal and orgasms. She can be told to use the vibrator alone so she can find out what feels good and to teach her husband how to use it. Annie denies that she is having any pain or fatigue so there is no need to pre-medicate before sexual activities. She was told to think about scheduling sexual activities with her husband that would take the pressure off her to perform at other times. This also will give her husband something to look forward to rather than guessing when they will be sexually active.

Vaginal lubricants that contain no petroleum products would be discussed to improve her comfort during sexual intercourse. If she has severe vaginal dryness with vaginal burning and itching, you would discuss vaginal moisturisers which are to be used twice weekly at night independent of frequency of sexual activity.

Since she doesn't feel comfortable being nude around her husband because of her breast scars, you would recommend that she wear a silk teddy or a camisole during sexual encounters. This would also enable her breasts to receive sexual stimulation while keeping them covered. She could also give her husband permission to touch her breasts. This would not hurt her, nor cause the cancer to spread or return.

You would also discuss what she does like about her body, not just what she doesn't like. She could also be sent to see a dietitian to talk about what foods are healthier for her and also direct her to some type of regular exercise programme like walking which could help her with weight control.

15.3.2 Case 2

Mr. Bill Barnes, a 58 year-old-married white male, was treated one year ago for rectal cancer. He had a colostomy, chemo-radiation and is now cancer-free, but has ED. He has tried sildenafil (Viagra®), but it was ineffective. He and his wife of 29 years had a very satisfying sex life and are continuing to be sexually intimate. Before his surgery, they would have sexual intercourse several times a week; now it is monthly or less. He remains orgasmic and continues to please his wife, but would like to participate in penile–vaginal intercourse, again. Since his surgery involved nerves around the rectum that also affect erections, it is highly unlikely that his erections will return spontaneously. With nerve involvement, it is important to use a mechanical means of creating erections such as the vacuum erection device or penile injections. Bill denies that he has any body image issues with his colostomy or any fatigue. The vacuum pump was demonstrated on a penile model and Bill had multiple questions about comfort and about how to remove the penile band after orgasm. Some men find it more comfortable to shave an area at the base of the penis to decrease the likelihood of pubic hair getting caught in the band. He was instructed not to leave the band on longer than 30 minutes. Penile injections were briefly discussed, but he was not interested in them. He was given a booklet of the option for treatment of ED which included penile implants, but he was not interested in surgery at this time. If his wife has vaginal dryness, vaginal lubricants could be recommended for comfort. Since some preparation time is necessary with the vacuum erection device, sexual activity will not be as spontaneous as before. The time to achieve an erection varies from man to man with the vacuum erection device.

15.4 Evidence on Efficacy

Oncology patients are very grateful when someone acknowledges sexuality dysfunction as a side effect of treatment or the cancer itself. Just knowing that they are not the only one with sexuality concerns helps to normalise their concerns. Evidence shows that a stronger bond is created between the health care provider and the patient and his/her partner after sexuality issues are addressed. Patients are willing to try anything to improve sexuality functioning if sexuality is important to them. If the intervention is ineffective, they are grateful that someone tried to help them.

15.5 Service Development

After a pilot study on sexuality dysfunction in patients referred to psychiatry, it was decided to address this important issue with all of our patients. One practitioner can be the designated person to deal with sexuality issues and get sexuality consults not only from oncologists, but other psychiatric colleagues. Word of mouth has kept consults coming, but only 10% of the patients are specifically referred for sexual dysfunction.

15.6 Summary

The importance of assessing and treating sexual dysfunction in oncology patients has been discussed in this chapter. Because of cancer treatments, treatment for sexual dysfunction often has to be modified so as not to interfere with this. When asked, both men and women are willing to discuss sexuality changes, but might be able to only describe the changes in their language rather than clinically. During active treatment, most patients do not feel like being very sexually active, but as treatments end quality of life issues surface. Patients are often hopeful that as they feel better physically, they will become more sexually active. If their hormones have been manipulated, this might not be the case. Despite cancer treatments being over, some patients suffer from chronic fatigue which is a big deterrent to sexuality. Both men and women who had a satisfying sexual relationship are eager to resume this and disappointed when it doesn't happen. Women are sometimes more willing to learn to live with sexual changes than men. Men are more persistent to find a way to solve sexuality problems. Oncologists are often relieved to have someone to refer the patient to with sexuality dysfunction since the oncologists want to focus on treating cancer.

15.7 Supporting Materials

15.7.1 Sexuality Web-Ography

Selected web sites for health care professionals and patients

American Association of Sex Educators, Counsellors and Therapists www.aasect.org

The Alexander Foundation for Women's Health www.afwh.org

International Society for the Study of Women's Sexual Health www.isswsh.org

National Vulvodynia Association (USA) www.nva.org (Information for women with genital pain)

SexualHealth.com (USA based site on sexuality and disability) www.sexualhealth.com

Sexuality Information and Education Council of the US www.siecus.org

Sexuality Information and Education Council of Canada www.sieccan.org

Society for Sex Therapy and Research www.sstarnet.org

http://www.cancerbackup.org.uk/Resourcessupport/ Relationshipscommunication/Sexuality. This web site is from the UK and provides comprehensive information about sexual changes after cancer.

Web sites for patients

http://www.mdanderson.org/topics/sexuality/

Sexuality may not be the primary focus for many cancer patients, but at some point, whether because of sexual changes, relationship issues or difficulties with fertility, patients' realise the impact of cancer on their sexuality. No matter the diagnosis or prognosis, you can take care of your sexual health.

http://www.uoaa.org/ostomy_info/

Organisation offers guidebooks and fact sheets about having sex for those with an ostomy.

http://www.cancerhelp.org.uk/help/default.asp? page=215

Tells you about sex and sexuality and how it can be affected when you have cancer.

http://www.cancer.net/patient/Coping/Emotional+and+ Physical+Matters/Sexual+and+Reproductive+ Health/Body+Image+and+Sexuality For both men and women, the physical changes brought on by surgery or chemotherapy can have a constant effect on their well-being and body image. There are some common worries related to sexuality that many people with cancer share.

http://www.livestrong.org/site/c.khLXK1PxHmF/ b.2660611/k.BCED/Home.htm Provides links to different physical effects, including sexual dysfunction in men and women and fertility.

http://www.caring4cancer.com/go/cancer/wellbeing/ physical-wellbeing/frequently-asked-questions-about-sexuality-and-cancer.htm Frequently asked questions about cancer and sexuality.

http://www.state.nj.us/health/ccr/resourcebook/ rb9929.htm

It is often very hard for the person with cancer to talk about what affect cancer or cancer treatment has on their sexual feelings or functioning. This site includes information regarding phases of sexual response, impact of cancer on sexuality and includes a listing of helpful readings.

Sexuality and reproductive issues

http://www.cancer.gov/cancer_information/ doc_pdq.aspx?viewid=829EA02D-5EB8-43E8-B0DB-54CB0B0F9BC1

This site addresses the impact cancer and cancer treatment can have on all aspects of an individual's sexuality, including sexual desire, and physical and psychological sexual dysfunction. You can select from two available versions: For the Patient or For the Health Professional.

Fertile Hope www.fertilehope.com (Advocates and provides information on cancer and infertility)

The Oncofertility consortium www.myoncofertility.org

Pregnant with Cancer ww.pregnantwithcancer.org (Information and peer support for women diagnosed during pregnancy)

http://www.bccancer.bc.ca/PPI/RecommendedLinks/ coping/symptomssideeffects/fertility.htm This gives links to web sites discussing fertility and cancer.

The sexuality, intimacy and communications

http://www.cancersupportivecare.com/sexuality.html

The material presented on this site will help to increase awareness of attitudes about sexuality to form a basis to begin to communicate sexual feelings and needs more directly.

Sexuality and cancer

http://www.cancer.med.umich.edu/share/ pro01sp04.htm

Common questions and answers about sexuality and cancer treatment.

Information about sexuality for women with cancer

Female Sexual Dysfunction www.femalesexual dysfunctiononline.org

http://www.medicalnewstoday.com/articles/
126327.php

This journal is devoted entirely to women's sexuality
and cancer

http://www.cancersa.org.au/aspx/Sexuality_for_
women_with_cancer.aspx

When you're first diagnosed with cancer, you usually
want to focus on getting well. You may not think
about the impact on your sex life, body image, relationships and self-esteem until treatment is over.

http://www.breasthealth.com.au/livingwithcancer/
sexuality.html Breast surgery, radiotherapy, hormonal therapy and chemotherapy often have a
significant effect on how women feel about themselves and their attractiveness. This can happen to
any woman, whether or not she has a partner.

**Sexuality and cancer: for the woman who has
cancer and her partner**

http://documents.cancer.org/6710.00/

This American Cancer Society booklet is an excellent
resource for patients and health care providers.

http://www.cnn.com/HEALTH/library/SA/00071.html

The most common physical sexual problem for women
after cancer is painful intercourse. It is most often
caused by hormonal changes that lead to vaginal
dryness. This site explains why this happens and
offers some possible solutions.

http://cancer.med.upenn.edu/coping/article.cfm?
c=4&s=42&ss=90&id=470

This site includes interviews with five women who
were diagnosed with breast cancer and underwent
different cancer treatments at various stages of life.
They share their experiences of diagnosis and treatment and changes in their sexuality.

The Mautner project: for lesbians with cancer

http://www.mautnerproject.org/ Founded in 1990, the
Mautner Project is the only organisation dedicated to
lesbians with cancer, their partners and caregivers.

Information about sexuality for men with cancer

Impotence.org www.impotence.org (a web site funded
by a major pharmacological manufacturer, but created by an independent group of experts and spon-
sored by AFUD)

International Society for Sexual and Impotence
Research (follow the links to 'The book *Erectile
Dysfunction* is online!') The ISSIR is an international professional organisation that studies ED
www.issir.org

Consortium for Improvement in Erectile Function
(CIEF). www.erectilefunction.org

http://www.prostate-cancer.org.uk/pdf/toolkit/
sexuality.pdf

This fact sheet is for men who have been diagnosed
with prostate cancer and their partners.

http://www.prostatehealth.org.au/newsitem.html?
notice_id=388

This web site describes alternative sexual activities for
men with prostate cancer and ED.

**Sexuality and cancer: for the man who has cancer
and his partner**

http://documents.cancer.org/6709.00/

This American Cancer Society booklet is an excellent
resource for patients and health care providers.

US Too, International: www.ustoo.com (Prostate
cancer support organisation)

This web site is for men who have had prostate cancer
and their partners. www.Phoenix5.com

Acknowledgements

Special thanks to Mark Morrow, B.S. for his editorial
assistance.

References

1. Thaler-DeMers, D. (2001) Intimacy issues: sexuality, fertility, and relationships. *Seminars in Oncology Nursing*, **17** (4),
255–262.
2. Schover, L., Montague, D. and Lakin, M. (1997) Sexual
problems, in *Cancer: Principles and Practices of Oncology*,
5th edn (eds V.T. Devita, S. Hellman and S.A. Rosenberg),
Lippincott-Raven, Philadelphia, pp. 2857–2871.
3. Schover, L.R. (2008) Premature ovarian failure and its consequences: vasomotor symptoms, sexuality, and fertility. *Journal of Clinical Oncology*, **26** (5), 753–758.
4. Leiblum, S.R., Baume, R.M. and Croog, S.H. (1994) The
sexual functioning of elderly hypertensive women. *Journal
of Sex and Marital Therapy*, **20** (4), 259–270.
5. Bober, S.L. (2009) From the guest editor: out in the open:
addressing sexual health after cancer. *Cancer Journal*, **15**
(1), 13–14.

6. Bruner, D.W. and Boyd, C.P. (1999) Assessing women's sexuality after cancer therapy: checking assumptions with the focus group technique. *Cancer Nursing*, **22** (6), 438–447.

7. Tomlinson, J.M. (2005) Talking a sexual history, in *ABC of Sexual Health*, 2nd (ed. J.M. Tomlinson), Blackwell Publishing, Inc., Malden, MA, pp. 13–16.

8. Maslow, A. (1943) A theory of human motivation. *Psychological Reviews*, **50**, 370–396.

9. Tierney, D.K. (2008) Sexuality: a quality-of-life issue for cancer survivors. *Seminars in Oncology Nursing*, **24** (2), 71–79.

10. Shell, J.A. (2007) Sexuality, in *Oncology Nursing* (eds R. Carroll-Johnson, L. Gorman and N. Bush), Mosby, St. Louis, MO, pp. 546–564.

11. Stausmire, J.M. (2004) Sexuality at the end of life. *American Journal of Hospice and Palliative Medicine*, **21** (1), 33–39.

12. Shifren, J.L., Monz, B.U., Russo, P.A. *et al.* (2008) Sexual problems and distress in United States women: prevalence and correlates. *Obstetrics and Gynecology*, **112** (5), 970–978.

13. Malcarne, V.L., Banthia, R., Varni, J.W. *et al.* (2002) Problem-solving skills and emotional distress in spouses of men with prostate cancer. *Journal of Cancer Education*, **17** (3), 150–154.

14. Masters, W. and Johnson, V. (1966) *Human Sexual Response*, 1st edn, Little Brown, Boston, MA.

15. Gregoire, A. (2005) Male sexual problems, in *ABC of Sexual Health*, 2nd edn (ed. J.M. Tomlinson), Blackwell Publishing, Inc., Malden, MA, pp. 37–39.

16. Basson, R. (2001) Human sex-response cycles. *Journal of Sex and Marital Therapy*, **27** (1), 33–43.

17. Kandeel, F.R., Koussa, V.K. and Swerdloff, R.S. (2001) Male sexual function and its disorders: physiology, pathophysiology, clinical investigation, and treatment. *Endocrine Reviews*, **22** (3), 342–388.

18. Katz, A. (2007) *Breaking the Silence on Cancer and Sexuality*, Oncology Nursing Society, Pittsburgh, PA.

19. Schiavi, R.C. and Segraves, R.T. (1995) The biology of sexual function. *Psychiatric Clinics of North America*, **18** (1), 7–23.

20. Sarrel, P. (1990) Genital blood flow and ovarian secretions. *The Journal of Clinical Practice in Sexuality*, (Special Issue), 14–15.

21. Zilbergeld, B., Ellison, C., Leiblum, S. and Pervin, L. (1980) Desire discrepancies and arousal problems in sex therapy, *Principles and Practice of Sex Therapy*, Guildord Press, New York.

22. Gallo-Silver, L. (2000) The sexual rehabilitation of persons with cancer. *Cancer Practice*, **8** (1), 10–15.

23. Maurice, W.L. (1999) *Sexual Medicine in Primary Care*, Mosby, St. Louis, MO.

24. Goldstein, I., Meston, C.M., Traish, A.M. *et al.* (2007) Future directions, in *Women's Sexual Function and Dysfunction: Study, Diagnosis, and Treatment*, Taylor & Francis, London, pp. 745–748.

25. Schover, L. (2007) Reproductive complications and sexual dysfunction in cancer sarvirors, in *Cancer Survivorship; Today and Tomorrow* (ed. P.A. Ganz), Springer, New York, pp. 251–271.

26. Derogatis, L.R. and Kourlesis, S.M. (1981) An approach to evaluation of sexual problems in the cancer patient. *CA: A Cancer Journal for Clinicians*, **31** (1), 46–50.

27. Schover, L.R. (2005) Sexuality and fertility after cancer. *Hematology: American Society of Hematology Education Program*, 523–527.

28. Wenzel, L., Dogan-Ates, A., Habbal, R. *et al.* (2005) Defining and measuring reproductive concerns of female cancer survivors. *Journal of the National Cancer Institute Monographs*, **34**, 94–98.

29. Schover, L.R. (1999) Psychosocial aspects of infertility and decisions about reproduction in young cancer survivors: a review. *Medical and Pediatric Oncology*, **33** (1), 53–59.

30. Schover, L.R. (2005) Motivation for parenthood after cancer: a review. *Journal of the National Cancer Institute Monographs*, **34**, 2–5.

31. Simon, B., Lee, S.J., Partridge, A.H. and Runowicz, C.D. (2005) Preserving fertility after cancer. *CA: A Cancer Journal for Clinicians*, **55** (4), 211–228; quiz 63–64.

32. Partridge, A.H., Burstein, H.J. and Winer, E.P. (2001) Side effects of chemotherapy and combined chemohormonal therapy in women with early-stage breast cancer. *Journal of the National Cancer Institute Monographs*, **30**, 135–142.

33. Fossa, S.D. and Dahl, A.A. (2008) Fertility and sexuality in young cancer survivors who have adult-onset malignancies. *Hematology/Oncology Clinics of North America*, **22** (2), 291–303, vii.

34. Dow, K.H. and Kuhn, D. (2004) Fertility options in young breast cancer survivors: a review of the literature. *Oncology Nursing Forum*, **31** (3), E46–E53.

35. Leonard, M., Hammelef, K. and Smith, G.D. (2004) Fertility considerations, counseling, and semen cryopreservation for males prior to the initiation of cancer therapy. *Clinical Journal of Oncology Nursing*, **8** (2), 127–131, 145.

36. Wallace, W.H., Anderson, R.A. and Irvine, D.S. (2005) Fertility preservation for young patients with cancer: who is at risk and what can be offered? *Lancet Oncology*, **6** (4), 209–218.

37. Lamb, M.A. (1995) Effects of cancer on the sexuality and fertility of women. *Seminars in Oncology Nursing*, **11** (2), 120–127.

38. American Society of Clinical Oncology (2006) ASCO Recommendations on fertility preservation in cancer patients: guideline summary. *Journal of Oncology Practice*, **2** (3), 143–146.

39. Oktay, K. and Sonmezer, M. (2004) Ovarian tissue banking for cancer patients: fertility preservation, not just ovarian cryopreservation. *Human Reproduction*, **19** (3), 477–480.

40. Carter, J. (2005) Cancer-related infertility. *Gynecologic Oncology*, **99** (3, Suppl. 1), S122–S123.

41. Katz, A. (2009) Gay and lesbian patients with cancer. *Oncology Nursing Forum*, **36** (2), 203–207.

42. Dibble, S., Eliason, M.J., Dejoseph, J.F. and Chinn, P. (2008) Sexual issues in special populations: lesbian and gay individuals. *Seminars in Oncology Nursing*, **24** (2), 127–130.

43. Boehmer, U., Potter, J. and Bowen, D.J. (2009) Sexual functioning after cancer in sexual minority women. *Cancer Journal*, **15** (1), 65–69.

44. Andersen, B.L. (2009) In sickness and in health: maintaining intimacy after breast cancer recurrence. *Cancer Journal*, **15** (1), 70–73.

45. Manne, S.L., Ostroff, J., Winkel, G. *et al.* (2005) Partner unsupportive responses, avoidant coping, and distress among women with early stage breast cancer: patient and partner perspectives. *Health Psychology*, **24** (6), 635–641.

46. Annon, J.S. (1976) The PLISSIT model: a proposed conceptual scheme for the behavioral treatment of sexual problems. *Journal of Sex Education and Therapy*, **2**, 1–15.

47. Hughes, M.K. (2000) Sexuality and the cancer survivor: a silent coexistence. *Cancer Nursing*, **23** (6), 477–482.

48. Smith, D.B. and Babaian, R.J. (1992) The effects of treatment for cancer on male fertility and sexuality. *Cancer Nursing*, **15** (4), 271–275.

49. Hughes, M.K. (1996) Sexuality changes in the cancer patient: M.D. Anderson case reports and review. *Nursing Interventions in Oncology*, **8**, 15–18.

50. Hughes, M., Holland, J., Greenberg, D. and Hughes, M. (eds) (2006) Sexual Dysfunction, *Quick Reference for Oncology Clinicians: The Psychiatric and Psychological Dimensions of Cancer Symptom Management*, IPOS Press, Charlottesville, VA.

51. Masters, W.H., Johnson, V.E. and Kolodny, R.C. (1992) *Human Sexuality*, HarperCollins, New York.

52. Notelovitz, M. (1990) Management of the changing vagina. *The Journal of Clinical Practice in Sexuality*, (Special Issue), 16–21.

53. Schover, L.R. (1993) Sexual rehabilitation after treatment for prostate cancer. *Cancer*, **71** (Suppl. 3), 1024–1030.

54. Guirguis, W.R. (1998) Oral treatment of erectile dysfunction: from herbal remedies to designer drugs. *Journal of Sex and Marital Therapy*, **24** (2), 69–73.

55. Hughes, M.K. (2008) Alterations of sexual function in women with cancer. *Seminars in Oncology Nursing*, **24** (2), 91–101.

56. Padma-Nathan, H., Hellstrom, W.J., Kaiser, F.E. *et al.*, Medicated Urethral System for Erection (MUSE) Study Group (1997) Treatment of men with erectile dysfunction with transurethral alprostadil. *New England Journal of Medicine*, **336** (1), 1–7.

57. Albaugh, J.A. (2006) Intracavernosal injection algorithm. *Urologic Nursing*, **26** (6), 449–453.

58. Kendall, A., Dowsett, M., Folkerd, E. and Smith, I. (2006) Caution: vaginal estradiol appears to be contraindicated in postmenopausal women on adjuvant aromatase inhibitors. *Annals of Oncology*, **17** (4), 584–587.

59. Greenwald, H.P. and McCorkle, R. (2008) Sexuality and sexual function in long-term survivors of cervical cancer. *Journal of Womens Health*, **17** (6), 955–963.

60. Heiman, J.R. (2008) Treating low sexual desire - new findings for testosterone in women. *New England Journal of Medicine*, **359** (19), 2047–2049.

16 Focused Family Therapy in Palliative Care and Bereavement

David W. Kissane and Talia I. Zaider

Department of Psychiatry and Behavioral Sciences, Memorial Sloan-Kettering Cancer Center, New York, NY, USA

The predominant models of psychotherapy are individual or group approaches in the main, a finding that is not surprising given the dominant research paradigms. Yet when psychiatric illness relapses, attention to family influences is vital to counter perpetuating factors contributing to the predicament. In the cancer setting, a focus on family-centred care seems imperative once it becomes clear that cure or disease containment is no longer achievable. This reality has encouraged the 20 years of research into families with cancer that has underpinned the Family Focused Grief Therapy (FFGT) model described in this chapter.

16.1 Theoretical Background

The functioning of the family proves highly determinative of the relapse of most mental illnesses, whether schizophrenia [1], bipolar disorder and depression [2] or complicated grief [3]. In serious mental illness, the presence of high 'expressed emotion' in the family contributes to relapse, and this is recognised by the presence of critical comments, hostility or emotional over-involvement, exemplified by excessive worry [4]. In bereavement care, the empirical model developed by our group identified cohesion, communication and conflict resolution, the three 'C's' of family relationships, as determinative of the family's adaptiveness [5, 6].

A typology of family functioning during palliative care and bereavement was assessed using the Family Environment Scale (FES) [7], which differentiates families into well functioning, intermediate and dysfunctional classes [5, 6]. From the 10 subscales comprising the FES, only three known as the Family Relationships Index (FRI), which are based on members' perceptions of the family's cohesiveness, expressiveness and capacity to deal with conflict, were found in cluster analyses to differentiate families for this typology [8].

Two family types are well functioning: *supportive* families are characterised by very high levels of cohesion, and *conflict resolvers* tolerate differences of opinion and deal with conflict constructively through effective communication. During advanced cancer care, about 50% of families are like these. They are resilient families, have low levels of psychosocial morbidity and do not need family therapy.

Two family types show dysfunctional relationships: *hostile* families are characterised by high conflict, low cohesion and poor expressiveness, and tend to reject help; *sullen* families also carry impairments in communication, cohesiveness and conflict resolution, but their anger is muted and they seek help. These dysfunctional families have high rates of psychosocial morbidity, including clinical depression. Fifteen to 20% of palliative care families are dysfunctional, the rate increasing to 30% during the initial phase of bereavement [3].

Between these well and poorly functioning groups remain one third of families, who exhibit moderate cohesiveness and remain prone to psychosocial morbidity. Their functioning has been termed *intermediate* and tends to deteriorate under the strain of death and bereavement.

FFGT is operationalised on the seminal observation that the two dysfunctional and intermediate classes carry the substantial psychosocial morbidity found during palliative care and bereavement and become the target of the intervention [9]. Rather than attempting to treat each family member individually, FFGT offers a cost effective, systemic approach, which can be applied preventively. We refrain from pathologising families in any way as our classification is not diagnostic, but only points to those 'at risk'. Given the importance we attach to assisting families as they care for their dying relative, these families carrying greater needs are invited to meet together for family sessions.

16.2 Target Groups of Patients

'At risk' families are identified through screening with the short form of the FRI [7], a 12-item, self-report measure that is completed independently by family members. The FRI's sensitivity is high, with 86% rate of detection of dysfunction against the FAD [10, 11]; an independent group reported 100% sensitivity to

detect family dysfunction and 88% to detect clinical depression [12]. The FRI is unlikely to miss those at risk, although its poorer specificity will generate some false positives. Threshold scores are shown in Figure 16.1.

16.3 Main Themes and Format of the Therapy

The therapy is focused and time-limited, comprising 6–10 sessions of 90 minutes duration, which are arranged flexibly across 9–18 months. FFGT is a manualised intervention, whose guidelines were published in a book, with a series of clinical illustrations [13]. The intervention aims to optimise cohesion, communication (of thoughts and feelings) and the handling of conflict while promoting the sharing of grief and mutual support. The story of illness with its associated losses and changes, both current and anticipated, is shared in the process.

		TRUE	FALSE
1.	Family members really help and support one another		
2.	Family members often keep their feelings to themselves		
3.	We fight a lot in our family		
4.	We often seem to be killing time at home		
5.	We say anything we want to around the home		
6.	Family members rarely become openly angry		
7.	We put a lot of energy into what we do at home		
8.	It is hard to "blow off steam" at home without upsetting somebody		
9.	Family members sometimes get so angry they throw things		
10.	There is a feeling of togetherness in our family		
11.	We tell each other about our personal problems		
12.	Family members hardly ever lose their tempers		

Cohesiveness = Q1 + Reverse Q4 + Q7 + Q10; Expressiveness = RQ2 + Q5 + RQ8 + Q11; Conflict = Q3 + RQ6 + Q9 + RQ12. FRI = sum of Cohesiveness + Expressiveness + Reverse Conflict scores. FRI scores of 10–12 = well functioning families; 8–9 = intermediate; 5–7 = sullen; 0–4 = hostile types. Modified and reproduced by special permission of Consulting Psychologists Press, Inc., Palo Alto, CA from the Family Environment Scale Form-R by Rudolf H. Moos.[7]

Figure 16.1 *The family relationships index (FRI).*

FFGT has three phases: *assessment* (one to two weekly sessions) concentrates on identifying issues and concerns relevant to each family and on developing a plan to deal with them (see Box 16.1 for checklist covering the content of these assessment sessions); *intervention* (typically three to six monthly sessions) focuses on the agreed concerns (see Box 16.2 for checklist covering the content of these sessions) and *termination* (one to two sessions spaced two to three months apart as booster sessions), in which gains are consolidated and response prevention for the future considered.

The number and regularity of sessions are adapted to suit the family. Where therapy can be commenced

---

Box 16.1 Checklist for Assessment Phase of FFGT

1. Welcome and introductions.
2. Orientation.
   a. Gather their expectations about the family meeting together.
   b. Add therapists' objectives for the family.
3. Data gathering.
   a. The story of illness:
      'What's happening? How serious is it?'
   b. Assess communication:
      'How openly do you talk about the illness?'
   c. Assess cohesiveness:
      'How well do you help and support each other?'
   d. Assess conflict:
      'Who fights with whom in your family and what happens?'
   e. Assess roles, rules and expectations:
      'Who does the caregiving? Who is effective at comforting one another? Are rules important? Is more mutual help needed?'
   f. Assess values and beliefs:
      'What distinguishes you as a family? Do you have a motto?'
4. Construct a family genogram, seeking to understand coping patterns with previous losses and what relational styles are evident across the generations.
5. Identify family strengths:
   Both group-as-a-whole and noteworthy individual contributions.
6. Summarise family concerns in the context of their functioning:
   Name the patterns of communication, teamwork and conflict resolution.
   Invite consensus.
7. Clarify options and agree on future management plan with dates for sessions.

Box 16.2 Checklist for Focused Treatment Phase of FFGT

1. Each session begins with a welcome and orientation:
   a. Use linear questions to connect with each person present.
   b. Remind family through use of a summary of their focused goals of therapy.
2. Review how the family is coping with the illness and their grief over losses or bereavement (if patient is deceased):
   Use circular questioning to ask members to comment on how they perceive others are coping with their grief.
3. Acknowledge losses and related grief, including any emergent strength in mutual support.
4. Remind the family of their prioritised concerns, including relevant aspects of communication, cohesiveness and conflict resolution, or other agreed targets of the work.
   a. Review what has been good progress since last meeting. Any examples?
   b. Identify any challenges since last meeting.
   c. Use group problem solving regarding declared concerns.
5. Unspoken concerns/palliative care themes.
   a. Identify any issues or themes that the family wishes to talk about.
6. Summarise what progress is evident, affirming strengths alongside any continuing targets for future effort.
   a. Affirm instances of shared grief as a family group.
   b. Affirm improved communication, cohesion or conflict resolution.
7. Arrange next session, locating it within the overall plan of time-limited therapy.

---

over approximately the last six months of the patient's life, generally four to five sessions are held with the patient actively involved and before the frailty of illness prevents his or her continued contribution. Therapists maintain regular telephone contact with the family over the days/weeks of the dying process, and the therapist attends the funeral to sustain their therapeutic alliance. Resumption of the family sessions can usually occur one to two months post death and then continue for another five to six sessions until the goals of therapy have been both accomplished and consolidated. Families with only intermediate disturbance to their functioning may gain by six sessions overall, whereas those with greater levels of dysfunctionality need around 10 sessions to adequately support the family.

16.4 Therapy Processes and Techniques

16.4.1 Key Theoretical Models Underpinning FFGT

Three theories have guided our development of FFGT: attachment theory [14], cognitive processing theory in adaptation to trauma [15] and group adaptation [16]. These will, in turn, guide the techniques and processes of therapy.

16.4.1.1 Attachment Theory

Grief resulting from relational losses can be understood to develop proportionately to the strength of the bonds of attachment. The most significant relationships that people have are generally found in families, whether nuclear, family-of-origin or extended family [17]. While family members share emotional expression about the many losses associated with the illness and death, restorative coping responses are triggered as the family strives to re-establish some order and continuity. Our FFGT model facilitates both elements of the dual-process model [18] through inviting sharing of grief alongside improved family functioning, in which communication, co-operation and mutual support are enhanced.

16.4.1.2 Cognitive Processing Theory

Beyond emotional expression, the related cognitive processing involves achieving an understanding of events in accordance with one's prior belief system, as well as the modification of this system, termed 'the assumptive world' [19, 20]. This is a schema of ideas, values, attitudes and beliefs that we each employ to organise our life in the world, including our adaptation to new events. Illness and death disrupt the assumptive world schema. At the family level, emotional disclosure and social sharing impact on members' assumptive world views [21, 22], leading to cognitive reappraisal as confrontation or avoidance strategies unfold within the family. Family functioning through the family's basic communication processes and negotiation of differences impacts dynamically on members' cognitions. Families challenge negative rumination and model how to find positive meaning, despite the sadness of the loss [23]. They guide a sensible and balanced regulation of grieving, recognising when some avoidance is healthy, but too much is detrimental. Families pursue cognitive reframing iteratively, using the diverse views of the membership to test out options, problem solve and mutually support each other in finding new meaning

and coping adaptively. The family is also well placed to counter the loneliness of bereavement.

16.4.1.3 Group Adaptation

The dynamics of any group discussion oscillate between enabling and restrictive solutions, as constructive suggestions are offered by some to resolve an issue, while others urge caution based on their fear of what could happen [16]. The group, in this case the family, grapples with these options. The resultant debate may generate consensus, with adaptive choices generally resulting from constructive views. Sometimes a dominant individual will impose a deleterious point-of-view or indecisive persons are led by the majority. Difference of opinion can create conflict, such disagreements dividing the group and reducing their sense of unity. The cohesiveness of a family is one hallmark of its effectiveness in promoting the development and maturity of its members.

16.4.2 Key Therapist Techniques in the Application of FFGT

Therapists should be trained in family therapy, can function as individual therapists and commonly come from the disciplines of social work, psychology and psychiatry. A co-therapy model is possible for therapists' training. The therapist interacts warmly and authentically, manifesting both interest and concern. Their first skill is to build a solid collaborative alliance, as this models the style of relating that is a prominent family objective. Secondly, the therapist promotes resilience by explicitly acknowledging family strengths through praise and affirmation. This reinforces what is proven to work well and prevents the family feeling criticised. Thirdly, by reaching agreement over identified 'issues' or 'concerns' (note that the word 'problems' is deliberately avoided), a treatment plan is negotiated to work collaboratively. The development of this shared agenda safeguards against the therapist acting directively and builds team solutions to the family's concerns.

One of the fundamental skills used by an effective clinician is the ability to ask the 'right' question, as this invites observation, reflection and consideration of change. As each family member responds, others listen and enter the discussion. Following Tomm's model, questions can be classified into linear, circular, strategic and reflexive [24] and are illustrated in Table 16.1. During assessment, therapists use more orienting and investigative types of questions, whereas later in the

Table 16.1	Types of orienting and influencing questions asked by therapists in FFGT	
Complementary types of questions	**Description of the function and purpose of each questioning style**	**Typical examples used in FFGT**
Linear (generally orienting and informative about individuals)	These generate a one-to-one conversation between the therapist and each individual, help to obtain information, join with and support individuals, prove useful when open-ended to take a history but are conservative in promoting family interaction.	What job do you have? What grade are you in at school? What sports do you like to play?
Circular (orienting and informative about family-as-a-whole dynamics)	These seek observations from one family member about others, asking each iteratively to step into the shoes of one another and share diverse views that stimulate family discussion and reveal relational dynamics.	How are your spouse and children coping? Who talks to whom? Who are you most worried about?
Reflexive (generally influencing without being directive)	These encourage mutual understanding and support via greater insight and awareness of the meaning of any individual responses, can include hypotheses about dynamics inserted into the wording of the question, and seek to promote reflection upon solutions and consideration of acceptance or change.	What are your expectations about the future? How might things look different in one year? If X were still alive, what would she ask of you? Why do you think he's become more irritable?
Strategic (both influencing and potentially more directive in intent)	These invite a search for a solution and aim to build consensus about future directions, including options for acceptance or change; if too directive, they may be constraining rather than generative.	How helpful might it be for dad to reach out to old friends? What benefits would come from talking about end-of-life care? Might more open sharing of feelings increase your sense of family connection?

active phase of therapy, questions become more influencing and generative in style [25].

Another essential skill is the therapist's use of summaries, which check that what the clinician has understood to have occurred, is agreed with or amended by the family. The clinician may also invite the family to add to the therapist's summary. Summaries serve as the main means of sustaining the focus of the therapy on family functioning, coping and grief work. In general, summaries are offered at the beginning of each session to link back to prior work and help set an ongoing agenda. Importantly, summaries at the close of each session ensure that the family integrates its understanding of gains and direction of effort. Sessions that have been busy, argumentative or chaotic and running over in time can derail a therapist from attending to this task, yet it is a fundamental step in the focused application of this model.

A final technique is the ability to encourage expression of genuine feelings. This depends on spotting cues, often non-verbal in nature. The clinician then seeks to understand what lies behind the feeling, thus fostering open sharing of distress and resultant mutual comfort. Rather than the direct, linear model of empathic validation or normalisation used in

individual therapy, the family therapist stays circular in asking others what the 'tears-in-the-eye' mean, thus fostering an empathic exchange between family members instead of solely therapist-to-individual.

16.4.3 Key Therapeutic Processes for the Family in FFGT

Challenging scenarios that arise when meeting with distressed families in palliative care include facilitating talk about death and dying and managing volatility in family sessions. The patterns described below come from observations of FFGT where direct quotes illustrate key processes, although identifying information has been changed to protect confidentiality. These therapeutic strategies recognise relationships as reciprocal and mutually influencing and look to harness relational sources of strength and resilience [26].

16.4.3.1 Facilitating Talk about Death and Dying

One fundamental goal of FFGT is to empower family members to openly share concerns about the threat of loss and its implications for the future. Paradoxically, family members' well-meaning protectiveness and loyalty can strongly inhibit frank discussion about death and dying. The role of the clinician is to recognise and gradually chip away at the relational constraints that block this conversation, while also respecting the emotional threshold, any cultural norms and pace of the family as they steer towards and away from this issue. These discussions ultimately diminish family members' isolation and help them better coordinate mutual support.

Because we view the family as a social unit, it is informative to draw from early theoretical writings that describe the process of dying as a social process. Glaser and Strauss [27], in a monograph entitled *Awareness of Dying* described how patients, relatives and hospital staff co-create a context of awareness. The movement from closed to open awareness of dying is socially coordinated so that patients, relatives and hospital staff negotiate what is said to whom and what is kept silent. Their emphasis was on the communication of medical information, as they were writing when most physicians did not provide much detail. Many societies (Japan, China, Italy, Spain and Latin America) that considered death talk taboo have been gradually moving to a more open stance. More recent theorists [28, 29] have emphasised that preparation for death involves more than the pursuit of information – which in this day and age is done more openly – because there is a kind of 'sentiment work' that needs to unfold, a processing of one's affective response to the predicament. In families, these factual discussions of illness, death or prognosis may be orchestrated to regulate and maintain a level of emotional intensity that feels manageable.

Evidence of the benefits of 'detoxifying death' [30] through open discussion has accumulated over recent decades. Hebert and colleagues noted that communication is the central pathway through which caregivers prepare for death [31]. This includes both patient–doctor and family communication about prognosis, future plans and concerns. Moreover, we know that caregivers who are poorly prepared for their relative's death are more likely to suffer morbid outcomes (e.g. increased depression, complicated grief) [32, 33]; that disclosure about cancer-related concerns is associated with better relationship functioning and lower distress among patients and their relatives [34]; and that open discussion about death, dying and bereavement with terminally ill patients and their caregivers is not perceived to add stress, but rather prove helpful to many [35]. This should always be developed at a culturally sensitive pace.

We turn now to a description of how talk about death and dying can unfold therapeutically in the context of FFGT.

16.4.3.2 The Entry Point: Inviting Discussion of Death into the Room

There are things that I feel we don't talk about and um...I understand why...but I feel like I – it's something I'd like to – I would like to use some of our time – if it's appropriate – in, um...[pause] We don't talk about me dying...and um...and I'd like to. (Patient)

I remember – my mother died of cancer...it was so difficult for everybody and...I somehow would like to make it a little better for us...we would talk to each other about my mother, but she was the one dying and then nobody talked to her about how – what they were experiencing...and it was very, very difficult. And I see a little bit of that now. (Patient)

We don't talk about the essence of it ...that this person that perhaps you love is not going to be here anymore. I hit the surface with you [turns to husband] but I can't really talk about it with you because you talk me out of it. (Patient)

In each of these statements, the patient expresses a wish to acknowledge and discuss the inevitability of loss, signalling an opportunity for the clinician to invite conversation about death and dying into the room. More often, clinicians may need to initiate this discussion themselves. Two guiding principles increase the likelihood of an effective entry into this discussion: (i) *Considering the hypothetical*: when the prognosis is unclear, or when some family members express a strong wish to preserve a positive outlook, the clinician can minimise the threatening nature of discussing death by asking the family to consider the threat of loss as a *hypothetical*, rather than imminent, scenario. Furthermore, explicitly asking permission of the family to reflect on this possibility, while it seems a small step, can set the course for a collaborative versus coercive process; (ii) *Maintaining Neutrality*: family members often adopt divergent views with respect to the patients' prognosis, with one member 'specialising' in a hopeful stance (e.g. advocating the pursuit of second opinions or alternative treatment strategies) and another in grief (e.g. acknowledging imminent loss). The tension between these positions can polarise family members, generating conflict and pulling the clinician into alignment with one or the other view. The principle of neutrality guides the clinician to give voice to the dilemma that exists for the family, thus making space for all points of view and avoiding the temptation to problem-solve or support one position. By staying neutral and curious [36], the clinician is able to contain and normalise differences in the family as a way of managing the ambiguity of their circumstances.

16.4.3.3 Talk about Prognosis

Discussions of death and dying often begin with an exchange of information about prognosis and the perceived seriousness of the disease. However, as the therapist elicits news of the patient's medical condition, treatment course and future outlook, the family is invited to observe one another's emotional response to this information. Doing so enables family members to become attuned to one another's coping, thus strengthening cohesiveness. In the following excerpt, the family expresses concern about one family member, Frank, who initially minimises his distress. The discussion that ensues highlights the value of conjoint family sessions, in which individuals who might not otherwise seek support or openly verbalise their distress are recognised and supported by those closest to them.

THERAPIST: How do you think your mom is doing...I want to check in with the three of you to see what your impressions are and how it's been going?

DAUGHTER 1: It's harder and sadder.

PATIENT: I think it's harder for Frank now; it just seems hard for me when I look at him.

THERAPIST: What have you been seeing?

FRANK: I'm alright, I'm okay, I'm going to be fine, one day at a time.

PATIENT (tearful): Basically that's it, yeah. I think it's harder for him for some reason.

DAUGHTER 2: Yeah, I think I know what you mean.

DAUGHTER 1: It's hard for all of us, like you said, but for Frank, I don't know, it might hit him a little harder.

THERAPIST: So Frank, your mom started crying when she saw you.

FRANK: I don't even know what to say honestly. I'm fine, I take it one day at a time, you know, I'm upset, you know, I don't know what else to say. I deal with it in my own way, but I'm strong.

THERAPIST: So how do you deal with it?

FRANK: How do I deal with it? I don't know, I get mad, sad, you know. I take it out on certain people I shouldn't take it out on, work-wise. I don't know. It's all inside and I don't know how to get out of it, but I'm okay. I'm okay. It's just weird.

16.4.3.4 Talk about 'Talk'

Families often discuss the process of talking together about the illness, their dynamic of choosing what they say to stay safe and not distress each other, their motivation to protect one another.

They're worried that I'll think they've made it final. (Patient)

The fact that she is still feeling like she wants to make it to one hundred makes it hard for me to discuss any more things about her dying...I don't want to take away that will that is making her fight. (Patient's daughter)

These statements hint at some of the concerns that constrain open communication about death and dying among family members. When talk about death and dying proves too difficult or anxiety provoking, the therapist attempts to 'slice it thinner' [37] by stepping back from painful content and inquiring instead about the process of talking itself (e.g. 'How is it to talk about this now?', 'Who has the hardest time talking about this?', 'Who is most comfortable talking about this?', 'Who is most helped by talking about this?'). This enables the family to clarify factors that enable or restrict conversations about illness, and to become familiar with the conditions needed to sustain open communication. Contributing factors might include trans-generational patterns of communication or differences in communication styles among its members that need to be acknowledged and accommodated. In addition, underlying premises held by family members about the dangers of talking openly about death and dying can be useful to explore. The process by which the therapist unpacks these constraining beliefs is illustrated below in an excerpt from an FFGT session. In the following segment, the family reconsiders the strongly held belief that open sharing of distress implies weakness:

THERAPIST: So it sounds like "strong' in this family means like you hold some of your emotions back to protect yourself and others?

DAUGHTER 1: To protect the other person!

THERAPIST: So what happens with Sarah?

SARAH: I guess I'm not that strong?

SON: She's very emotional, she gets upset.

SARAH: I can't, I can't hold it in. I don't know, it's just... but when I know I have to be, I guess I can do it. I don't know if that's the right word, strong, then, maybe that's the wrong word.

THERAPIST: I don't know, I mean we've all been saying strong, but I wonder if keeping your feelings in really means that you're strong or does it just mean...?

DAUGHTER 2: Tough?

SON: Well, I act all tough around here, but when I get home, I'm crying on my wife's shoulder.

THERAPIST: It sounds then like everyone in this family can get upset sometimes, while also feeling strong. Is it possible to do both?

16.4.3.5 Talk about Future Needs

I don't want you to think that, after 6 months, everything is forgotten... people do that, out of sight, out of mind – I'll go to a meeting, then come home to an empty house. (patient's husband to his adult children)

She [patient] is the glue that holds everything together... between me and my dad. I'm worried about that. (patient's daughter)

Once family members are able to consider the real or hypothetical threat of losing their loved one, the process of preparing for a future without this person begins. The therapist asks the family to anticipate concerns about vulnerable family members, and/or vulnerable relationships that are likely to be disrupted by loss. Future-oriented questions are used to both identify future needs, and generate strategies for mobilising support. In the excerpts that follow, the therapist asks the family to anticipate ways they might recognise one another's grief and plan support accordingly. In addition to the pragmatic value of shoring up resources, this process also builds empathic attunement among family members:

Case 1

DAUGHTER 1: But how are we all going to deal with Brenda's depression when mommy does pass?

THERAPIST: So that's the question, if there is a point one or two months down the line when we do lose mom... what approaches would we take then to share that grief and to get help?

BRENDA: I wish my old therapist was still active, I could give her a call.

THERAPIST: But who in the family could you pick up the phone to and say, 'It's been a month since mommy died and I'm really missing her?'

BRENDA: I'm not sure.

THERAPIST (to family): Who would Brenda be likely to turn to first?

DAUGHTER 1: I think she's most comfortable confiding in our brother, Don.

Case 2

THERAPIST (to Patient's Husband): Bill, how will you know when Kate (daughter) is overwhelmed and anxious? What are the signs?

HUSBAND: She's unable to function in certain ways ... I mean she can work, she can take care of Johnny, but she can't do anything else.

THERAPIST: And what's helpful for her at that time, what helps pull her out of that?

HUSBAND: Nothing...

THERAPIST: Nothing? Anne (Patient), Can we turn to you? What helps Kate?

PATIENT: Well, it's not the time to bring it up, her room is a mess, not the time to go after her about her room. You have to just sit with her, put your arm around her and say, 'I know how you're feeling' and even then she might say, 'No you don't', but if you're just sitting with her and stay present, she'll appreciate it.'

As is described above, helping at-risk families talk about end-of-life concerns and sharing feelings involves guiding them through multiple phases of discussion, but this can be achieved within the scope of a brief intervention. Key processes include facilitating mutual disclosure of information and emotional response, creating awareness of family rules and patterns that restrict talk, and inviting family members to anticipate and strategise ways of addressing future needs. As noted by Hebert and colleagues [31], 'good communication is dependent on more than simple information exchange', but also involves changing the '*permeability* of channels available for the exchange of information' [38].

16.4.4 Key Challenges in the Application of FFGT

Careful attention is needed to the engagement of significant family members, setting appropriate goals for the intervention, running sessions in the home, and meeting the challenges that mixed cultures can bring to the family scene.

16.4.4.1 Problems with Engagement of the Family

Clinicians can be told that an individual will attend a planned session, only to discover later that the invitation was not extended. Generally, the less cohesive the family, the more active the therapist needs to be in personally inviting each member to attend. Planning ahead calls for active consideration of any barriers to involvement in the family's work.

16.4.4.2 Limits to Therapeutic Goals

Chronic mental illness, longstanding personality difficulties and subsystem issues (for instance, marital difficulties for the children of the dying person) lie outside the goals of care in our time-limited intervention. Nevertheless, across several months, how much commands attention in families is striking – job loss, study problems, alcohol and drug abuse, pregnancy, miscarriages, infidelity, relationship breakdown and accidents are exemplars. Families may need to talk about these events, but the therapist must monitor overall family functioning as stories unfold, and deal with them in that context. Sustaining focus is crucial to the success of a brief intervention, as is the setting of realistic goals that are achievable within the time frame.

16.4.4.3 Therapy in the Home

Palliative care is increasingly community-based. If they so wish and are able, patients are empowered to stay with their families, receive treatment in familiar settings and die in their own homes. Disability and failing health, including cancer-induced paraplegia, significant frailty and imminent death make this venue an asset to members being able to attend. The patient can more readily contribute when therapist and family come, metaphorically, to the bedside. The home is not, however, necessarily the best location for every family. Those with a history of conflict are better served in a neutral location, such as the therapist's office, since they are then on equal terms and the therapist is more readily perceived as not 'taking sides'. Approximately two-thirds of therapy can occur safely in the home.

Before starting home-based therapy, 'guidelines' are established to both protect and empower the

process. These include stipulating the duration of the session and creating an appropriate setting by determining seating arrangements, switching off radio or television, avoiding disruptive telephone calls and visitors, settling pets and deferring refreshments.

16.4.4.4 Cross Cultural Challenges

Many families blend cultural backgrounds such that the rituals and traditions of each may come into tension at times of stress and illness. Therapists may lack insight into these historical influences upon the family and need to inquire as to what earlier generations did. Putting a name to the difference evident in these approaches can help families to evaluate their respective value and make choices to better suit their mutual needs.

Various cultures, including Asian, Italian and Hispanic ethnic groups, have strong family traditions and welcome a family-centred model of care and decision-making. Nevertheless, dysfunction can still occur and be aided by FFGT. Moreover, culture should not require automatic acceptance of requests to withhold discussion of the prognosis or negative news from the patient. In our experience, families carry diverse views about these culturally-determined approaches, and by therapists asking each member how they perceive the seriousness of the patient's illness to be, we find that someone often introduces concern such that the topic is opened up for family discussion. Commonly the patient will ask to discuss the very issues that others have tried to avoid. Hence the therapist's neutrality can be preserved through an open inquiry which lets the family choose its words and depth of discussion.

16.4.4.5 Families with Young Children

When cancer afflicts a parent of younger children, concern emanates about prematurity of death before the parenting task is complete. Feeling deprived of that role is a source of additional grief. The family may also be rendered insecure through losing a material provider. Caring for families with younger children and adolescents is common and inevitable. Genuine sharing of innermost feelings helps younger family members mature into sensitive people, but the process does not necessarily come easily. Protective barriers are readily erected to shield children from harm, with the attendant risk of denying them an authentic experience of family grief. Our model promotes open sharing of thoughts and feelings to foster mutual support, and commonly helps a surviving parent grow in confidence in their support of their children. (Further description of therapy programmes for patients with dependent children is also outlined in Chapter 19 by Lewis).

16.4.4.6 Ethical Issues

An ethic of care is at the heart of FFGT. The intimate relationships within families correspond with the feminist contribution to ethics that stresses that sense of responsibility for others over any individual rights [39]. Core notions of caregiving, parenting, being responsible for and protecting others capture this state of relationships. Traits such as compassion, sympathy, fidelity, trust, discernment, sensitivity and love take precedence over rules, impartiality and rights.

An ethical quandary in FFGT can arise from the competing needs of family members. Should all members be treated equally, the needs of the dying made paramount, or might one member be occasionally privileged over others? In general, the therapist strives to be neutral and treat all equally, but pragmatic factors do prevail in circumstances of exceptional vulnerability for one family member, warranting greater attention at this time. Family decision-making exists in some balance with individual choice; mindfulness about these tensions serves to ensure careful attention to all.

16.5 Supporting Materials

FFGT does not make use of formal homework beyond giving families encouragement to work on the issues or concerns that have been discussed. However, follow-up sessions always seek news of progress with these endeavours. Referral to parallel forms of psychological or psychiatric care are appropriate, when needed, be this individual or couple therapy for family members, or for pharmacology to address specific symptoms.

16.6 Overview of Evidence on Efficacy

Modest initial evidence exists from the Australian randomised controlled trial for the ability of this intervention to reduce distress and depression among family members in bereavement [40]. Randomisation of some 81 families (363 individuals) was in a 2 to 1 ratio, placing 53 families (233 individuals) in the FFGT therapy arm, with 28 families (130 individuals) receiving usual care. Assessments occurred at baseline, 6 and 13 months after the patient's death. Primary outcome measures were the Brief Symptom Inventory (BSI), Beck Depression Inventory (BDI) and Social Adjustment Scale (SAS). Family Adjustment Device (FAD) was a secondary outcome measure of family functioning. Analyses, allowing for correlated family data, employed generalised estimating equations (GEEs), controlled for site and were based on intention-to-treat. The overall impact of FFGT revealed a significant reduction in distress (BSI) at 13 months ($p = 0.02$). Significant improvement in distress and depression were demonstrated for individuals with high BSI and BDI baseline scores. Intermediate and sullen families tended to improve overall, whereas depression was less influenced in the most dysfunctional (hostile) families.

The generalisability of this model was evidenced through the successful training of 15 therapists, 86% of whom demonstrated the capacity to adhere faithfully to the core elements of the model [41]. Therapist competence was evidenced by a strong therapeutic alliance for 94%, affirmation of family strengths in over 90% and focus on agreed themes in 76% of sessions observed in a substudy on the fidelity of application of the model.

Interestingly, expression of normal grief was equivalent across family types as an outcome measure and a measure of complicated grief was not available when the initial study was commenced. An American replication study will provide future evidence of impact on complicated grief, as well as the dose responsiveness of FFGT to different levels of family dysfunction.

16.7 Case Examples

Figure 16.2 shows the genogram for a family in whom the mother was dying from advanced breast cancer and aware that her husband was drinking more to mask his fear of loss. The therapist worked to engage the sons more with their father, while helping to contain tension between the father and his daughter, who still resided at home. Although depressive disorders still need individual management, including antidepressants, conjoint family therapy helps reduce overall conflict, which might otherwise perpetuate the depression and sustain the dependence on substances like alcohol.

Joe had spent ten years in an orphanage as a child, leaving him with a vulnerability to abandonment that had been assuaged by his marriage to Sheila. Her death cast Joe back into a lonely state, despairing, 'It feels like a flood and I have to swim through it,

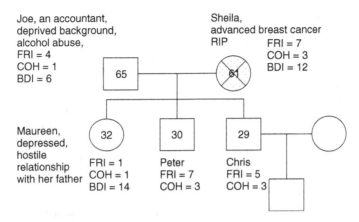

Figure 16.2 *Genogram of a family whose father abused alcohol to cope, while becoming conflictual with his depressed daughter (FRI, family relationships index; COH, Cohesiveness; BDI, beck depression inventory (short form, where BDI > 5 suggests caseness for depression)).*

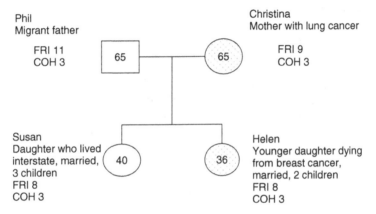

Figure 16.3 *Genogram of a family burdened by the occurrence of double cancer (FRI, family relationships index; COH, cohesiveness).*

and I cry and feel ashamed of this. My uselessness! A timeless life! I am withered up. I have nothing. I think of suicide'. The daughter, Maureen, was also bereft as the remaining woman of the household. Both sons, Peter and Chris, had created independent lives away from the family home. Therapy gave them insight into the need to support Joe and Maureen, visiting regularly and engaging with them until the pain of grief began to ease. The therapy contained their distress, and although Joe and Maureen declined referral for individual treatment, the family sessions guided them supportively across 18 months until they both re-engaged in life again.

Figure 16.3 illustrates a family burdened by cancer afflicting two family members simultaneously, bringing a cumulative emotional strain upon them.

A family-centred approach to care has great wisdom in the presence of 'double cancers'.

Intense grief was found in this family in which both mother and daughter had cancer. The parents came from different backgrounds: Christina's family was close, whereas Phil had lost contact with his through migration. Curiously, one daughter, Susan, lived interstate and was perceived as the 'black sheep' compared to her sister, Helen, mum's close confidante. The threat of these illnesses drew the families together, with the therapist involving sons-in-law to expand the circle of mutual support. Exploring ways to lay down memories for the grandchildren became another focus of discussion. A strengthened reconnection emerged for Susan, who eventually provided helpful support for both her bereaved father and brother-in-law.

16.8 Service Development

Deployment of the FFGT model to clinical services is dependent upon the employment of clinicians with training in the conduct of family therapy in oncology and palliative care programmes, including bereavement services. The model allows for excellent continuity of care for the bereaved family and is essentially preventative in its orientation. For some institutions, a cultural shift in service orientation is needed to incorporate this family-centred model of care alongside the predominant pattern of individual patient care. We are confident that this orientation enriches all programmes of care.

The introduction of routine screening of family functioning by palliative care clinical teams is a key step to permit recognition of 'at risk' families. Hospice programmes have struggled to do this well, often with nurses making the first clinical assessment in the home and asking to defer the administration of the 12-item FRI to the programme's social workers, who may not visit all families, or may not visit them from the outset. Programme leadership must want to embrace family-centred care before these turf issues can be resolved.

Our model grew empirically from observational data of families on this journey. Merit exists in its further adaptation to meet the specific needs of paediatric families, by incorporating age-appropriate features suitable as shared family activities into sessions when young children are present. Further replication across a variety of cultural groups is also important.

16.9 Summary

Oncology and palliative care services need to offer a range of psychosocially-oriented programmes as there will always be the need for individual counselling and group support alongside family therapy. Developing clear guidelines for the adoption of different therapies would be helpful. Our work has introduced a preventive model that targets families at increased risk clinically to develop bereavement morbidity, and it engages with these families early during palliative care, sustaining continuity into bereavement until family functioning has improved and active mourning has begun to wane. A key premise is that bereavement care begins at entry to the palliative care or hospice programme. Our ongoing work has been to normalise the screening of family functioning as the means to initiating family-centred care, and the further refinement of the model in response to specific family features and needs. We are very optimistic about the long term future of FFGT as an integral component of psychosocial care – family mourning involves the sharing of grief, a pivotal step in empowering its healing.

Acknowledgement

This research has been supported by the National Cancer Institute grant **R01CA115329** (PI: D.W. Kissane) and grant **R03CA138131** (PI: T.I. Zaider). We are grateful to our research staff and the many therapists, supervisors, clinicians and families who have contributed to this research.

Recommended Reading

Kissane, D.W. and Bloch, S. (2002) *Family Focused Grief Therapy: A Model of Family-centred Care During Palliative Care and Bereavement*, Open University Press, Buckingham.
This book is a clinically oriented account of how to deliver Family Focused Grief Therapy, providing extensive illustration with a multitude of clinical examples. It serves as a comprehensive manual for FFGT and has been translated into several languages.

References

1. Leff, J.P. and Vaughn, C.B. (1985) *Expressed Emotion in Families*, Guilford Press, New York.
2. Keitner, G.I. and Miller, I.W. (1990) Family functioning and major depression: an overview. *American Journal of Psychiatry*, **147** (9), 1128–1137.
3. Kissane, D.W., Bloch, S., Onghena, P. *et al.* (1996) The Melbourne family grief study II: psychosocial morbidity and grief in bereaved families. *American Journal of Psychiatry*, **153**, 659–666.
4. Leff, J., Berkowitz, R., Shavit, N. *et al.* (1989) A trial of family therapy v. a relatives group for schizophrenia. *British Journal of Psychiatry*, **154**, 58–66.
5. Kissane, D.W. (1994) Grief and the family, in *The Family in Clinical Psychiatry* (eds S. Bloch, J. Hafner, E. Harari and G. Szmukler) Oxford University Press, Oxford, pp. 71–91.
6. Kissane, D.W. and Bloch, S. (1994) Family grief. *British Journal of Psychiatry*, **164**, 728–740.
7. Moos, R.H. and Moos, B.S. (1981) *Family Environment Scale Manual*, Consulting Psychologists Press, Stanford, CA.
8. Kissane, D.W., Bloch, S., Dowe, D.L. *et al.* (1996) The Melbourne family grief study, I: perceptions of family functioning in bereavement. *American Journal of Psychiatry*, **153**, 650–658.
9. Kissane, D.W., Bloch, S., McKenzie, M. *et al.* (1998) Family grief therapy: a preliminary account of a new model to promote healthy family functioning during palliative care and bereavement. *Psycho-Oncology*, **7**, 14–25.
10. Kissane, D.W., Bloch, S., Burns, W.I. *et al.* (1994) Perceptions of family functioning and cancer. *Psycho-Oncology*, **3**, 259–269.

11. Kissane, D.W., McKenzie, M., McKenzie, D.P. *et al.* (2003) Psychosocial morbidity associated with patterns of family functioning in palliative care: baseline data from the Family Focused Grief Therapy controlled trial. *Palliative Medicine*, **17**, 527–537.

12. Edwards, B. and Clarke, V. (2004) Validity of the family relationships index as a screening tool. *Psycho-Oncology*, **14** (7), 546–554.

13. Kissane, D.W. and Bloch, S. (2002) in *Family Focused Grief Therapy: A Model of Family-centred Care During Palliative Care and Bereavement*, Open University Press, Buckingham.

14. Bowlby, J. (1969) *Attachment and Loss*, Attachment, Vol. **1**, Basic Books, New York.

15. Creamer, M., Burgess, P. and Pattison, P. (1992) Reaction to trauma: a cognitive processing model. *Journal of Abnormal Psychology*, **101** (3), 452–459.

16. Whitaker, D.S. and Lieberman, M.A. (1964) *Psychotherapy Through the Group Process*, Adline, Chicago, IL.

17. Shaver, P. and Tancredy, C. (2001) Emotion, attachment and bereavement: a conceptual commentary, in *Handbook of Bereavement Research: Consequences, Coping and Care* (eds M. Stroebe, R. Hansson, W. Stroebe and H. Schut), US: American Psychological Association, Washington, DC, pp. 63–88.

18. Stroebe, M. and Schut, H. (2001) Models of coping with bereavement: a review, in *Handbook of Bereavement Research: Consequences, Coping and Care* (eds M. Stroebe, R. Hansson, W. Stroebe and H. Schut), APA Books, Washington, DC, pp. 375–403.

19. Parkes, C. (1972) *Bereavement: Studies of Grief in Adult Life*, Tavistock, London.

20. Parkes, C. (1998) *Bereavement Studies of Grief in Adult Life*, 3rd edn, International University Press, Madison, CT.

21. Janoff-Bulman, R. (1989) Assumptive worlds and the stress of traumatic events: applications of the schema construct. *Social Cognition*, **7**, 113–136.

22. Janoff-Bulman, R. and Berg, M. (1998) Disillusionment and the creation of value: from traumatic losses to existential gains, in *Perspectives on Loss: A Sourcebook* (ed. J. Harvey), Brunner Mazel Inc., Philadelphia, PA.

23. Folkman, S. and Moskowitz, J.T. (2000) Positive affect and the other side of coping. *American Psychologist*, **55** (6), 647–654.

24. Tomm, K. (1988) Interventive interviewing: part III. Intending to ask lineal, circular, strategic or reflexive questions? *Family Process*, **27**, 1–15.

25. Dumont, I. and Kissane, D. (2009) Techniques for framing questions in conducting family meetings in palliative care. *Palliat Support Care*, **7** (2), 163–170.

26. Rolland, J. (1994) In sickness and in health: the impact of illness on couples' relationships. *Journal of Marital and Family Therapy*, **20** (4), 327.

27. Glaser, B.G. and Strauss, A.L. (1965) *Awareness of Dying*, Weidenfeld & Nicolson, London.

28. Mamo, L. (1999) Death and dying: confluences of emotion and awareness. *Sociology of Health and Illness*, **21** (1), 13–36.

29. Timmermans, S. (1994) Dying of awareness: the theory of awareness contexts. *Sociology of Health and Illness*, **16** (3), 322–336.

30. Spiegel, D. and Spira, J. (1991) *Supportive-expressive Group Therapy: A Treatment Manual of Psychosocial Intervention for Women with Metastatic Breast Cancer*, School of Medicine, Stanford University, Stanford, CA.

31. Hebert, R.S., Prigerson, H.G., Schulz, R. and Arnold, R.M. (2006) Preparing caregivers for the death of a loved one: a theoretical framework and suggestions for future research. *Journal of Palliative Medicine*, **9** (5), 1164–1171.

32. Barry, L.C., Kasl, S.V. and Prigerson, H.G. (2002) Psychiatric disorders among bereaved persons: the role of perceived circumstances of death and preparedness for death. *American Journal of Geriatric Psychiatry*, **10** (4), 447–457.

33. Valdimarsdottir, U., Helgason, A., Furst, C. *et al.* (2004) Awareness of husband's impending death from cancer and long-term anxiety in widowhood: a nationwide follow-up. *Palliative Medicine*, **18** (5), 432–443.

34. Porter, L.S., Keefe, F.J., Hurwitz, H. and Faber, M. (2005) Disclosure between patients with gastrointestinal cancer and their spouses. *Psychooncology*, **14** (12), 1030–1042.

35. Emanuel, E.J., Fairclough, D.L., Wolfe, P. and Emanuel, L.L. (2004) Talking with terminally ill patients and their caregivers about death, dying, and bereavement: is it stressful? Is it helpful? *Archives of Internal Medicine*, **164** (18), 1999–2004.

36. Cecchin, G. (1987) Hypothesizing, circularity, and neutrality revisited: an invitation to curiosity. *Family Process*, **26**, 405–413.

37. Johnson, S.M. (2003) The revolution in couple therapy: a practitioner-scientist perspective. *Journal of Marital and Family Therapy*, **29** (3), 365–384.

38. Gurman, A.S. (1988) Issues in the specification of family therapy interventions, in *The State of the Art in Family Therapy Research: Controversies and Recommendations* (ed. L.C. Wynne), Family Process Press, New York, p. 132.

39. Gilligan, C. (1982) *In a Different Voice*, Harvard University Press, Cambridge, MA.

40. Kissane, D., McKenzie, M., Bloch, S. *et al.* (2006) Family focused grief therapy: a randomized controlled trial in palliative care and bereavement. *American Journal of Psychiatry*, **163**, 1208–1218.

41. Chan, E.K., O'Neill, I., McKenzie, M. *et al.* (2004) What works for therapists conducting family meetings: treatment integrity in Family Focused Grief Therapy during palliative care and bereavement. *Journal of Pain and Symptom Management*, **27**, 502–512.

Section D

Therapies Across the Life Cycle

17 Therapy in the Setting of Genetic Predisposition to Cancer

Mary Jane Esplen[1,2] and Jonathan Hunter[1,3]

[1]Department of Psychiatry, Faculty of Medicine, University of Toronto, Toronto, ON, Canada
[2]University Health Network, Toronto, ON, Canada
[3]Mount Sinai Hospital, Toronto, ON, Canada

17.1 Background

Clinical genetic testing for disease susceptibility is becoming widespread, leading the way to revolutionary cancer prevention and treatment options. Identifying that one is at substantially increased risk for cancer may help individuals prepare both medically and psychologically. However, difficult emotional reactions can be stimulated by the testing procedure and outcomes. Such reactions can impact not only on individuals but on other family members as well. This chapter will describe the process of genetic susceptibility testing, associated emotions and the current state of knowledge about supporting individuals psychologically through this process. A case example serves to integrate the information presented. Given the psychosocial challenges that can arise during genetic testing, there is a need to integrate psychological care into genetics services.

17.1.1 The Process of Genetic Testing

When a concern about a family history of cancer is identified, individuals are frequently referred to speciality clinics. One or more pre-test counselling sessions by a genetic counsellor or geneticist occurs to assess the genetic (and non-genetic) risk factors for the cancer, to determine eligibility for the genetic test and to help individuals decide whether or not to proceed with the test. Information is provided on the potential meaning of test results, be they 'positive' (indicating the presence of a susceptibility mutation), 'negative' (indicating the absence of such a mutation) or 'uninformative' (not allowing a definite risk to be assigned). Family implications are raised from the outset. If testing goes forward there is a waiting period while laboratory DNA analysis occurs. A post-test counselling session is then provided, wherein the test result and its impact is fully explored. This includes an assessment of the individual's understanding of their risk for disease, their assimilation of this new information and how it compares to their previous expectations. Specific surveillance and prevention recommendations are discussed, and follow-up appointments for screening tests or consultations with specialists who can address such options as prophylactic surgery are scheduled. The implications of the test for family members are also discussed, including an exploration of potential issues around communicating the new genetic information to relatives. Typically a follow-up appointment is booked, either in person or via telephone, within one to four weeks, in order to assess the individual's ongoing adjustment, their perceptions and decisions about surveillance and prevention, family communication problems, and to determine if any additional support is required. This process is often discussed in the literature as if it was purely factual, but it is frequently highly emotional. Standard clinic processes, such as constructing a family tree depicting the cancer diagnoses or deaths of loved ones across generations can result in profound emotional reactions. In fact, receiving information about the presence of a genetic mutation is life-altering, as revealed by patients' frequent description of 'my

Handbook of Psychotherapy in Cancer Care, First Edition. Edited by Maggie Watson and David W. Kissane.
© 2011 John Wiley & Sons, Inc. Published 2011 by John Wiley & Sons, Inc.

self before genetic testing', phrasing that emphasises the test as a significant juncture in their lives.

17.1.2 Emotional Factors in Genetic Testing

Genetic testing often precipitates awareness of a state of threatened health, and there are frequently fears about developing the disease, feelings of anger (towards those who transmitted the disease) or guilt (about the potential transmission of the gene mutations to offspring) [1]. These emotional reactions can affect the person's well-being and can also interfere with family relationships or the dissemination of genetic information to at-risk family members [2]. Even before testing occurs there are emotional variables that influence who comes forward for the testing. A consistent predictor of interest in testing is *perceived risk*, regardless of an individual's actual risk level [3, 4]. Individuals who feel vulnerable due to family experience with illness, or a cognitive style that involves the monitoring of health-threat information are often interested in attending a genetics centre [5–7]. These individuals frequently have beliefs and associated emotions regarding their destiny [8]. For instance, women with one first-degree relative with breast cancer frequently overestimate their risk [9–11], believing, for example, that illness is inevitable, as revealed by perceptions of being at 'high' risk or having a '100% chance' of developing the disease. These overestimations of risk are common and often persistent, making them difficult to modify with information-oriented interventions alone [7,12–15]. Factors that have been identified as being associated with elevated risk perception include: having a family history of disease, beliefs about the disease and risks, previous loss of a family member from the disease, over-identification with a family member who has had the disease and media representations [7]. Once the test occurs emotional reactions may be organised by the type of result obtained.

17.1.2.1 A Test Result Indicating the Presence of a Genetic Mutation

Reactions to a positive test understandably include a feeling of vulnerability to disease. Individuals may also wrongly assume that the illness is inevitable and not treatable [16]. Some individuals may underestimate their emotional reactions following receipt of their results [17]. Commonly, responses after testing positively include the sense of 'feeling like a walking time bomb' and a belief that 'it is just a matter

of time before the disease occurs'. Having younger children and a history of previous losses to cancer may contribute to emotional distress [18, 19]. Individuals often understand that they did not intentionally pass along a gene mutation, but can still develop feelings of guilt or worry concerning offspring [17, 20, 21]. The expectation of having a negative test result and a coping style that is primed towards the monitoring of health information, as well as lower levels of social support, are associated with greater distress [22]. Additional factors associated with distress following the disclosure of a positive test result include: the level of penetrance (the probability of developing the disease) associated with the gene mutation, the perception of the immediacy of risk (proximity in age to perceived disease onset) [23] and the perception of control over the disease (including the number of prevention/treatment options) [24, 25].

In the case that a positive test result brings forward serious and difficult decisions, anticipated or not, additional psychological burden can arise, due to a reduced sense of control and increased feelings of isolation. These issues include: decision-making around increased surveillance, prophylactic surgery or chemoprevention, test result notification to extended family members and offspring, and decisions that bear on marriage and childbearing [18, 21, 26]. In some cases a person may feel 'ambushed' by unanticipated consequences, such as being at increased risk for ovarian cancer if BRCA1/2 positive [21], and having to decide about prophylactic oopherectomy. After testing positively individuals must weigh the potential costs of an intervention against its benefits. For instance, those that undergo prophylactic procedures do report satisfaction and the benefit of a decreased sense of vulnerability and concern about cancer risk following prophylactic surgery [18, 27, 28], but reports also indicate negative impact on psychological functioning, body image, sexual functioning and self-concept [18, 26, 28]. It is also important to note that genetic information does not always lead to behavioural change. One study of female carriers in BRCA 1/2 families failed to demonstrate optimal level of adherence to recommendations one year after receiving positive test results [29].

For some individuals, ongoing family and personal reactions can persist, with individuals experiencing emotional distress [21, 30] and changes in relationships [18, 23, 31]. Amongst risk counselled individuals with elevated distress approximately 10–25% demonstrate levels consistent with a clinical diagnosis of depression or anxiety [22, 32, 33]. Studies that have utilised standardised disease-specific measures of distress (e.g. a cancer worry scale) have demonstrated even higher rates [34, 35]. However, evidence suggests that most carriers of genetic mutations do not become more distressed over time [36]. By one year post-test psychological functioning among the majority of positive individuals is similar to those receiving negative test results [30,36–38], suggesting the effectiveness of genetic counselling and the role of time in facilitating adjustment. Most individuals identify specific benefits to testing [39, 40], which are important in counteracting the emotional costs. Increased certainty concerning disease risk and close monitoring contributes to relief. Individuals frequently note that their deceased or older relatives were not afforded such opportunities as intense surveillance or the chance to participate in trials of risk-reducing interventions. Others indicate a sense of feeling 'empowered' by the test result, describe 'knowing their body well' and believing that through self and medical monitoring they will detect the disease early and survive [41]. Others express hope for the development of future medical technology that will address disease risk and effectively treat illness.

Additional quality of life benefits to genetic testing include the opportunity for an individual to examine his/her health behaviours and life decisions. The existential threat associated with testing positive can be a powerful motivator, enabling an individual to adopt healthier life style behaviours, such as changes in diet, exercise habits or smoking cessation. The experience of feeling 'life is vulnerable' often results in an individual examining his/her life in an honest and authentic manner. For example, individuals may connect more in relationships, and spend more time in desired activities or with valued others [21]. Genetic information can also be used to make career choices, plans for retirement or to obtain life insurance and for medical decision-making [42]. Opportunities to support others have direct impact to buffer a stress response facilitating active coping [21]. Such outcomes can occur spontaneously, but for others psychological and behavioural interventions that examine the full range of reactions to a genetic test can encourage this perspective. Lastly, the feeling of altruism, enacted through participation in health research that may assist future generations (including one's own relatives) is a frequently identified benefit [21].

17.1.2.2 A Test Result Indicating the Absence of a Genetic Mutation

The news that one does not carry a genetic mutation is generally associated with improved psychological functioning, decreases in worry about disease risk and a sense of relief [43, 44]. However, there is evidence that testing negatively can result in some individuals experiencing difficulty in adjusting to their risk status, especially when the result puts them at odds with others in the family.

This occurs in two ways. Some individuals have integrated a sense of being at increased risk into their self-concept [16, 18]. They have a sense of 'merger' or a strong identification with the relative(s) affected by the disease. The negative test then creates a separation from this loved one, which is experienced as reduced affiliation which in turn causes distress [21]. Alternatively, an individual can test negatively, but siblings are notified that they are carriers. In this case the negative test recipient may feel guilty about being spared the legacy of the familial disease, a response consistent with 'survivor guilt' [31]. Such a feeling conflicts with the relief that usually accompanies a favourable test result.

17.1.2.3 Ambiguous Test Results

A third type of result is possible, the ambiguous or 'inconclusive' test. In this case the individual has a family history that suggests a genetic risk, but there is no affected individual to test, the protocol that has the highest yield for detecting an abnormality. The presenting individual is then screened for the genes that are most frequently linked to the disease. If these are not detected, it is still possible that unknown or rare variants not tested for may be contributing to the familial pattern, thus preventing an absolutely firm conclusion of no genetic contribution to disease risk. Such a result causes concern to clinicians who fear that the individual is falsely reassured. The individual's comprehension of an inconclusive test result must be examined during follow-up, particularly in relation to compliance with surveillance and preventive options [45–47]. In addition, an individual who misunderstands his/her inconclusive test result may communicate inaccurate information to family members [45, 47].

17.1.2.4 The Impact of Genetic Testing on the Family

Not surprisingly, the familial context of the genetic test results plays an important role in an individual's psychological adjustment [48]. Some individuals describe feeling closer to family members who carry the same genetic mutation. But, as noted above, relationships among siblings, parents and offspring can be complicated by individuals receiving different test results. Other family relationships are also affected. Spouses can have difficulty adjusting and have demonstrated high levels of distress and loss as well as concern for their partner [49]. In addition, a parent who carries a genetic mutation needs to decide when and how to inform adolescent or adult offspring. Women with BRCA1 and 2 mutations in a group support programme reported that one of their greatest challenges was informing an adult daughter of the mutation. The mothers were torn between wanting their adult daughter to have close surveillance and a wish to have her maintain her sense of youthful invulnerability and its associated sense of freedom in having a complete and uncomplicated future [21]. Even when parents decide to delay telling younger children about a genetic mutation, the parents still need to explain absences or changes due to medical appointments or procedures [50]. For example, a woman with the BRCA1 mutation who chooses to undergo prophylactic surgery must find a way to communicate to her children the necessity for a surgical procedure, while reassuring them that she is not currently ill or dealing with a disease.

Families also can have challenges around notifying family members they may not know well, or whom they fear burdening with unwanted or unexpected risk knowledge [20, 51]. Individuals may feel they are 'opening a can of worms' or feel ill-equipped to discuss a sensitive topic when relatives are unfamiliar or relationships are strained. In contrast, some family members feel a strong pressure to encourage siblings or other family members to be tested, even when these individuals may not be interested, precipitating conflict. These family communication challenges may require guidance or support by health care professionals in order to minimise additional stress and to facilitate family adjustment.

17.2 Counselling and Psychotherapeutic Interventions

17.2.1 Optimal Clinic Process

Genetic testing clinics should integrate complementary psychological care to guarantee optimal conditions for information processing and to enhance adjustment to genetic testing [8, 52]. Although most individuals will adapt over time with normal clinical process and acquire accurate comprehension around their risk and options [18, 36, 37, 53], others will maintain inaccurate risk perception and elevated distress following genetic counselling [11, 13, 54, 55]. Optimally, psychosocial support is integrated in order to address problems before they interrupt medical care.

The first step is to screen individuals for psychological distress or disorders, and identify those at risk for adjustment difficulties [56]. Recently, psychosocial instruments have been designed and tested specifically for cancer risk populations [57]. They identify empirically derived psychological risk markers related to the heritable cancer experience and genetic testing. They can be used either in lieu of, or in addition to global measures of mood or anxiety symptoms. When screening it is important to note that a significant group will not meet criteria for a psychiatric disorder per se, but will nevertheless suffer with a variety of thoughts, emotions and behaviours that need to be understood within their personal and historical contexts. These individuals are often described as the 'worried well' and are helped by psychological intervention. Relevant risk factors for emotional distress detected by these measures are detailed in Box 17.1 [56, 58–60].

Box 17.1 Factors Associated with Psychological Risk or Adjustment Difficulties with a Positive Test

- Sociodemographic
  - Age/developmental level/proximity to age of affected family member
  - Gender
  - Culture/ethnicity
  - Socioeconomic status
  - Having young children
- Medical
  - Penetrance
  - Severity/nature of disease
  - Prevention options and risk-reducing procedures
- Psychosocial
  - Loss of relative to disease (especially parent)
  - Care-giving of family member with disease
  - Prior history of additional life losses/trauma
  - Premorbid psychological history/condition
  - Current level of psychological functioning (e.g. presence of depression, anxiety, disease-specific worry)
  - Current life stressors (e.g. job stress, divorce)
  - Expectation of receiving a negative test result
  - Coping style (e.g. anxious preoccupied, health monitoring)
  - Social support level (low level).

Once the level of distress is identified, it is helpful to utilise interventions along a continuum, matched to the intensity of need (see Box 17.2). For example, for individuals who experience low levels of worry that do not interfere with daily functioning, straightforward educational materials are indicated. The empirical literature

---

Box 17.2 Psychosocial and Psychotherapeutic Interventions Recommended for Distress Levels

Low level of distress	Moderate level of distress	High level of distress
Educational Pamphlets, CDs Internet information	Cognitive-behavioural (e.g. stress management, coping strategies for living with uncertainty) Interactive CD ROMS Manual and computer-based decisional aids Telephone counselling and follow-up counselling Peer support (1 : 1; group)	Individual psychotherapy/ supportive counselling Professionally led support groups Family counselling Psychotropic medication

---

to date has concentrated on these genetic counselling approaches or psycho-educational tools. Individualised in-person or telephone-based counselling approaches [13–15, 61–64], and decisional aids [63, 65–68] have demonstrated improvements in knowledge and awareness of screening options.

Individuals with moderate levels of anxiety that interrupts sleep, and interferes with coping and decision-making will additionally benefit from 1 : 1 sessions with a genetic counsellor or a mental health professional, individual or group peer support, or cognitive-behavioural interventions designed to manage anxiety and uncertainty [15]. When depressive symptoms or anxiety interferes with daily functioning or self-care, or when a person feels hopeless or suicidal, specialised services offered by a skilled mental health professional are necessary. Potential interventions for this highly distressed group include individual psychotherapy to address unresolved grief issues, psychotropic medication directed at a current psychiatric syndrome, professionally led support groups and longer follow-up.

The use of social support, such as ongoing connections with the genetic clinic or a peer support group [21, 69, 70] can augment any of these levels of interventions. Groups have shown improvements by decreasing cancer worry, anxiety or by improving coping strategies [21, 62]. They also facilitate decision-making around genetic testing or prevention, as well as assisting communication with family [65, 71].

Despite often numerous attempts using information-oriented interventions and genetic counselling techniques to reduce distress, some individuals continue to overestimate their cancer risk or have difficulties coping, often experienced as frequent intrusive thoughts about their cancer risk [13]. These individuals benefit from additional therapy to address pathological self-beliefs, to build on existing coping strategies and to address any unresolved grief issues. The research on

more intensive psychotherapeutic interventions can be summarised by type of therapy.

17.2.2 Cognitive and Behavioural Strategies

In general settings, behavioural interventions are frequently utilised to reduce anxiety and facilitate stress management. Relaxation or distraction [72] techniques can reduce the ongoing, and indeed lifelong, stress associated with frequent screening visits and appointments. One technique known to facilitate quality of life and stress management in a variety of clinical populations, including cancer, is mindfulness based stress reduction [73]. Strategies to assist adoption of healthy life style behaviours, such as regular exercise and diet can enhance the feeling of control in minimising disease risk. Alternatively, a therapist might help develop communication skills via role-play or mental rehearsal of scenarios to assist in discussion of issues with a doctor, or risk information in the family.

Cognitively oriented strategies, such as those employed in cognitive-behavioural therapy (CBT), have also been included in treatment of distress or in decision-making interventions addressing genetic risk. They may be used in individual or group formats. An initial focus is on distorted or over-inflated personal cancer risk estimates [72, 74], which can be addressed by the use of structured learning exercises to teach patients to identify and monitor 'catastrophic' thinking or 'dysfunctional' thoughts, or to help an individual learn about the connections amongst thoughts, moods and behaviours [75]. Techniques such as role-play, self-reflective journal exercises, the use of guided imagery and thought analyses can identify self-beliefs or rigid thoughts that are contributing to anxiety or mood difficulties. Homework assignments and thought records can be used to elicit the person's inaccurate cognitions and to encourage more realistic interpretations of their circumstance.

Such explorations help individuals identify their theories of themselves, and lead to greater awareness of how their behaviours and thought patterns occur in relation to past experiences with cancer. This can help them to clarify their current risk, or understand what gets in the way of family communication. In particular, individuals can explore self-beliefs, many of which are entrenched as a result of past traumatic experiences during times of illness in the family and that can obstruct uptake of positive health strategies. For instance, Wellisch and Lindberg, and Wellisch *et al.* [15, 33], have highlighted the unique issues that are highly relevant in young women who lost a mother to cancer, particularly during their adolescence. Regardless of her objective risk level, a woman with such a history can develop a sense that it is inevitable that she will suffer and die from cancer, just as her mother did. Identifying this 'catastrophic' belief about herself and comparing it to her objective risk can help her adapt more functionally in the current day. The past is not the only focus of CBT in at-risk populations. Mentally constructing one's future health and developing hope can motivate a person to adopt screening and important lifestyle changes, or facilitate challenging medical decision-making.

17.2.3 Psychodynamic Strategies

A psychodynamic therapy, by contrast, would emphasise emotions more than cognition, and utilise the alliance between the therapist and the individual as a means of understanding that person and creating change. The aim is to acquire insight by appreciating how early life experience, such as previous relationships and bereavements – particularly those related to cancer in the family – relate to current distress. To illustrate by building on the example above of the adolescent girl whose mother dies, a dynamic therapy would explore beyond the event itself, perhaps to how the subsequent unavailability of the surviving parent due to their own grief resulted in the woman's distrust of others' capacity to support her, a sense of being unworthy of love, and the subsequent development of a strong sense of self-reliance in order to avoid such a painful experience again. Once this self-awareness is established, the way it interacts with her beliefs about the need to be independent or the reliability of the genetics staff or psychotherapist can be explored and modified towards better adaptation. Reflection upon these distressing past events within the context of a trusted therapeutic relationship can develop an appreciation of how the consequences of the early experience impacts on their current emotional reaction to the genetic risk, testing, recommended procedures and family communication.

A current dynamic approach reported in other patient populations focuses on identifying the *attachment style* of people. Attachment style refers to the fundamental beliefs and behaviours that were formed in childhood about relationships, and that persist into adulthood for most people [76, 77]. This approach has the benefit of being easy to understand and apply, and even if one is not engaged in a formal therapy, it can provide insight into what motivates an individual's behaviours. For instance, knowledge of attachment style allows one, with some certainty, to predict the person's capacity to trust others, regulate anxiety, process fearful information and tolerate uncertainty, all functions that pertain to the genetic risk counselling circumstance [76].

Another style of psychodynamic therapy that has promise in at-risk populations is Interpersonal therapy (IPT). This is a structured, manualised, short-term therapy, with good evidence of efficacy in depression, including that associated with medical illness [78, 79]. Although not specifically tested in this population, IPT concentrates on grief, role transitions, interpersonal role disputes and deficiencies, domains that are highly pertinent to the emotional struggles of the individual in a genetic clinic [79].

The most widely studied psychodynamic approach in at-risk populations [11, 80] is Supportive-Expressive group therapy (SEGT) [81–83]. This approach brings together 5–10 individuals who share an issue – such as a family history of cancer – within a mutually supportive group, typically for 90-minute sessions once a week for eight weeks, followed by four monthly 'boosters'. It also includes a one time family session, when group participants are invited to bring a family member or two to the group to explore and discuss some of the family impacts. The goals of SEGT in an at-risk population include the acquisition of an accurate cancer risk, enhanced quality of life by appreciating the relevance of the here-and-now (as opposed to preoccupation with the past), and encouragement to live life 'authentically' [11, 21, 80]. This later goal, which emphasises the legitimacy of a full range of emotion and the centrality of relationships in giving value to life is taken from existential psychotherapy and is a valued outcome of SEGT [81, 82]. SEGT has been used with women at risk for breast cancer as well as women who are known carriers of BRCA1/2 mutations. It has strong empirical proof of efficacy, having been proven to facilitate coping, the expression and working through of grief and improved psychological functioning [11, 21, 81].

In the sessions participants can talk openly about their experiences and their emotional reactions to their cancer risk. The two group leaders typically have backgrounds in mental health and genetics and are trained in the management of affect. They promote shared support, group cohesion and normalisation of the at-risk or cancer experience. They also fluidly focus the group on certain important topics that will benefit participants. For example, domain topics include medical decision making, grief and loss, feeling vulnerable to cancer, impact on self and family impacts [21]. These strategies provide a safe place that permits and encourages role-modelling and expressions of past and current grief, fears and emotions, within a non-judgemental environment.

The inclusion of women who have survived cancer with younger women who are at risk but not affected creates the opportunity for a direct exchange between these two subgroups of women. They can then test out assumptions, such as how a daughter might react to genetic information, or if cancer inevitably results in death. This in turn introduces the group member to a broader rage of outcomes than occurred in her particular case, which can 'detoxify' cancer [82, 83] or cancer risk, resulting in a greater sense of control and improved quality of life. Having often lived life without peers who share or understand their experience of parental loss or fear of illness, women find themselves in a room of others who share and intuitively appreciate their experience, resulting in decreased isolation and increased mastery. Sharing the emotional impact of their family history in the context of mutual support diminishes its intrusiveness, freeing the individual to consider and assimilate risk/genetic information and consider the decisions that they must make with less emotional burden.

17.3 Case Example

Although described as separate approaches for the sake of clarity, the psychotherapies described above are not mutually exclusive, and multiple approaches are often employed, such as the use of educational materials and group therapy. The following case illustrates such a multi-therapeutic approach. This woman was adjusting fairly well in life prior to genetic testing. Her belief that she was at high risk for breast cancer brought her to the genetic clinic, where she learned she was overestimating her risk. Following the initial consultation she felt unable to adjust to being at 'lower risk' and

began to have more questions around her risk and ability to cope. She engaged in a 'stepped care' approach to therapy, increasing the intensity of the interventions as required by her level of distress. These steps were crucial in her eventually finding a new sense of freedom and peace in her life. She became able to manage the emotional turmoil triggered by the genetic counselling, and ultimately used her newfound insight to increase her quality of life.

Janet (not her real name) is a married woman whose mother developed breast cancer when Janet was a young child, eventually dying when Janet was 10 years of age. Janet was very close to her mother, often crawling on to her bed to be with her and recalls fondly (but painfully) how her mother believed Janet was smart and would be very successful. Janet's father was somewhat involved in administering care to his wife, but the two girls (Janet has an older sister, Mary) provided most of the assistance to their mother and were almost constantly with their mother until her death at home.

Janet recalls a large family funeral where she felt great sadness, but that after only a couple of days she and her sister were expected to return to school. Janet did so, but with difficulty. When tearful at school a teacher told her 'You must be strong... your mother would want that', leading her to suppress her tears. Her father was very quiet and rarely spoke about her mother's death. Janet soon focused on her hobbies and school and spent most of her time alone. She excelled at school, attended university and became a successful health professional. She dated men in her 20s, but felt her relationships were shallow and would often end them after a few months. She did marry in her 30s and describes her husband as 'supportive and caring'. She made a conscious decision to not have children, stating, 'I knew I would not be there for them', and 'Why would I do what my mother did to me? ... it would be devastating'.

Following her consultation for genetic testing, the genetic counsellor referred her to a six month group therapy programme, as she was having difficulty accepting that she was at a lower risk than she had expected, despite having seen the usual educational materials. In fact, Janet believed 'it was just a matter of time before she would develop breast cancer'. She entered the group with other women who had a first degree relative with breast cancer. The SEGT utilised a psychodynamic approach in which the group members revisited their familial experience of cancer focusing on what happened, what losses occurred and examining their emotional consequences. The group acknowledged the women's risk perceptions, but the group leaders helped members to examine how their experiences impacted on their current life patterns and sense of risk. Emphasis was placed on the recognition and expression of affect during the group sessions.

Initially Janet wanted to leave the programme as she found the focus on the time of her mother's illness uncomfortable. As well, Janet highly valued her self-reliance, and therefore felt ambivalent about participating in group therapy. With encouragement, Janet persisted and became increasingly intrigued by the other women's experiences. They provided a sense of validation to her and decreased her emotional isolation, providing a normalisation and corrective experience for the silencing and solitude imposed on her during her bereavement as a child. She recognised her profound sense of vulnerability to cancer and her very strong belief that she would have her mother's life and would therefore inevitably die from cancer. She also started to feel that her sense of aloneness and fears were not unusual for someone with her past experience. When Janet recognised the lack of opportunity as a youngster to grieve her mother she felt fear, grief and anger.

The group highlighted how the death of her mother had played a role in many of her life decisions, including her decision not to have children. She also wondered if she was afraid to get closer to her husband 'in case she would die'. She also related this fear to her history of shallow contacts with men in her 20s, recognising that she prevented them from becoming closer by abruptly ending the relationships. The consequence of this reflection raised other issues for her, such as dealing with the anger of not having children, knowing that she was now too old to do so.

Despite these insights, Janet continued to have difficulty sleeping, stayed worried about her cancer risk, felt immense anxiety during routine surveillance and the days leading up to her appointments, and struggled with feelings of emptiness and depression. Following the group programme, Janet found herself feeling there was more to explore and felt unsettled, and at times more depressed. She still struggled to acknowledge the possibility that she might not develop cancer. Although difficult for her to do, given her tendency to be self-reliant, she requested an individual therapist.

Within the one-to-one therapy sessions Janet built a therapeutic relationship. She received education about the aetiology and treatment options for depression. Eventually, with encouragement she was able to accept a trial of medication to address her low mood, insomnia and decreased occupational functioning.

During the individual therapy CBT was also employed to address her core negative self-beliefs, and the distorted thinking around her 'threatened' life course. CBT approaches were also used to augment her rigid coping strategies. For example, she often used an avoidant coping style and was less skilled with techniques such as positive reappraisals to regulate her emotions. She maintained a journal and also joined a course to train in mindfulness-based stress reduction to assist her in managing her anxiety.

In addition to CBT, psychodynamic techniques were utilised to build insights related to her early family patterns, her relationship with and over-identification with her mother. She was able to recognise that she needed to further grieve her mother and recognised her guilt at being able to have a life that her mother could not. She also realised that her inflexible independence was an adaptation to the disruptions caused by the tragic loss of her mother and the subsequent lack of support. Janet felt for the first time that this played a role in her current inability to feel close to or 'allow' herself to be close with others.

During the weekly individual sessions Janet was becoming more aware of and increasingly dissatisfied with, her life choices. She also recognised that she resisted being too close to women, choosing instead to 'take care of herself' and avoid becoming 'too dependant'. She became increasingly angry and saddened about 'not being allowed to be a child' after her mother died. She regretted not having children. She learned that she tended to repress painful feelings, eventually carrying them as an unmetabolised burden inside herself. Guided imagery was another technique that assisted Janet's bereavement by imagining discussions or interactions with her mother as either a young girl or as an adult. These exercises helped to resolve aspects of their relationship and reflect on attributes that she shared (or did not share) with her mother.

Relationships with the women from the group, many of whom had lost mothers too, helped her to realise she was not alone, especially when the contact was maintained following the group. Over time Janet developed insight into how the loss of her mother had affected most of her life decisions and her past and current relationships, including the lack of closeness with her husband.

By the end of her multi-modal treatment, Janet realised that her successful job was producing little real satisfaction. She began to take risks in relationships and to try out new activities exploring the arts, mindfulness meditation and different work opportunities that would be less demanding, but provide her with more solace and leisure time. She increased closeness with her husband, and trusted him enough to allow his support. He also began to believe that she might not die from cancer and together they imagined and planned for retirement and other future-oriented life goals. Janet also was able to better tolerate and manage the stress and anxiety she experienced during routine surveillance and requested less 'extra' appointments when she felt frightened. Each of these interventions (education, SEGT, CBT, guided imagery, psychotropic medication, and psychodynamic psychotherapy) increased her mood and quality of life and renewed her hope that she might attain a healthy future. She was able to enjoy life more fully in the here-and-now and feel that she could enjoy life without guilt, despite the tragedy of her mother's interrupted life.

17.4 Evidence on Efficacy

There is clear evidence that genetic predisposition testing is acutely stressful for an individual and their family, and that a sub-population of patients will have ongoing distress. However, the use of psychotherapeutic interventions to help at-risk genetic populations is still in an early stage. The empirical evidence to date has been focused on psycho-educational approaches or decisional-aids to facilitate genetic counselling and decision-making about medical interventions. With respect to psychotherapy, proper empirical evidence supports SEGT as facilitating adjustment to risk, psychological coping and the expression and working through of grief. Studies are ongoing to examine specific counselling approaches, such as cognitive-behavioural strategies, to address coping challenges. Research testing family interventions, IPT or attachment informed therapy is yet to be done.

17.5 Service Development

Genetic health care providers offer some important basic psychosocial support to the majority of individuals undergoing testing, but additional psychological intervention is warranted in cases where screening detects a particular vulnerability or when persistent adjustment difficulties exist. To address this need, mental health professionals are increasingly being asked to function as consultants to genetic services. This approach provides a comprehensive 'biopsychosocial' assessment, the development of treatment plans to address identified psychological concerns, (especially those that may impact on relevant decision-making), and assists in the management of co-morbid disorders, including the use of psychotropic medications if required. Furthermore, this approach guarantees the opportunity for neutral reflection on genetic technologies and the consideration of options while maintaining a view 'from outside' the intensely scientific forum of genetic medicine.

17.6 Summary

Genetic knowledge of disease predisposition resulting from this new and constantly evolving field has the potential to provide many benefits. But such knowledge in and of itself does not translate directly into desired positive changes in health behaviours. Rather, evidence suggests that psychosocial, emotional, personal historical and familial contextual factors play an important role in an individual's capacity to assimilate genetic information, manage the emotions precipitated by the knowledge of their genetic risk, and maintain or improve their quality of life. Adverse psychological and behavioural reactions are reduced when genetic testing is provided within an integrated psychological framework that identifies and pre-empts or addresses emotional distress. Programmes should present clear information and emotional support throughout the genetic testing process. A number of promising approaches, both individual and group focused are available to provide such support. Such a biopsychosocial model of care facilitates a comprehensive range of preventive health care, and enhances the well being of individuals and their families, thereby encouraging the optimal use of this new medical technology.

17.7 Supporting Materials

- www.facingourrisk.org associated with 'Willow', a Canadian breast cancer support group, provides information that individuals can access on their own.

- The Zane Cohen Centre for Digestive Diseases is a state of the art facility for both clinical and genetic research in digestive diseases at Mount Sinai Hospital in Canada. http://www.mountsinai.on.ca/care/ddcrc/ddcrc-main

- National Center for Biotechnology Information (NCBI), GeneReviews http://www.ncbi.nlm.nih.gov/bookshelf/br.fcgi?book=gene&part=hnpcc

References

1. Lerman, C., Daly, M., Masny, A. *et al.* (1994) Attitudes about genetic testing for breast-ovarian cancer susceptibility. *Journal of Clinical Oncology*, **12**, 843–850.

2. Appleton, S., Fry, A., Rees, G. *et al.* (2000) Psychosocial effects of living with an increased risk of breast cancer: an exploratory study using telephone focus groups. *Psychoon-cology*, **9**, 511–521.

3. Bowen, D., McTiernan, A., Burke, W. *et al.* (1999) Participation in breast cancer risk counseling among women with a family history. *Cancer Epidemiology Biomarkers and Prevention*, **8**, 581–585.

4. Codori, A.M., Petersen, G.M., Miglioretti, D.L. *et al.* (1999) Attitudes toward colon cancer gene testing: factors predicting test uptake. *Cancer Epidemiology Biomarkers and Prevention*, **8**, 345–351.

5. Rees, G., Fry, A. and Cull, A. (2001) A family history of breast cancer: women's experiences from a theoretical perspective. *Social Science and Medicine*, **52**, 1433–1440.

6. Leventhal, H., Kelly, K. and Leventhal, E. (1995) Population risk, actual risk, perceived risk, and cancer control: a discussion. *Journal of National Cancer Institute Monographs*, **25**, 81–85.

7. Kash, K.M. and Lerman, C. (1998) Psychological, social, and ethical issues in gene testing, in *Psycho-Oncology* (ed. J.C. Holland), Oxford University Press, New York, pp. 196–207.

8. Stiefel, F., Lehmann, A. and Guex, P. (1997) Genetic detection: the need for psychosocial support in modern cancer prevention. *Support Care Cancer*, **5**, 461–465.

9. Black, W.C., Nease, R.F. Jr. and Tosteson, A.N. (1995) Perceptions of breast cancer risk and screening effectiveness in women younger than 50 years of age. *Journal of National Cancer Institute*, **87**, 720–731.

10. Durfy, S.J., Bowen, D.J., McTiernan, A. *et al.* (1999) Attitudes and interest in genetic testing for breast and ovarian cancer susceptibility in diverse groups of women in western Washington. *Cancer Epidemiology Biomarkers Prevention*, **8**, 369–375.

11. Esplen, M.J., Toner, B., Hunter, J. *et al.* (2000) A supportive-expressive group intervention for women with a family history of breast cancer: results of a phase II study. *Psychooncology*, **9**, 243–252.

12. Kash, K.M., Holland, J.C., Halper, M.S. *et al.* (1992) Psychological distress and surveillance behaviors of women with a family history of breast cancer. *Journal of the National Cancer Institute*, **84**, 24–30.

13. Lerman, C., Lustbader, E., Rimer, B. *et al.* (1995) Effects of individualized breast cancer risk counseling: a randomized trial. *Journal of the National Cancer Institute*, **87**, 286–292.

14. Edwards, A., Gray, J., Clarke, A. *et al.* (2008) Interventions to improve risk communication in clinical genetics: systematic review. *Patient Education and Counseling*, **71**, 4–25.

15. Wellisch, D.K., Gritz, E.R., Schain, W. *et al.* (1991) Psychological functioning of daughters of breast cancer patients. Part I: daughters and comparison subjects. *Psychosomatics*, **32**, 324–336.

16. Marteau, T.M. and Senior, V. (1997) Illness representations after the human genome project: the perceived role of genes in causing illness, in *Perceptions of Illness and Treatment Current Psychological Research and Implications* (eds K. Petrie and J. Weinman), Harwood Academic Press, Amsterdam, pp. 41–66.

17. Dorval, M., Patenaude, A.F., Schneider, K.A. *et al.* (2000) Anticipated versus actual emotional reactions to disclosure of results of genetic tests for cancer susceptibility: findings from p53 and BRCA1 testing programs. *Journal of Clinical Oncology*, **18**, 2135–2142.

18. van Oostrom, I., Meijers-Heijboer, H., Lodder, L.N. *et al.* (2003) Long-term psychological impact of carrying a BRCA1/2 mutation and prophylactic surgery: a 5-year follow-up study. *Journal of Clinical Oncology*, **21**, 3867–3874.

19. Esplen, M.J., Urquhart, C., Butler, K. *et al.* (2003) The experience of loss and anticipation of distress in colorectal cancer patients undergoing genetic testing. *Journal of Psychosomatic Research*, **55**, 427–435.

20. Lerman, C., Peshkin, B.N., Hughes, C. *et al.* (1998) Family disclosure in genetic testing for cancer susceptibility: determinants and consequences. *Journal of Health Care Law and Policy*, **1**, 352–371.

21. Esplen, M.J., Hunter, J., Leszcz, M. *et al.* (2004) A multicenter study of supportive-expressive group therapy for women with BRCA1/BRCA2 mutations. *Cancer*, **101**, 2327–2340.

22. Vernon, S.W., Gritz, E.R., Peterson, S.K. *et al.* (1997) Correlates of psychologic distress in colorectal cancer patients undergoing genetic testing for hereditary colon cancer. *Health Psychology*, **16**, 73–86.

23. Meiser, B., Gleeson, M.A. and Tucker, K.M. (2000) Psychological impact of genetic testing for adult-onset disorders. An update for clinicians. *Medical Journal of Australia*, **172**, 126–129.

24. DudokdeWit, A.C., Tibben, A., Duivenvoorden, H.J. *et al.*, Rotterdam/Leiden Genetics Workgroup (1998) Distress in individuals facing predictive DNA testing for autosomal dominant late-onset disorders: comparing questionnaire results with in-depth interviews. *American Journal of Medical Genetics*, **75**, 62–74.

25. Codori, A.M., Slavney, P.R., Young, C. *et al.* (1997) Predictors of psychological adjustment to genetic testing for Huntington's disease. *Health Psychology*, **16**, 36–50.

26. Lloyd, S.M., Watson, M., Oaker, G. *et al.* (2000) Understanding the experience of prophylactic bilateral mastectomy: a qualitative study of ten women. *Psychooncology*, **9**, 473–485.

27. Metcalfe, K.A., Esplen, M.J., Goel, V. *et al.* (2004) Psychosocial functioning in women who have undergone bilateral prophylactic mastectomy. *Psychooncology*, **13**, 14–25.

28. Elit, L., Esplen, M.J., Butler, K. *et al.* (2001) Quality of life and psychosexual adjustment after prophylactic oophorectomy for a family history of ovarian cancer. *Familial Cancer*, **1**, 149–156.

29. Lerman, C., Hughes, C., Croyle, R.T. *et al.* (2000) Prophylactic surgery decisions and surveillance practices one year following BRCA1/2 testing. *Preventive Medicine*, **31**, 75–80.

30. Watson, M., Foster, C., Eeles, R. *et al.* (2004) Psychosocial impact of breast/ovarian (BRCA1/2) cancer-predictive

genetic testing in a UK multi-centre clinical cohort. *British Journal of Cancer*, **91**, 1787–1794.

31. Smith, K.R., West, J.A., Croyle, R.T. *et al.* (1999) Familial context of genetic testing for cancer susceptibility: moderating effect of siblings' test results on psychological distress one to two weeks after BRCA1 mutation testing. *Cancer Epidemiology Biomarkers and Prevention*, **8**, 385–392.

32. Coyne, J.C., Benazon, N.R., Gaba, C.G. *et al.* (2000) Distress and psychiatric morbidity among women from high-risk breast and ovarian cancer families. *Journal of Consulting and Clinical Psychology*, **68**, 864–874.

33. Wellisch, D.K. and Lindberg, N.M. (2001) A psychological profile of depressed and nondepressed women at high risk for breast cancer. *Psychosomatics*, **42**, 330–336.

34. Trask, P.C., Paterson, A.G., Wang, C. *et al.* (2001) Cancer-specific worry interference in women attending a breast and ovarian cancer risk evaluation program: impact on emotional distress and health functioning. *Psychooncology*, **10**, 349–360.

35. Coyne, J.C., Kruus, L., Racioppo, M. *et al.* (2003) What do ratings of cancer-specific distress mean among women at high risk of breast and ovarian cancer? *American Journal of Medical Genetics A*, **116A**, 222–228.

36. Schwartz, M.D., Peshkin, B.N., Hughes, C. *et al.* (2002) Impact of BRCA1/BRCA2 mutation testing on psychologic distress in a clinic-based sample. *Journal of Clinical Oncology*, **20**, 514–520.

37. Butow, P.N., Lobb, E.A., Meiser, B. *et al.* (2003) Psychological outcomes and risk perception after genetic testing and counselling in breast cancer: a systematic review. *Medical Journal of Australia*, **178**, 77–81.

38. Meiser, B. (2005) Psychological impact of genetic testing for cancer susceptibility: an update of the literature. *Psychoncology*, **14**, 1060–1074.

39. Struewing, J.P., Lerman, C., Kase, R.G. *et al.* (1995) Anticipated uptake and impact of genetic testing in hereditary breast and ovarian cancer families. *Cancer Epidemiology Biomarkers and Prevention*, **4**, 169–173.

40. Cappelli, M., Surh, L., Humphreys, L. *et al.* (1999) Psychological and social determinants of women's decisions to undergo genetic counseling and testing for breast cancer. *Clinical Genetics*, **55**, 419–430.

41. Esplen, M.J., Stuckless, N., Hunter, J. *et al.* (2009) The BRCA self-concept scale: a new instrument to measure self-concept in BRCA1/2 mutation carriers. *Psychooncology*, **18**, 1216–1229.

42. Cappelli, M., Surh, L., Walker, M. *et al.* (2001) Psychological and social predictors of decisions about genetic testing for breast cancer in high-risk women. *Psychology, Health and Medicine*, **6**, 323–335.

43. Lerman, C., Narod, S., Schulman, K. *et al.* (1996) BRCA1 testing in families with hereditary breast-ovarian cancer. A prospective study of patient decision making and outcomes. *Journal of the American Medical Association*, **275**, 1885–1892.

44. Marteau, T.M. and Croyle, R.T. (1998) Psychological responses to genetic testing. *British Medical Journal*, **316**, 693–696.

45. Maheu, C. and Thorne, S. (2008) Receiving inconclusive genetic test results: an interpretive description of the BRCA1/2 experience. *Research in Nursing and Health*, **31**, 553–562.

46. Ardern-Jones, A., Kenen, R., Lynch, E. *et al.* (2010) Is no news good news? Inconclusive genetic test results in BRCA1 and BRCA2 from patients and professionals' perspectives. *Hereditary Cancer in Clinical Practice*, **8**, 1.

47. Dorval, M., Gauthier, G., Maunsell, E. *et al.* (2003) Are women with an inconclusive BRCA1/2 genetic test result falsely reassured? *Psycho-Oncology*, **12**, 166.

48. Foster, C., Watson, M., Moynihan, C. *et al.* (2004) Juggling roles and expectations: dilemmas faced by women talking to relatives about cancer and genetic testing. *Psychology and Health*, **19**, 439–455.

49. Williams, J.K., Schutte, D.L., Holkup, P.A. *et al.* (2000) Psychosocial impact of predictive testing for Huntington disease on support persons. *American Journal of Medical Genetics*, **96**, 353–359.

50. Tercyak, K.P., Peshkin, B.N., Streisand, R. *et al.* (2001) Psychological issues among children of hereditary breast cancer gene (BRCA1/2) testing participants. *Psychooncology*, **10**, 336–346.

51. Evers-Kiebooms, G., Welkenhuysen, M., Claes, E. *et al.* (2000) The psychological complexity of predictive testing for late onset neurogenetic diseases and hereditary cancers: implications for multidisciplinary counselling and for genetic education. *Social Science and Medicine*, **51**, 831–841.

52. Decruyenaere, M., Evers-Kiebooms, G., Denayer, L. *et al.* (2000) Predictive testing for hereditary breast and ovarian cancer: a psychological framework for pre-test counselling. *European Journal of Human Genetics*, **8**, 130–136.

53. Braithwaite, D., Emery, J., Walter, F. *et al.* (2004) Psychological impact of genetic counseling for familial cancer: a systematic review and meta-analysis. *Journal of the National Cancer Institute*, **96**, 122–133.

54. Watson, M., Lloyd, S., Davidson, J. *et al.* (1999) The impact of genetic counselling on risk perception and mental health in women with a family history of breast cancer. *British Journal of Cancer*, **79**, 868–874.

55. Michie, S., Marteau, T.M. and Bobrow, M. (1997) Genetic counselling: the psychological impact of meeting patients' expectations. *Journal of Medical Genetics*, **34**, 237–241.

56. Thewes, B., Meiser, B., Tucker, K. *et al.* (2003) Screening for psychological distress and vulnerability factors in women at increased risk for breast cancer: a review of the literature. *Psychology Health and Medicine*, **8**, 289–303.

57. Kasparian, N.A., Wakefield, C.E., Meiser, B. (2007) Assessment of psychosocial outcomes in genetic counseling research: an overview of available measurement scales. *Journal of Genetic Counseling*, **16**, 693–712.

58. Tercyak, K.P., Demarco, T.A., Mars, B.D. *et al.* (2004) Women's satisfaction with genetic counseling for hereditary breast-ovarian cancer: psychological aspects. *American Journal of Medical Genetics A*, **131**, 36–41.

59. van Oostrom, I., Meijers-Heijboer, H., Duivenvoorden, H.J. *et al.* (2007) Comparison of individuals opting for BRCA1/2 or HNPCC genetic susceptibility testing with regard to coping, illness perceptions, illness experiences, family system characteristics and hereditary cancer distress. *Patient Education and Counseling*, **65**, 58–68.

60. van Oostrom, I., Meijers-Heijboer, H., Duivenvoorden, H.J. *et al.* (2007) Prognostic factors for hereditary cancer distress six months after BRCA1/2 or HNPCC genetic susceptibility testing. *European Journal of Cancer*, **43**, 71–77.

61. Graves, K.D., Wenzel, L., Schwartz, M.D. *et al.* (2010) Randomized controlled trial of a psychosocial telephone counseling intervention in BRCA1 and BRCA2 mutation carriers. *Cancer Epidemiology Biomarkers and Prevention*, **19**, 648–654.

62. McInerney-Leo, A., Biesecker, B.B., Hadley, D.W. *et al.* (2004) BRCA1/2 testing in hereditary breast and ovarian cancer families: effectiveness of problem-solving training as a counseling intervention. *American Journal of Medical Genetics A*, **130A**, 221–227.

63. Miller, S.M., Roussi, P., Daly, M.B. *et al.* (2005) Enhanced counseling for women undergoing BRCA1/2 testing: impact on subsequent decision making about risk reduction behaviors. *Health Education and Behaviour*, **32**, 654–667.

64. Appleton, S., Watson, M., Rush, R. *et al.* (2004) A randomised controlled trial of a psychoeducational intervention for women at increased risk of breast cancer. *British Journal of Cancer*, **90**, 41–47.

65. Wakefield, C.E., Meiser, B., Homewood, J. *et al.* (2007) Development and pilot testing of two decision aids for individuals considering genetic testing for cancer risk. *Journal of Genetic Counseling*, **16**, 325–339.

66. Stacey, D., O'Connor, A.M., DeGrasse, C. *et al.* (2003) Development and evaluation of a breast cancer prevention decision aid for higher-risk women. *Health Expectations*, **6**, 3–18.

67. van Roosmalen, M.S., Stalmeier, P.F., Verhoef, L.C. *et al.* (2004) Randomized trial of a shared decision-making intervention consisting of trade-offs and individualized treatment information for BRCA1/2 mutation carriers. *Journal of Clinical Oncology*, **22**, 3293–3301.

68. van Roosmalen, M.S., Stalmeier, P.F., Verhoef, L.C. *et al.* (2004) Randomised trial of a decision aid and its timing for women being tested for a BRCA1/2 mutation. *British Journal of Cancer*, **90**, 333–342.

69. Wellisch, D.K., Hoffman, A., Goldman, S. *et al.* (1999) Depression and anxiety symptoms in women at high risk for breast cancer: pilot study of a group intervention. *American Journal of Psychiatry*, **156**, 1644–1645.

70. Karp, J.B.K., Sullivan, M.D. and Massie, M.J. (1999) The prophylactic mastectomy dilemma: a support group for women at high genetic risk for breast cancer. *Journal of Genetic Counseling*, **8**, 163–173.

71. Wang, C., Gonzalez, R., Milliron, K.J. *et al.* (2005) Genetic counseling for BRCA1/2: a randomized controlled trial of two strategies to facilitate the education and counseling process. *American Journal of Medical Genetics A*, **134A**, 66–73.

72. Phelps, C., Bennett, P., Iredale, R. *et al.* (2006) The development of a distraction-based coping intervention for women waiting for genetic risk information: a phase 1 qualitative study. *Psychooncology*, **15**, 169–173.

73. Carlson, L.E., Speca, M., Patel, K.D. *et al.* (2003) Mindfulness-based stress reduction in relation to quality of life, mood, symptoms of stress, and immune parameters in breast and prostate cancer outpatients. *Psychosomatic Medicine*, **65**, 571–581.

74. Bennett, P., Wilkinson, C., Turner, J. *et al.* (2007) The impact of breast cancer genetic risk assessment on intentions to perform cancer surveillance behaviors. *Journal of Genetic Counseling*, **16**, 617–623.

75. Beck, A.T. (1976) *Cognitive Therapy and The Emotional Disorders*, International Universities Press, New York.

76. Hunter, J.J., Maunder, R.G. and Gupta, M. (2007) Teaching consultation-liaison psychotherapy: assessment of adaptation to medical and surgical illness. *Academic Psychiatry*, **31**, 367–374.

77. Maunder, R.G. and Hunter, J.J. (2008) Attachment relationships as determinants of physical health. *Journal of American Academy of Psychoanalysis and Dynamic Psychiatry*, **36**, 11–32.

78. Weissman, M.M. and Markowitz, J.C. (1998) An overview of interpersonal psychotherapy, in *Interpersonal Psychotherapy* (ed. J. Markowitz), American Psychiatric Press, Washington, DC, pp. 1–33.

79. van Straten, A., Geraedts, A., Verdonck-de Leeuw, I. *et al.* (2010) Psychological treatment of depressive symptoms in patients with medical disorders: a meta-analysis. *Journal of Psychosomatic Research*, **69**, 23–32.

80. Esplen, M.J., Toner, B., Hunter, J. *et al.* (1998) A group therapy approach to facilitate integration of risk information for women at risk for breast cancer. *Canadian Journal of Psychiatry*, **43**, 375–380.

81. Spiegel, D. and Spira, J. (1991) *Supportive-Expressive Group Therapy: A Treatment Manual of Psychosocial Intervention for Women with Recurrent Breast Cancer*, Psychosocial Treatment Laboratory, Stanford University School of Medicine, Sanford, CA.

82. Spiegel, D., Bloom, J.R., Kraemer, H.C. *et al.* (1989) Effect of psychosocial treatment on survival of patients with metastatic breast cancer. *Lancet*, **2**, 888–891.

83. Leszcz, M. and Goodwin, P.J. (1998) The rationale and foundations of group psychotherapy for women with metastatic breast cancer. *International Journal of Group Psychotherapy*, **48**, 245–273.

18 Psychotherapy with Paediatric and Adolescent Cancer Patients

Julia Kearney[1] and Abraham S. Bartell[2,3]

[1]Department of Psychiatry and Behavioral Sciences and Department of Pediatrics, Memorial Sloan-Kettering Cancer Center, NY, USA
[2]Department of Psychiatry and Behavioral Sciences and Department of Pediatrics, Memorial Sloan-Kettering Cancer Center, NY, USA
[3]Weill Cornell Medical College, Cornell University, NY, USA

18.1 Introduction

Any conversation about therapeutic interventions in children with cancer begins with a review of the factors that make this a unique group and how they impact the therapy, therapist and therapeutic relationship. Our approach to the population does not favour one particular type of psychotherapy, but a therapeutic method, that is individualised, flexible, multi-disciplinary and inclusive/comprehensive, including all members of a child's social system who may be impacted by the illness.

Approaching a therapeutic intervention for any patient begins with a thorough evaluation, which must include an assessment of the characteristics of the patient, the psychopathology or diagnosis, the background of illness and the therapy being considered. The depth and accuracy of the assessment and how these factors impact on each other often drives the choices of therapy and therapist, allowing for optimal conditions for a successful therapeutic relationship.

18.2 Assessment

18.2.1 Patient Factors

When working with children, with or without medical issues, there are important considerations that come into play. Children are not autonomous and rarely does therapy happen without the involvement of, or at least the influence of, their family, however it is defined. The question of who the identified patient is must be addressed; in paediatrics the concept of a 'vicarious patient' is common and widely accepted and often factors significantly into defining the identified patient. It may be the child, the individual parent or caregiver, the parental dyad, the sibling or the family either in its entirety or some combination of its parts or the wider 'family' including friends and community. While it may be somewhat expected that parents or caregivers are involved in treatment it is important to remember the influence siblings and friends have on children's lives – especially in the adolescent stage, and inclusion of these 'family' members can be appropriate and have an even greater impact than only individual treatment.

The 'paediatric cohort' encompasses patients from birth to young adulthood and spans the ages of days old to 21 years and often slightly older if they are students or have adolescent issues. These years can be understood as an individual trajectory spanning several developmental stages across different domains of development (see Table 18.1).

Each stage of development can be described by its milestones, capacities that represent typical progress in many different domains: language, cognitive, social-emotional (including attachment and psychosexual development, and others) and physical. Thus the therapist must have a good sense of developmental theories and experience with normative child development to make a thorough and ongoing developmental assessment of each child. It is crucial not to fall victim to the notion that chronologic age equals developmental stage. Development is a

Table 18.1	Major child developmental theories				
Age (years)	Developmental milestones	Mahler	Erikson	Freud	Piaget
0–1	Rapid socioemotional, language and motor development	Autistic / Symbiotic	Trust vs. mistrust	Oral phase	Sensorimotor
2	Walking, talking, toilet training	Separation-individuation	Autonomy vs. shame and doubt	Anal phase	
3	Plays, picture books, sibling rivalry	Object constancy, gender identity	Initiative vs. guilt	Phallic phase (oedipal phase)	Preoperational
4	Numbers, shapes, symbolic play, uses 'I'	Increasing Internalisation			
5–6	Mastery through games, sports, academics	Differentiated self-object relations	Industry vs. Inferiority	Early latency phase	Concrete operations
7–11				Late latency phase	
12–15	Puberty, adolescence		Identity vs. identity diffusion	Phallic phase	Formal operations

complex web-like mosaic, that is constantly changing and the different developmental lines can be impacted in different ways by a traumatic life experience such as a cancer diagnosis. For instance, the same child whose cognitive ability to understand medical facts may be developmentally accelerated could have attachment issues related to early life threats and separations due to treatment, or an arrested/disrupted psychosexual development due to bodily integrity issues from surgery during a vulnerable window of time.

18.2.2 Presenting Problem Factors

Careful consideration of the nature of psychopathology is a given in any treatment situation. In children and

adolescents with cancer, this begins with understanding the onset of issues. Did the psychopathology precede the cancer diagnosis or was onset after the diagnosis and initiation of treatment? Although both pre-existing and reactive issues need to be addressed they may have to be addressed with different interventions, different therapists, different therapies and different settings.

The nature of the issues is important to examine as well. Are the issues psychological or psychiatric in nature and best described as psychopathology or are they developmental in nature? Are the issues specific to the individual child or are they family concerns? Do the issues manifest as emotional/social in nature or educational/cognitive in nature? These questions drive both the evaluation and the therapeutic intervention processes.

18.2.3 Medical Illness and Treatment Factors

The patient's illness narrative is a critical part of the psycho-oncology assessment. Every characteristic of the illness can impact the patient's experience, but when taking a medical history it is important to assess for acuity and stage of illness (acute, chronic, recurrent, end of life and survivorship) and type of cancer (location, stage and characteristics of the tumour, solid versus liquid tumours). Further considerations should focus on the treatment and examine the type of treatment (chemotherapy, surgery, immunotherapy, radiation therapy, stem cell/bone marrow transplantation and combinations of one or more of them), nature of (how available, how refined, standard care vs. experimental, what phase experimental, safety and efficacy, how new, how experienced is treating team with the treatment, how invasive, how tolerable, duration of treatment) and intent of treatment (curative vs. palliative). In paediatrics, a therapist may hear one story of the illness from the patient and a completely different version of events from a parent or sibling, depending on the person's understanding, defences and attitude about the illness and individual experience in their own role. All the perspectives help to synthesise a true picture of how the illness has impacted the patient and family.

18.3 Service Development

With the goal of delivering care, that is individualised, flexible, multi-disciplinary and inclusive, there are special considerations about treatment setting and treatment provider that guide the development of the Paediatric Psycho-oncology Service. Some promising research has shown the utility of universal screening tools, to identify families at risk for need of higher levels of care, with the goals of early identification and introduction of services, crisis and trauma prevention and conservation of resources [1, 2].

18.3.1 Treatment Setting

Special attention can be paid to the discussion of the treatment setting in paediatric psycho-oncology. Treatments may occur in the community (i.e. private practices, clinics and counselling centres) or hospital settings (at the cancer centre). A patient who is undergoing multiple cycles of high dose chemotherapy is unlikely to be able to attend twice a week psychodynamic psychotherapy, but may be very amenable to bedside supportive or expressive therapy offered by the hospital consultation liaison service.

The distance from home, family and community may be influenced by the type and duration of cancer treatment and may further influence the type of psychotherapy that will be effective. Even when distance is not an issue there are scheduling constraints based on the frequency and duration of the cancer treatment and how treatment is tolerated. Many paediatric patients feel that they are 'always at the doctor' and do not want to have 'another doctors appointment' or take another medication regardless of what type of doctor or therapy may be offered. In other cases being able to provide care during the cancer treatment obviates the need for a separate appointment but has its own inherent challenges and limits that affect scheduling, content and treatment adherence.

When psychotherapy can be done at the bedside, an effort should be made to create a 'therapeutic space' or routine that protects the patient's confidentiality and autonomy. Giving the patient control over when, where and how often the therapy occurs within some therapeutic guidelines, can go a long way in establishing a trusting relationship with appropriate boundaries. Creating rituals and routines around therapy, such as favourite games, special toys from your office or even predictable checking-in questions (for instance about mood, sleep or family coping) can set the therapeutic interaction apart from the hundreds of other caregiver-patient transactions that happen each day for a hospitalised patient.

18.3.2 Treatment Providers

At most cancer centres, the child in cancer treatment interacts with multiple support people throughout the treatment course. A well-staffed and well-rounded psychosocial team is the best defence against the preventable stressors involved in treatment, but is not always possible. Each member of the team has a role and provides important, complementary skills to the child and family. A therapist with medical training may be able to offer skilful symptom management, for instance with nausea, pain or fatigue, as first line, which for some families may be a more easily accepted service. Once the relationship is established, the psychiatrist can approach more sensitive, well-guarded subjects such as coping with a recurrence or fear of uncertainty. A therapist trained in play therapy may be perfect for younger children struggling to understand and express their experience. Social workers often provide the first line of support for families, helping them realise their experiences and reactions are normal and expected. An experienced social worker also becomes a valued guide for family problem solving around the inevitable challenges that come with cancer treatment, whether the nature is financial, time management, childcare, transportation or a myriad of other common concerns.

Child life specialists are experts in child development, who promote effective coping through play, education and self-expression activities. They provide emotional support and guidance for families, and encourage optimum development of children. They also serve as an interface with others involved in a child's care and are important in informing the process. In this role child life staff are an invaluable part of paediatric cancer centres and often become the everyday companions and comforters of children in treatment. The recreation programming they provide is critical to combat the boredom and lack of stimulation that comes with waiting for doctors, prolonged infusions and especially long term hospital isolations.

Complementary therapies can be wonderful additions to treatment or can be primary interventions in cases where a child or family doesn't need or want traditional psychiatric/psychological services. These include creative/expressive therapies such as art, dance and music therapy; relaxation focused therapies such as meditation, reiki or massage and even pet therapy with therapeutic animal companions. The question of who should be included in the psychosocial support team can be answered either narrowly or broadly and some centres include anyone involved in the day to day care of the child who has the ability to affect positively quality of life. Representatives from school tutoring, nursing staff, nutrition services, chaplaincy and physical and occupational therapy all play a part in supporting parents, motivating children and maximising quality of life. A team approach has been recognised as ideal, for optimal care of the child and family as well as burnout prevention for staff [1, 3, 4].

Any primary therapist in this setting will develop a way of engaging parents and children in psychological services. It is common for families to be taken aback at the suggestion to involve a psychiatrist or psychologist, arguing their child is 'not crazy'. However, most usually come to understand and appreciate the role of the professional in supporting the patient and parents through treatment. Indeed, most young children have no difficulty understanding why a cancer centre might have a 'feelings doctor' on staff, and can usually be easily engaged around commonly expressed feelings about the cancer experience.

18.4 Treatment Selection: Methods, Techniques and Efficacy

The process of treatment selection is not significantly different for children and adolescents with a cancer diagnosis than it is in the healthy paediatric population. All modalities of treatment should be considered including various types of individual, group and family therapies. Any available therapies should be considered; however the nature of the therapy including frequency, duration, goals and expectations may have to be modified to accommodate the physical limitations resulting from the cancer treatment.

Patients who require intervention around diagnosis and initiation of treatment often need basic supportive therapy until the patient and family get accustomed to the experience. An eight session, individual intervention for mothers, soon after a child's cancer diagnosis, targeted improved problem-solving and was shown to be effective in decreasing symptoms of depression and anxiety in English and Spanish speaking populations [5]. Medical play and art therapy tend to be helpful during the early phases of treatment with younger children. With children and teens educational interventions are often helpful to address their fears and concerns, identify misinformation or myths and provide targeted reassurance. Educational interventions have been shown to be an important part of many therapeutic trials, from cognitive behavioural therapies (CBTs), to family, to group interventions [6, 7].

Once treatment has progressed and things settle in it may be necessary to reassess the treatment choice and give consideration to behavioural therapies (BTs) and CBT as discreet issues arise. Behavioural techniques such as hypnosis, yoga breathing, guided imagery, distraction, other relaxation techniques, coaching by parent/clinician have been shown to be useful in the reduction of physical symptoms like nausea or pain, including procedure related pain and the accompanying distress or anxiety [8–13]. Further addition of cognitive techniques such as education, self monitoring, problem-solving, enlisting support, exploring role changes and family stressors and reshaping negative or self-defeating thought patterns are all effective in working with cancer patients to reduce anxiety, depression or post traumatic symptoms.

With the pre-teen and teen population as well was with parents and caregivers the group therapy options can be very effective. As with any group therapy the options vary based on the age of the patients, diagnoses or symptoms being targeted as well as the setting in which the group is held. In almost all cases it is very effective to address the angst that the patients are somehow different, unique or alone in their experience. It is both comforting and therapeutic to encounter other patients with similar diagnoses or experiences. Initially the interaction helps normalise the experience. Practically, group therapies may help children problem solve and gain from others' experiences – both successes and failures. It can be enormously helpful, for similar reasons, for caregivers and siblings although it is often difficult to get an adequate size group of siblings for the group to be effective. Many of the same types of interventions and techniques used in individual therapy (education, monitoring, reframing, exploring roles) can be effective in group therapy as well [14, 15].

The cancer diagnosis in the paediatric population presents an opportunity and need for family and friends to connect, rally in mutual support and express their concern for the sick child. Amid sources of social support, the family is one of the most important. All child and adolescent consultations are done with the family system as an integral part of the assessment, engagement, treatment and discharge planning. We generally accept that children and adolescents are not independent or autonomous, but rather highly dependent entities within a family. It further stands to reason that parents, family members and the family unit as a whole are of paramount importance to a child in almost all situations, and that reliance is multi-faceted. Children depend on their parents for nurturance, guidance and support, both emotional and financial. That reliance increases significantly at times of stress, and especially in the face of a cancer diagnosis.

Research on the impact of childhood illness on the family shows a 'reciprocal relationship' whereby the child's illness affects parent coping and parent's coping affects the child's adaptation [16]. Parents have routinely answered that the most difficult role they must perform is that of emotional support for their sick child. The medical setting presents parents and families with the additional role of guardian, medical decision maker and legal proxy. The latter role changes for adolescents where the importance of the patient's assent and the process of actual consent become increasingly pertinent.

However some situations really do call for a specific family level intervention, with individual family members or the family as a whole. Family therapy goals are rooted in understanding family interactions and dynamics and use the family's strengths to address problems by restructuring any maladaptive behaviours, improving communication and optimising problem solving skills. Problem solving approaches include behavioural, structural, psycho-educational and strategic–systemic models. Trans-generational and developmental approaches, such as Beavers and McMaster [17–22], include the family life cycle, psychodynamic and experiential models.

Parenting therapies can focus on providing guidance and support to parents as they navigate the new and unfamiliar experience of having a child with cancer. Parents often have the tendency to see their child's world through their own eyes, leading parents to identify issues where none exist or amplifying the ones that do. They may project their own fears onto their child, or have unrealistic expectations of how their child copes with illness. It should be made clear that parents and children have different experiences, understanding and expectations which impact each of them very differently. In some cases it may necessitate a parent completing their own psychological evaluation and entering into treatment. Research is ongoing in this area of developing interventions for parents in order to support and stabilise the family system, including CBT and problem solving interventions in either groups or individual settings [5, 23].

It is worth briefly noting that neuropsychological issues often arise during or after cancer treatment. The evaluation and remediation of neuropsychological issues is often important in the school re-entry experience whether that occurs during the treatment, often in the chronic or maintenance stages, or post treatment. Neuropsychological testing and educational planning may become an issue requiring the attention of all clinicians involved in a child's cancer treatment in an effort to help the child, their parents, the school, and often the community at large adjust to, and accommodate to, the return of a sick child to the school and community.

18.5 Issues in Treatment

18.5.1 Common Diagnoses

Once in treatment the commonly encountered psychopathology in Paediatric Oncology span a fairly broad range. In the case of pre-existing psychopathology there is no diagnosis excluded. Children with any, or all, disorders get cancer and when they do those issues must be managed. It is not uncommon for pre-existing issues to be exacerbated by the stress of a cancer diagnosis and treatment. Often children undergoing cancer treatments are in the hospital or clinic a great deal and the likelihood of adherence to treatment increases if the psychological therapy can take place in the same setting as their cancer treatment. Community providers may become overwhelmed emotionally by the cancer diagnosis and burden of treatment, or just lack the experience to manage new issues and the impact on old issues that cancer treatment may have. The transfer of care to a psycho-oncologist, at least during cancer treatment, is often advisable. Many community clinicians maintain contact during that transfer of care and, that is often helpful both as a support during treatment and for transition back to the community provider after treatment.

In the case of new issues or psychopathology that arises as a result of the diagnosis or cancer treatment there is also a broad range. It is common to encounter issues of mood, anxiety, bereavement and issues related to death and dying. In many children the issues are transient and fall under the heading of an adjustment disorder, which may settle once they get through the initial shock and impact of diagnosis and the new experience of treatment. Treatment is often long and cyclic in nature so that after a cycle or two both the children and their caregivers become more accustomed to the treatment and know what to expect. Much of the reactive symptomatology resolves with education and supportive therapy. Issues related to death and dying, symptom management of the treatment side effects and issues related more specifically to the illness itself, often persist and require more targeted therapy.

Paediatric Medical Traumatic Stress has evolved as a useful concept to understand common reactions of the patient and family to the experience of illness and treatment. It is defined as: 'a set of psychological and physiological responses of children and their families to pain, injury, serious illness, medical procedures and invasive or frightening treatment experiences' [7, 24–26]. The range of acute and post-traumatic symptoms can be present in both children and adolescent patients and their parents, and research has identified interventions that help reduce traumatic symptoms by reframing beliefs about cancer, modifying adversity belief systems and improve problem solving [7].

18.5.2 Impact of Child Development on Understanding Illness and Death

Assorted internal and external variables affect a child's comprehension, including developmental stage and cognitive abilities associated with that stage (see Table 18.2). For a full discussion of this important

Table 18.2	Variables affecting a child's understanding and coping with illness and death

Child's personality and life experience
Child's loss history, including, for example: illness, death, trauma, separation, parental divorce, geographical moves
How parents convey their cognitive and spiritual understanding of death
How parents and other family members convey their emotions and ways of coping
Style and patterns of communication in the family
Availability of social support to child and family
Cultural attitudes and beliefs around illness and death
Developmental stage influencing cognitive and emotional ability to understand death

topic, full of rich clinical material, see Barbara Sourkes' books [27, 28] and the online resources of the Initiative for Paediatric Palliative Care [29]. When talking about death with children it is helpful to concentrate on major themes that may be points of misunderstanding or confusion for children, including irreversibility, non-functionality, universality and causality. Regression is the rule for children under stress, so older children can often demonstrate behaviours and even cognitive frameworks typical for a 'younger' developmental stage. Most research on how children understand death and illness has been done with bereaved children, not sick or dying children but it is generally thought to apply to children suffering from illness themselves [6, 30]. As with all therapy, listening for the child's own perspective and ideas about how the illness occurred, why it happened to them, how it will be fixed and what happens if medicines don't work, is more important than lecturing the child with 'developmentally appropriate' explanations. Even with the youngest children, it is best to provide truthful but simple explanations that give reasons for the symptoms and changes the child experiences in their body, or sees in the body of a loved one (i.e. 'the leukaemia cells were making you so tired', or 'we didn't know your brother had a tumour in his bone until he got kicked on the soccer field'). It is important not to use euphemism and metaphor with young children who often take things literally. Exploring with children what they have heard from well-meaning friends and family is useful as well, since many people are uncomfortable talking about death, illness or uncertainty with young children.

Adolescent to late adolescent children have achieved formal operational thinking and understand the realities of death and even the realities of survival, in terms of late effects of treatment and the impact of cancer on their lives. They experience the full range of existential issues described in adult patients, including feeling cheated out of a future, feeling anxious about whether their life has had meaning and feeling anxious about whether they have fulfilled their human potential or purpose ('existential guilt'). Feeling that 'life is interrupted' is a common cry of teens and efforts to keep connected to that life through social networking media, special arrangements for visitors and day passes to participate in key events like graduations, can go a long way to fighting against depression and isolation. With adolescent patients there is the impact on autonomy to consider. As adolescents they strive for individuation and autonomy and now they are reliant on family and the medical community. Often despite being given the opportunity to participate in the decision making process they feel as though there are really no choices. This often leads to anger and conflict with caregivers, parents and doctors.

18.5.3 Illness-Specific Issues in Therapy

The illness and treatment are the day to day reality for the paediatric oncology patient, and so the psychotherapist working with paediatric oncology patients is wise to develop an understanding of the basic illnesses and treatment regimens their patients are experiencing. If the therapist is not embedded in the oncology practice setting, an ongoing relationship with the primary team will help support the therapist by providing accurate knowledge of decisions that need to be made, prognosis and treatment planning. This knowledge establishes the therapist as the patient's resource for exploring, understanding and sharing the physical and emotional impact of the disease and treatment.

Specific issues that arise in the context of chemotherapy often have to do with toxic side effects. Many children experience anticipatory nausea or anxiety when they know they will receive chemotherapy with nausea-genic side effects and will need symptomatic relief or a relaxation strategy from the minute they wake up on treatment day. CBT and hypnosis have been found to be useful for anticipatory and procedural symptoms [9–11, 31, 32]. For younger children, the concept of 'side effects' is a bit of a difficult one, especially if they were asymptomatic or less symptomatic before diagnosis of their cancer and are now feeling severely ill from treatment side effects. It is easy to see how a child would feel the 'doctors made me sick' or the 'chemo makes me sick' and refuse to come to appointments or to get certain treatments. Working with Child Life and/or the

therapist to explain and review models of disease and treatment through play, video/cartoon media or art can often help even children as young as three or four years of age to grasp this concept and thus feel some predictability in their physical experience and some mastery over the hospital environment. Even paging through a picture encyclopaedia of the body can lead children to share their fears and questions about their disease, treatments and side effects. One child was eager to see the blood vessel pictures 'where my IV goes when the needle goes in'; another who was hospitalised with pancreatitis was very relieved to see a diagram of a pancreas in the belly of the person that correlated with her pain.

Other treatments have unique issues that can be explored and supported in therapy. Immunotherapy for neuroblastoma, for instance, can be a painful systemic infusion that children endure daily for many courses. However, most children have found coping skills through therapeutic support including rocking, watching videos, directing parents in massage or using dance and movement with music to face this difficult treatment with remarkable grace and mastery. Stem cell transplant is a particularly challenging treatment for young children to face because of the prolonged isolation required during engraftment. Even for adolescents, who have described this experience as having 'life on hold', this isolation is distressing and disruptive to their relationships and sense of self. Particular interventions useful in transplant include structured daily schedules of nursing care requirements (mouth care, weight check), scheduled interventions with physical therapy, school tutoring; limited and carefully screened visits with family and friends; supportive therapy; aggressive symptom management; recreational play. Parents are also affected, showing elevated levels of anxiety, Posttraumatic stress disorder (PTSD) and depression. Parents may benefit from intervention and support from paediatric psychosocial support staff during transplant, which in turn helps children by allowing the parent to be more emotionally available.

One aspect of treatment that colours most discussions about the illness experience is the intent of the treatment – curative or palliative. It is important to understand what the treatment team thinks, what the parents think and finally, what the child thinks about this, especially if a child has a progressive disease, that is not in remission and is still receiving disease-modifying treatments. Understanding what has been explicitly stated to parents and to the child will help the therapist recognise patient and parent's wishes, fears and fantasies about the outcomes of treatment, often brought up in subtle or ambiguous ways. Recognising the myriad of ways and reasons people can misunderstand or misconstrue this type of painful information the therapist can be helpful in sorting through the emotions that make decision-making more confusing and painful than necessary, and help a family prioritise quality of life, relationships and legacy building.

All ages and diagnoses may confront the uncertainty of treatment efficacy. Those fears and concerns are often amplified if there are modifications or changes made to the treatment plan regardless of whether the changes are made based on the efficacy of the treatment or how treatment is tolerated. There is often the natural tendency to ask 'what if' questions. The 'what ifs' may be fuelled by the thoughts and concerns stemming from diagnosis, doubts or regrets about treatment choices made along the way, or focused on the uncertainty of the future either relapse or post-treatment. These questions and the medical community's inability to answer them often lead to frustration anxiety and uncertainty as well as anger.

There are issues that emerge once treatment is completed. Often in the early post treatment period there is the difficulty accepting that treatment is really over. Questions and fears linger regarding the adequacy and effectiveness of the treatment. Some patients are afraid to stop, as they are no longer actively doing something to prevent the cancer from recurring. Even if the concerns are simpler they often struggle with whether or not they can really believe that the cancer is gone and question 'Am I really cured?' Further, once treatment is completed there is often a period of surveillance that may be intrusive and anxiety provoking and may create new feelings or feed into the existing fears of treatment effect and adequacy.

For many there is the hope or wish of 'getting back to normal' and anxiety, anger or disappointment when they realise that they can never go back and but must only move forward to a new normal.

18.5.4 Counter Transference and Burnout

In a field where a therapist engages daily in sessions with seriously ill children about the physical and emotional suffering they endure from their disease, counter transference can be a major issue in the therapeutic encounter and the long term efficacy and mental health of the therapist. Self-care is tantamount to this work and it starts with a thorough examination of one's own relationship to the job. There are many reasons why a person chooses to work with seriously ill and dying

children – one study interviewed 30 American paediatric oncologists and found that 57% of them had a serious childhood or adolescent illness themselves [33]. It is the task for each caregiver to understand their own expectations of the job and work on setting limits (emotional boundaries and workload limits), creating balance in their life and preventing burnout. Teams and workplace leaders can also do a lot to help prevent and respond to early stages of clinician burnout. Burnout has been defined by the International Society of Pediatric Oncology (SIOP) as having four stages [3, 34], starting with physical and emotional exhaustion and progressing through further destructive stages of indifference, sense of failure as a clinician and a person and finally, feeling 'dead inside', a stage associated with abandoning the profession and contemplating suicide. Severe reactions can be prevented through awareness and recognition of the early stages, fostering a sense of common mission among teams and co-workers, building caring and responsive leadership educated in burnout prevention. Individuals can learn to ask for help when overwhelmed by the work, set limits and participate more deeply in social support with peers. Psychological counselling should be sought when a professional or team is struggling with these tasks, in order to restore a sense of efficacy and worth.

18.6 Case Discussion: a Multidisciplinary Team Approach

Jason[1] is a 15 year old young man with Aplastic Anaemia who became transfusion dependant and due to iron overload required a bone marrow transplant. Due to the complexity of his social situation and his history of poor adherence to care, a couple of small centres with Bone Marrow Transplantation (BMT) programmes felt they could not successfully transplant him and he was referred to a large transplant centre with a multidisciplinary psychosocial care team. After several weeks experience of medical management and the preliminary pre-transplant process, and based on his history, the BMT team felt they could only move forward with transplant if a multi-disciplinary evaluation intervention was completed and the patient and his family were successful in adhering to treatment and showing they could manage the rigours of transplant and post-transplant follow up.

Jason lives with his biological mother and stepfather, his biological younger brother and stepbrother,

---

[1] The patient's name has been changed to protect confidentiality.

who is approximately the same age as Jason. His biological father is involved in his life but there have been tensions between his biological parents since divorcing. His biological father lives in a neighbouring state. Child protective services have been involved with Jason for various reasons, including allegations of physical abuse, medical neglect and educational neglect. Services have been provided in both states with minimal help.

Psychiatric evaluation reveals that Jason is depressed with irritability and at times aggressive behaviour. He smokes cigarettes but denies other drugs and has not attended school regularly for some time. His mother has a long history of depression and is on medication but not followed regularly and not in therapy. She often would disappear to go and take naps at the residence, leaving Jason alone in the hospital or clinic, which escalated his anger towards her withdrawal. His step brother has behavioural issues and a history of aggression and there have been multiple physical altercations at home.

The multidisciplinary team met and formulated the following plan.

Jason would be followed by child psychiatry and agree to try antidepressant medication as well as behavioural and supportive talk therapies. He should agree to attend a weekly teen group co-led by a Child Life specialist and social worker and participate in a smoking cessation programme. Jason's mother would agree to weekly therapy with the team social worker and attend regular meetings with a psychiatrist to manage her medications. Jason would begin school with the hospital's high school teacher. Both Jason and his mum were to participate in joint sessions, with other family members' involvement as needed, to initiate a behaviour programme and family therapy intervention. Jason and his mother were to reside at the Ronald McDonald House and agree to a structured weekly schedule that included various medical, school, psychological and psychiatric appointments. If Jason and his mother could successfully adhere to this multidisciplinary plan for six weeks the Bone Marrow Transplant team would move forward with transplant.

Adherence to the plan would be reviewed weekly at a team meeting with all members of the team updating the patient's and his mother's progress. Additionally, as a part of the pre-transplant work up, various medical evaluations including pulmonary, cardiology evaluations, physical therapy and nutritional evaluations would be completed and adherence to those appointments was also to be reviewed.

18.6.1 Roles

- **Social work**: provide support for family/practical problem solving for logistical issues; explore barriers to improved family care; meet one to one with the patient's mother for supportive psychotherapy, liaise with Ronald McDonald House staff regarding behaviour and function there;

- **Child and adolescent psychiatry**: to engage the patient in a talking therapy, psychotropic medications, symptom management and smoking cessation; co-lead family meetings with social work, advise/support team members with counter-transference; direct behavioural programme/consequences;

- **Physical therapy and occupational therapy**: provide healthy and appropriate exercise, provide feedback for team regarding behaviour during sessions;

- **Psychiatry**: Evaluate and meet with the patient's mother regarding her psychotropic medications;

- **Child life**: provide entertainment and engagement and lead an open out-patient teen group weekly; give feedback to the team regarding the patient's participation;

- **Teacher**: meet for regularly scheduled sessions and give feedback to the team regarding the patient's participation;

- **BMT team**: schedule pre-transplant medical workup and monitor adherence to medical treatment;

- **Physical therapy**: complete a pre-transplant evaluation and initiate weekly meetings to address the patient's needs;

- **Nutrition**: Provide guidance regarding healthy and appropriate foods, prepare the patient for post-transplant dietary requirements.

Both the mother and the patient benefitted from the medications and both depressions improved. The patient stopped smoking, the mother had much better energy and was able to participate in his care, decreasing the conflict in their relationship. The structure provided by the team allowed the mother to be more present at Jason's bedside, with brief visits home to address issues there more efficiently. In the therapy, both Jason and his mother began to appreciate the impact their chaotic lifestyle had on each other and the family functioning. Biological parents were able to plan visitation better and the father was able to visit Jason in the hospital during the mother's scheduled trips home. Despite concern and doubt on the part of the BMT team, based on the initial interaction, the patient and his mother adhered to the plan and after four weeks the transplant was scheduled and the patient was successfully transplanted.

18.7 Summary

Psychotherapy in children with cancer is influenced by the factors that make this a unique group. It is crucial to identify these factors and how they impact on the therapy, therapist and therapeutic relationship. A thorough and inclusive evaluation drives the process of designing a therapeutic intervention; the characteristics of the patient, the psychopathology and the nature and history of the medical illness must be assessed. In children developmental stages and abilities must be evaluated and taken into consideration throughout the process. Families must be assessed and their needs addressed as well. Interventions may include all modalities and durations of time and often changes as the needs and issues in this population evolve through the course of treatment and even in to the post-treatment period.

The treatment setting is unique and the demands of cancer treatment may require seeing a child in several different settings to provide consistency in therapy. Additionally the nature and content of therapy will change in response to the fluctuating acuity, needs and demands of the child and family throughout the treatment course. Given the variability of diagnosis and developmental issues within the paediatric cohort, consideration should be given to a multi-disciplinary approach to intervention whenever possible. Finally it is important to recognise the impact of working with this population on the therapist, which puts the therapist at risk for burn-out and vicarious traumatisation and contributes to counter-transference in the therapy.

References

1. Kazak, A.E., Rourke, M.T., Alderfer, M.A. *et al.* (2007) Evidence-based assessment, intervention and psychosocial care in pediatric oncology: a blueprint for comprehensive services across treatment. *Journal of Pediatric Psychology*, **32** (9), 1099–1110.
2. Pai, A.L., Patino-Fernandez, A.M., McSherry, M. *et al.* (2008) The psychosocial assessment tool (PAT2.0): psychometric properties of a screener for psychosocial distress in families of children newly diagnosed with cancer. *Journal of Pediatric Psychology*, **33** (1), 50–62.
3. Spinetta, J.J., Jankovic, M., Masera, G. *et al.* (2009) Optimal care for the child with cancer: a summary statement from the SIOP working committee on psychosocial issues in pediatric oncology. *Pediatric Blood and Cancer*, **52** (7), 904–907.
4. Rourke, M.T., Reilly, A., Kersun, L.S. *et al.* (2006) Understanding and managing challenging families in pediatric oncology. Poster presented at the American Psychosocial Oncology Society (APOS) Conference, Amelia Island, FL.
5. Sahler, O.J., Fairclough, D.L., Phipps, S. *et al.* (2005) Using problem-solving skills training to reduce negative affectivity in mothers of children with newly diagnosed cancer: report of a multisite randomized trial. *Journal of Consulting and Clinical Psychology*, **73** (2), 272–283.
6. Christ, G.H. and Christ, A.E. (2006) Current approaches to helping children cope with a parent's terminal illness. *CA: A Cancer Journal for Clinicians*, **56** (4), 197–212.
7. Pai, A.L. and Kazak, A.E. (2006) Pediatric medical traumatic stress in pediatric oncology: family systems interventions. *Current Opinion in Pediatrics*, **18** (5), 558–562.
8. Powers, S.W. (1999) Empirically supported treatments in pediatric psychology: procedure-related pain. *Journal of Pediatric Psychology*, **24** (2), 131–145.
9. Liossi, C., White, P. and Hatira, P. (2009) A randomized clinical trial of a brief hypnosis intervention to control venepuncture-related pain of paediatric cancer patients. *Pain*, **142** (3), 255–263.
10. Miller, D.L., Manne, S. and Palevsky, S. (1998) Brief report: acceptance of behavioral interventions for children with cancer: perceptions of parents, nurses, and community controls. *Journal of Pediatric Psychology*, **23** (4), 267–271.
11. Nash, M.R., Perez, N., Tasso, A. and Levy, J.J. (2009) Clinical research on the utility of hypnosis in the prevention, diagnosis, and treatment of medical and psychiatric disorders. *The International Journal of Clinical and Experimental Hypnosis*, **57** (4), 443–450.
12. Zeltzer, L. and Lebaron, S. (1984) The Role of psychotherapy in the treatment of children with cancer. *Psychotherapy in Private Practice*, **2** (3), 45–49.
13. DuHamel, K.N., Redd, W.H. and Vickberg, S.M. (1999) Behavioral interventions in the diagnosis, treatment and rehabilitation of children with cancer. *Acta Oncologica*, **38** (6), 719–734.
14. Baider, L. and De-Nour, A.K. (1989) Group therapy with adolescent cancer patients. *Journal of Adolescent Health Care*, **10** (1), 35–38.
15. Heiney, S.P., Ruffin, J., Ettinger, R.S. and Ettinger, S. (1988) The effects of group therapy on adolescents with cancer. *Journal of the Association of Pediatric Oncology Nurses*, **5** (3), 20–24.
16. Brown, R.T., Wiener, L., Kupst, M.J. *et al.* (2008) Single parents of children with chronic illness: an understudied phenomenon. *Journal of Pediatric Psychology*, **33** (4), 408–421.
17. Epstein, N., BIshop, D. and Levin, S. (1978) The mcmaster model of family functioning. *Journal of Family and Marital Counseling*, **4**, 19–31.
18. Beavers, W.R., Hampson, R. and Halgus, Y. (1985) Commentary: the beavers systems approach to family assessment. *Family Process*, **24**, 385–398.
19. Beavers, W.R. and Voeller, M.N. (1983) Family models: comparing and contrasting the Olson Circumplex model with the Beavers systems model. *Family Process*, **22** (1), 85–98.
20. Lee, C. (1988) Theories of family adaptability: toward a synthesis of Olson's Circumplex and the Beavers systems models. *Family Process*, **27** (1), 73–96.

21. Ravenstock, K. (1996) Family therapy, in *Child and Adolescent Psychiatry: A comprehensive Textbook* (ed. M. Lewis), Williams and Wilkins, Baltimore, pp. 850–868.

22. Johnson, G., Kent, G. and Leather, J. (2005) Strengthening the parent-child relationship: a review of family interventions and their use in medical settings. *Child: Care, Health and Development*, **31** (1), 25–32.

23. Sahler, O.J., Varni, J.W., Fairclough, D.L. *et al.* (2002) Problem-solving skills training for mothers of children with newly diagnosed cancer: a randomized trial. *Journal of Developmental and Behavioral Pediatrics*, **23** (2), 77–86.

24. Pediatric Medical Traumatic Stress (2010) National Child Trauma Stress Network. Available from www.nctsn.org; http://www.nctsn.org. Access year 2010.

25. Kazak, A.E. and Baxt, C. (2007) Families of infants and young children with cancer: a post-traumatic stress framework. *Pediatric Blood and Cancer*, **49** (Suppl. 7), 1109–1113.

26. Kazak, A.E., Kassam-Adams, N., Schneider, S. *et al.* (2006) An integrative model of pediatric medical traumatic stress. *Journal of Pediatric Psychology*, **31** (4), 343–355.

27. Sourkes, B. (1996) *Armfuls of Time: The Psychological Experience of a Child with a Life Threatening Illness*, 1st edn, University of Pittsburgh Press, Pittsburgh, PA.

28. Sourkes, B. (1982) *The Deepening Shade: Psychological Aspects of a Life Threatening Illness*, University of Pittsburgh Press, Pittsburgh, PA.

29. Initiative on Pediatric Palliative Care. Available from www.ippcweb.org. Access year 2010.

30. Skeen, J.E. and Webster, M.L. (2004) Speaking to children about serious matters, in *Psychosocial Aspects of Pediatric Oncology* (eds S. Kreitler and M.W. BenArush), John Wiley & Sons, Ltd, West Sussex, pp. 281–312.

31. Jay, S., Elliott, C.H., Fitzgibbons, I. *et al.* (1995) A comparative study of cognitive behavior therapy versus general anesthesia for painful medical procedures in children. *Pain*, **62** (1), 3–9.

32. Burish, T.G., Carey, M.P., Redd, W.H. and Krozely, M.G. (1983) Behavioral relaxation techniques in reducing the distress of cancer chemotherapy patients. *Oncology Nursing Forum*, **10** (3), 32–35.

33. Fanos, J.H. (2007) "Coming through the fog, coming over the moors": the impact on pediatric oncologists of caring for seriously ill children. *Journal of Cancer Education*, **22** (2), 119–123.

34. Spinetta, J.J., Jankovic, M., Ben Arush, M.W. *et al.* (2000) Guidelines for the recognition, prevention, and remediation of burnout in health care professionals participating in the care of children with cancer: report of the SIOP working committee on psychosocial issues in pediatric oncology. *Medical and Pediatric Oncology*, **35** (2), 122–125.

19 Therapy for Parental Cancer and Dependent Children

Frances Marcus Lewis[1,2,3]

[1]University of Washington, Seattle, USA
[2]Public Health Sciences Division, Fred Hutchinson Cancer Research Center, Seattle, USA
[3]University of Pennsylvania, Philadelphia, USA

19.1 Background

Annually, multiple thousands of dependent children are impacted by newly diagnosed cancer in a parent. Estimates of affected children vary by country, by type and stage of cancer and by gender of parent. Conservative estimates available in the United States are that 22–30% of newly diagnosed patients with breast, prostate or colorectal cancer will be a parent of a dependent child. This estimate does not include thousands of other children impacted by other types of parental cancers, such as lymphoma, leukaemia or skin cancers and it does not reflect the staggering numbers of potentially affected children in other countries. It also does not include adult children or children of a dying parent. This latter group of children constitutes a special population with unique issues; see Christ [1–3]. Despite the magnitude of the numbers of potentially affected children, most therapies, services and programmes in cancer are focused on the diagnosed patient, not on the family or children [4, 5]. When a parent is diagnosed with cancer, evidence is that the children are treated with benign neglect, even in high functioning families with a well intended parent [4–6]. There is a conspiracy of respectful silence: parents do not want to scare the child by talking about the cancer; the child does not want to add to the burden of an already over-burdened parent. This is true for young school age children and for adolescent children. When the child's outward behaviour is like it was before the parent's diagnosis, parents and family members do not know the child's inner questions, concerns, worries or issues [7]. Children or adolescents, as will be seen in a summary of studies below, are often on their own to interpret and manage the impact of their parent's cancer on their lives [8]. It is the internal world of the child and ways to help them that deserve the attention and response of the parent and providers.

This chapter aims to:

1. summarise the theoretical and evidence-based rationale for a cancer parenting programme;

2. describe the operational components of a five-session educational counselling programme for the diagnosed parent that was designed to be responsive to the evidence;

3. summarise research evidence on the efficacy of the programme;

4. summarise the training programme for the cancer parenting programme that is now available to health professionals.

The chapter concludes with a description of current as well as future directions and applications of the cancer parenting programme in diverse provider settings.

19.2 Theoretical and Evidence-Based Rationale

The Enhancing Connections (EC) Programme is an evidence-based cancer parenting programme that focuses on five factors that are known from research to affect the quality of a child's adjustment to parental cancer: parental mood and anxiety; parenting skills; parenting confidence; the quality of the parent-child relationship and the child's cancer-related concerns. The ultimate outcome of the programme is to enhance

Handbook of Psychotherapy in Cancer Care, First Edition. Edited by Maggie Watson and David W. Kissane.
© 2011 John Wiley & Sons, Inc. Published 2011 by John Wiley & Sons, Inc.

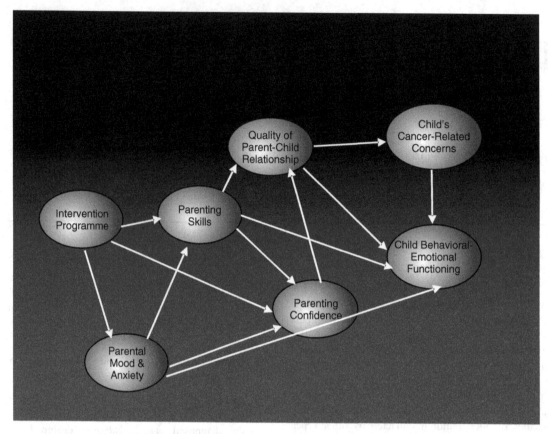

Figure 19.1 *Theoretical model of Enhancing Connections programme and outcomes.*

the child's behavioural-emotional functioning (see Figure 19.1). The five factors are potentially mutable through programmatic intervention or therapy, regardless of the prior history of parenting, regardless of concurrent events in the lives of the ill parent and child and regardless of the ill parent's treatment and demographic characteristics. Most studies to date that link the child's or adolescent's adjustment to parental cancer have involved mothers with breast cancer and their dependent children. This means that most of what is known may be confounded by threats to maternal attachment, not merely to parental cancer. An analysis of the published studies related to the six concepts in Figure 19.1 follows. The text moves from left to right in the figure.

19.2.1 Parental Mood and Anxiety

Women with breast cancer are known to experience high rates of depressed mood and affective problems for up to, or longer than, two years after diagnosis [9–11]. Depressed mothers are known to show

impaired parenting characterised by less psychological availability, communicativeness, supervision, consistency of discipline and initiative, as well as increased hostility, irritability and coerciveness [12, 13]. The link between parental clinical depression and problems with emotional or physical accessibility and child dysfunction is well documented in prior research [13–15]. However, only a beginning literature exists on the effects of short-term situational depressed mood in a parent on the child's or adolescent's adjustment.

19.2.2 Parenting Skills

Parenting skills are the interactional behaviours the parent uses to assist or interact with the child about the cancer. Data-based studies show that the ill parent is in a highly challenged position to effectively parent the child about the cancer in ways that minimise the threat to the child and help the child manage what is happening for the child. The reality is that diagnosed parents, even highly educated and credentialed parents, report they do not know what to do or say to help their child [16]. When the ill parent does talk to their child about the cancer, research shows they do one of three things. They overly disclose medical details in language that is more appropriate for an adult, not a child. They do not respond or attempt to elicit the child's worries, questions or concerns. Alternatively, they wait until their child asks a question about the cancer but do not initiate discussions with the child. The parent's over-disclosure is motivated by their belief that they want and need to 'be honest' and not 'hide' anything from their child. This means that the ill parent tells the child all that the parent knows. With rare exception, ill parents do not plan in advance what will be said to the child about the cancer and may instead blurt it out during the height of the parent's own fear and anxiety [16]. In studies with families dealing with maternal breast cancer, mothers commonly rely on the child's questions as the stimulus to talk about the cancer. When a child is silent, withdrawn, or does not ask questions, ill mothers do not know how to respond to help their child [op cit]. 'My older son (10 years) really got very quiet and didn't want to talk about the breast cancer at all. He wouldn't ask questions. He wouldn't talk about it.' Another ill mother said, "She didn't really ask questions. And I thought that she understood what was going on... but she really didn't..." Another mother said, "We were talking about chemotherapy and the ramifications of cancer. And I remember that he (12 years) just literally exploded and was very upset and tearful... didn't know how to express himself... didn't know how to ask questions. Didn't know what was going to happen. Just didn't understand any of what was going on or why it was happening" [op cit].

When ill mothers are asked what keeps them from being able to help the child, they claim their own anxiety, distress, fears about the cancer and symptoms (nausea, vomiting, extreme fatigue) often keep them from parenting their child in the ways they want. They claim to be in 'survival mode' and must put energy into themselves, not their child. Even when they recognise their child is having difficulty, they feel unable to reach out to help. As one mother shared, "I would say, 'Okay, this is horrible on (eight year old daughter), but I can barely get out of bed certain days.'" [op cit].

19.2.3 Parenting Confidence

Parenting confidence is the extent to which parents think and believe they have the requisite skills to successfully support and interact with their child about their cancer. The overriding evidence is that parents report a lack of confidence in knowing what to say or do to help their child, even as they admit to watching the child struggle. Results from case intensive interviews with ill mothers reveal that mothers emphasise a biomedical model of the illness when interacting with their child about the cancer [17]. Rarely does the ill parent attend to the affective or emotive concerns of the child, comfort the child about the illness and its related threats, or address the attributions, including partial or misunderstandings of the child, about the ill parent's cancer. The ill mothers describe themselves as being too emotional, centred around themselves and struggling with the breast cancer to assist their child. Mothers also report they are reticent or unable to talk about the cancer and feel unclear about what to say to the child [16]. They do not want to dwell on it, do not feel confident they can allay the child's concerns or deal with their child's emotional state, or do not want to face the child's questions, especially about death [18].

19.2.4 Quality of Parent-Child Relationship

The quality of the relationship between the child and the mother is a significant protective factor of the child's functioning [19, 20]. Parent-child relations characterised by parental withdrawal, indifference and unreliability have demonstrated links to behavioural, social and self-esteem problems [21] whereas responsive care giving assists the child's emotional regulation and confidence that supportive care is available [22]. In a series of path analytic studies involving parents with cancer and dependent children, parenting quality consistently related to adolescents' and school age children's scores on standardised measures of adjustment in households impacted by maternal breast cancer [23–25]. In a comparative study of adolescents of mothers with breast cancer, data obtained from 210 study participants revealed that adolescent self-esteem was significantly predicted by parenting quality in data from the ill mothers (Beta $= -.52$; p $= <.001$) [24]. (Self-esteem scores denoted *lower* self-esteem using Rosenberg's Self-esteem scale.)

19.2.5 Child's Cancer-Related Concerns

Children directly experience cancer-related pressures and concerns. Serious medical illness in a parent threatens the child in at least two ways. The child believes that the parent may not survive or that the child themselves may not survive either because of abandonment or because of vulnerability to the same illness [26]. The most direct evidence of attachment threat comes from qualitative interview studies with both school age and adolescent children of mothers with breast cancer in which the child discloses their concerns, fears or worries related to their parent's cancer [7, 8]. During stressful times like parental cancer, earlier ways of thinking, including poor hypothesis-testing and magical thinking, may reappear [27]. This means that we cannot assume an adolescent will be able to reason or problem-solve when a parent is diagnosed with cancer. Because strong emotional states may make it more difficult for the child to sort out what is happening, the upset child may experience more threat than she or he might otherwise. This temporary regression in judgement diminishes the child's capacity for self-comforting or using support from others. In the absence of information, children will also develop their own images and explanations – sometimes erroneous ones – of the changes in the ill parent's behaviour that they observe. Children may think they caused the parent's cancer or did something to make it worse. Left to independently interpret what is happening, the child or adolescent might misinterpret the parent's affective state or physical symptoms as something the child said, did or felt. Sadly, there is suggestive evidence that children may internalise their ill parent's behaviour as the child not being lovable or valued [28].

Even as children experience concerns, they tend to protect or hide their thoughts and feelings from the ill parent. This nine-year old girl reported, 'I went on the couch in front of the TV so she'd think that I'd been watching it, but I closed my eyes and I was thinking about her illness'. Some children thought it was their job to work things out on their own. In the words of this child, 'I know she's sick and I have to do things without her. I try not to bug her. I just try to figure it out myself, or I skip it . . .' [8]. Children report they are often on their own to manage and to cope with the impact of their mothers' breast cancer. In a seminal study with 35 school age children, only 46% reported receiving any parental assistance with the mother's cancer and an additional 26% reported that virtually no one helped them deal with their mother's illness, not even their own parents [8]. Children fear that the ill parent will die from the cancer. Results from a semi-structured interview study of 8–12 year olds revealed that 81% of the children believed their mother would die from the breast cancer, even though it was recently diagnosed as early stage disease [7]. Example quotes from these children are illustrative. An eight year old son said, "I thought about that she might die. And that I might die. And that a whole bunch of people might

die. Kind of pictured everybody just dying off because of the cancer. It was kind of hard". Another eight-year old son spoke of what it was like for him. "I wondered would I grow up without a mom? I was just mostly worried about how it would affect how I grew up". A 12-year-old girl said, "I was thinking about what would happen. I was actually planning for her to die . . . And I just went through all this mental imaging and I just assumed the worst. Which was a bad thing for now because I really made myself depressed".

Evidence of the child's fear of the parent dying from a cancer diagnosis has also been documented in an interview study of diagnosed mothers [16]. "The kids honestly thought I was going to die . . . I think that was their greatest fear . . . that they were going to have to watch me deteriorate . . . My eight year old daughter would lie there at night and worry about whether or not I was going to die . . . she would go through stages where at night she'd call me in and she'd double check to make sure that I was still OK, or, 'Are you gonna die, Mommy?'" Another mother said, "I was lying in bed . . . I could hear my daughter (12 years) tell my son (10 years) to be quiet, because Mom was going to die."

19.2.6 Child's Behavioural-Emotional Adjustment

There is inconsistent evidence on the level, degree or duration of behavioural-emotional disruption that occurs in a child when a parent has cancer and there are no prospective studies that enable us to unconditionally attribute the child's adjustment to parental cancer. However, studies using comparative designs or comparative analyses help build a compelling case that cancer impacts the child's adjustment, especially during the early period of diagnosis, treatment and early recovery. (Data on children of dying parents are a special case.) Specific problems shown by children of mothers with cancer include regression, withdrawal, anxiety about family stability and integrity and anti-social behaviour [26, 29–31]. In a case intensive interview study, diagnosed mothers of 36 children were asked to describe the difficult times the mothers had in parenting the child about the breast cancer [16]. Data were striking in the consistency with which the mothers reported detailed examples of distress and behavioural disruption in their child that the mothers attributed to the cancer. Eighty-three per cent of the children were described as having a difficult time with the breast cancer.

The most extensive set of studies on the impact of parental cancer on adolescents were conducted by

Compas' team [32–35]. Using standardised measures of adolescent adjustment, they examined the impact of parental cancer on adolescents close to the time of diagnosis, averaging two months. Measures of adolescent adjustment included the Child Behaviour Checklist (CBCL) and Youth Self Report (YSR), both measures of behavioural problems [36–38]. Results showed that adolescents of parents with cancer were at high risk for both anxiety and depression compared to normative samples. Further studies by Compas' team concluded that adolescents whose parents had cancer showed greater morbidity than did pre-adolescents. In addition, later research supported their initial finding that girls whose mothers had cancer were at greater risk for anxiety and depression than girls whose fathers had cancer or boys with either parent with cancer [34, 35]. Unfortunately, more recent investigators have published methodologically flawed studies in which measures of adolescent or child adjustment have been inappropriately aggregated across parents' stage of cancer, time since diagnosis, or both. Such aggregation has resulted in biased estimates [39].

Results from the most recent research with adolescents suggest two extreme patterns: adolescents' adjustment may be due to their own developmental challenges, not to their parent's cancer [40]. Alternatively, it may be attributable to parental cancer, including the parent's preoccupation with the illness [41–43]. Even when scores on standardised measures of adjustment do not reach or exceed a clinical level, there is current documentation that adolescents' lives are disrupted and the child must rely on their own ways to manage the cancer's impact [43]. Despite evidence of the seriousness of the ill parent's cancer for the child, there is only one evidence-based, theory-driven intervention that has been scientifically evaluated in a multi-state randomised clinical trial. This intervention, the Enhancing Connections Programme, was designed to be responsive to the evidence above and is described next [44].

19.3 Components of the Programme

The EC Programme evolved from descriptive and hypothesis-testing research conducted by multiple research teams studying the impact of cancer on parents and children: [19, 23, 24, 26, 28, 29, 45–49] (see [50–52] for recent reviews of descriptive research). Even when the level of morbidity in the child did not reach or exceed a clinical level of distress, the dominant pattern in completed studies was for children to be worried or concerned about their

parent's cancer. Children tended to hold back from expressing these worries and concerns and struggled unnecessarily and often alone in making sense out of what was happening to the parent and to their family because of the cancer. Commonly children's models of the parent's cancer were punctuated by frightening or horrific images. Parents concurrently struggled with what to do or say to help their child, even as they themselves were in survival mode and trying to get through the treatment. Parental mood and affect were elevated and often parenting behaviour (skills, quality, confidence) worked against the parent being a nurturing caretaker of their child. There are five components to the EC Programme:

1. five scripted patient educational counselling sessions delivered at two week intervals to the ill parent;

2. a specially designed interactive booklet about cancer to be read by the parent to the child;

3. a workbook that contains didactic text as well as in-session and at-home scripted assignments to be carried out by the ill parent, most of them with the child;

4. the child's 'My Story' booklet for drawing and adding information about the child's interests and ways of dealing with stress;

5. access by phone pager to the patient's counsellor 12 hours each day for contact as needed between the scheduled sessions.

The EC Programme can be delivered in the clinic, over the telephone or in the home setting by specially trained counsellors (clinical psychologists, advanced practice nurses, social workers, certified patient educators, mental health counsellors and chaplains, among other health professionals). Each session lasts approximately 45–60 minutes and is fully manualised. See Table 19.1 for a summary of each intervention session.

The internal structure of each intervention session has four parts: (i) a self-care part; (ii) session-specific didactic material; (iii) one or more skill-building exercises and (iv) presentation and rehearsal of an at-home assignment that the ill parent is to complete with the child between sessions. At the end of each intervention session, the counsellor gives the ill parent a copy of the printed material that was read aloud to the patient during the session. This printed material, along with the in-session and at-home exercises, are put into the ill parent's workbook. In that way, the parent is free to listen to the counsellor during the

Table 19.1	Session descriptions of the enhancing connections programme

Session 1: Anchoring yourself to help your child
This session helps the mother define the child's experience with the breast cancer as distinct from the mother's own experience and add to the mother's ways to manage her cancer-related emotions so that they do not emotionally flood her or her child. This session positions the mother to be a more attentive listener to her child as well as add to the mother's self-care skills.
Rationale: Mothers can attentively listen to their child if they are able to emotionally control their own affect. An overly emotive mother is unable to fully attend to the child's words, maintain healthy interpersonal boundaries, or be emotionally accessible to the child. Overly charged interactions can emotionally flood the child, risking further disconnection.

Session 2: Adding to your listening skills
This session assists the mother develop skills to deeply listen and attend to the child's thoughts and feelings, helping her complement her tendency to be a teacher, not a deep listener, of her child's thoughts, concerns, worries or understandings.
Rationale: In the absence of intervention, mothers proffer biomedical facts about the cancer to their child and tend to disclose highly charged information that is not developmentally appropriate. By focusing on the child's view of the cancer, the ill parent is more informed and able to strategically support the child in ways that are more articulate with the child's views and concerns.

Session 3: Building on your listening skills
This session builds on Session 2 and adds to the mother's abilities to elicit and help the child elaborate the child's concerns or feelings, even with a reticent child. It is one thing to engage a talkative child; it is another to help a child talk who is not forthcoming
Rationale: Session 2 entrains the ill parent to gain listening and attending skills but this session goes further to equip the ill parent with additional skills that enable her to engage and draw out a reticent, withdrawn or upset child.

Session 4: Being a detective of your child's coping
This session helps the mother focus on and non-judgmentally interpret her child's coping behaviour related to the breast cancer. It includes exercises that assist the mother to give away negative assumptions about the child's behaviour related to the parent's cancer. By giving away negative assumptions, the session enables the mother to positively interpret, not negatively evaluate, their child's behaviour. Concurrently the session offers the ill parent ways to elicit their child's report of what the parent can do to support and assist the child cope with the child's cancer-related pressures.
Rationale: Listening and drawing out the child's concerns is one thing; engaging in interpersonal behaviour that the child finds supportive is a different skill. All are important skills that the mother can use to reduce cancer-related distress in the child.

Session 5. Celebrating your success
This session focuses on the gains the ill parent made in prior sessions and what the parent was able to accomplish, in her own words, as a result of her participation in the programme. Both self-monitoring and self-reflection are key elements of efficacy enhancement. The session also assists the ill parent to identify the available resources she can use after programme completion in order to maintain the mother's newly acquired gains from the programme.
Rationale: This final session helps the mother internalise a new view of the self as a skilled and confident parent. Through the ill parent's self-report of her own behaviour and the gains she attributes to her participation in the programme, this self reflective session anchors the mother's new identity as an efficacious parent, not just a mother with new skills.

session, take the material home and re-read it, and is guided through the at-home assignments by the counsellor in advance of the parent's needing to do the assignment with the child. The content of each intervention session relates to the data-based studies that were previously summarised, including the ill parent's expressed difficulties in helping the child with the cancer; the child's most difficult times with the mother's cancer; and ways to interact with the child to diminish the child's worries and concerns and to enhance the child's emotional security.

Bandura's Social Cognitive Theory (SCT) is the theoretical basis for the structure and ways in which the ill parent is assisted by the counsellor to engage in the intervention and materials [53–55]. The theory emphasises the importance of changing behaviour, in this specific case parenting behaviour, through skill- and efficacy-enhancing exercises. The theory posits

that self-efficacy increases by adding to the person's knowledge and behavioural skills. Higher levels of self-efficacy have been linked in prior research with persistence at tasks, even when difficulties occurred, and the initiation of new activities, even when they are difficult or demanding.

In SCT self-efficacy levels are increased through four mechanisms: vicarious experience or modelling (learning from others); performance enactment (learning by doing); persuasion (being convinced by valued others) and minimising emotional arousal (learning without causing additional fear or anxiety). Each intervention session incorporates the three most powerful mechanisms: modelling, performance enactment and minimising emotional arousal. (Persuasion is effective for short-term change, not long-term changes in parenting behaviour.) The scripted exercises in each intervention session include modelling the parenting behaviour

Table 19.2	Outcomes of enhancing connections programme on standardised questionnaires
Outcome variable	**Standardised questionnaire**
Child behavioural-emotional functioning	Total problems (CBCL)***
	Externalising score (CBCL)***
	Internalising score (CBCL)+
	Child depression scale-CDI (total score)+
	Child depression scale-CDI (ineffectiveness)**
Quality of parent-child relationship	Disclosure of negative feelings (FPRQ)+
Maternal mood and anxiety	Center for Epidemiologic Studies-Depression Scale (CES-D)*
	State-Trait Anxiety Inventory (STAI)*
Parenting confidence	Cancer Self-Efficacy (CASE):
	Help child subscale+
	Deal and manage subscale+
Parenting skills	Connecting and coping skills*
	Elicitation skill+

$^+p < 0.10$; $*p < 0.05$; $**p = 0.01$; $***p < 0.009$;

of relevance to that specific session. Each intervention session also includes scripted exercises for the ill parent to engage in, both with the counsellor as well as at-home with her child. The in-session and at-home exercises and assignments are focused on achievable work that enables the ill parent to have a positive outcome and to reflect on these positive accomplishments with the patient counsellor. By focusing on achievable parenting behaviours and by having sessions designed so that the ill mother completes each session successfully, the intervention minimises emotional arousal.

19.4 Evidence for Efficacy

The EC Programme has been evaluated for efficacy in a recently completed six-state randomised clinical trial funded by the National Cancer Institute, National Institutes of Health in the United States.[1] Participating states included (alphabetical): Arizona, California, Indiana, Minnesota, Pennsylvania and Washington. Study participants were recruited from the medical practices of surgeons, radiation oncologists and haematology oncologists as well as through self-referral. Study participants were eligible if they were diagnosed with Stage 0–3 breast cancer within six months, had a school age child between 8 and 12 years of age, were able to read and write English, and lived within 100 miles of each state's study centre. Participants randomised to the control group were mailed a one-time printed mailing of educational

material that was available through the public domain on how to support the child when a mother was diagnosed with breast cancer. The control group also received a one-time phone call by a specially trained Masters educated nurse who used a script to review the key points in the booklet with the mother. In that way, the goal was to help mothers in the control group derive the most benefit from the booklet.

Outcome measures used to evaluate efficacy had extensive prior psychometric testing with comparable populations. Criterion validity (both predictive and concurrent), construct validity and stability and internal consistency reliability are high in study samples of comparable populations [23, 47–49, 56]. Scores on both sub-scales and total scales reached or exceeded internal consistency and stability reliabilities of 0.82; many were 0.90 and higher. Respondent burden was well tolerated and instruments were non-sensitising.

It was hypothesised that mothers and children would show improved functioning at two and 12 months post-baseline compared to controls on all study measures. See Table 19.2 for a summary of outcomes.

Compared to controls, there were significant improvements in mothers' and child's outcomes at both 2 and 12 months post-baseline. More specifically, children randomised to the EC Programme had significantly improved behavioural-emotional functioning (both diminished Total Problems and Externalising scores) compared to controls. Mothers randomised to the intervention group had significantly lower anxiety and depressed mood at two months, compared to controls. There were also statistical tendencies for intervention children to have fewer Internalising problems at two months and for intervention mothers

[1] The principal investigator for the study was Principal Investigators were Patti A. Brandt and Barbara B. Cochrane. Site Co-Investigators were (alphabetical): Marcia Grant, California; Joan A. Haase, Arizona and Indiana; Arlene Houldin, Pennsylvania, and Janice Post-White, Minnesota.

to have improved parenting quality at 2 months, improved parenting skills at 2 and 12 months and increased parenting self-confidence at 2 and 12 months, compared to controls. At one year follow-up, children randomised to intervention also tended to be less depressed (CDI total scale) and have significantly diminished scores on the ineffectiveness subscale of the Child Depression Inventory (CDI), compared to controls.

19.5 Summary of the Training Programme

19.5.1 Training for Delivering the Enhancing Connections Programme

Based on the evidence for efficacy, the study team is now training health care professionals working in diverse practice settings. The training is completed in three days, the goal of which is to enable the health professional to understand the underlying rationale of the programme and to be able to deliver each of the five fully scripted (manualised) intervention sessions at the same dosage and fidelity that were attained in the clinical trial.

Part 1 of the training introduces the intervention model (Figure 19.1) and provides the empirical and theoretical rationale for each component of the intervention. Anchoring the training in the underlying theory enables the trainee to understand the session's rationale but also enables the trainee to know areas that can or cannot be modified in order to translate and disseminate the programme into the trainee's practice setting.

Part 2 of the training engages the trainees in reading through and watching skilled counsellors carry out each of the intervention sessions. This includes the counsellors' efficient use of the printed Patient Educator Manual, including the in-session exercises and at-home assignments. The trainee also observes skilled counsellors engage a 'mock' ill parent in each session's skill-building and efficacy-enhancing exercises.

Part 3 of the training engages each trainee in practising the delivery of each intervention session. Concurrently, a skilled counsellor sits behind the trainee, coaching on the use of the scripts and materials. At the end of each training session, the trainee is invited to ask questions. In addition, other participants in the training concurrently observe the training session and evaluate the dosage and fidelity of the intervention session with a performance checklist of the trainee's behaviour. These performance checklists are the same as those used to evaluate dosage and fidelity in the completed clinical trial.

Training has been completed with diverse health professionals, including, PhD clinical psychologists, PhD nurses, Masters prepared nurse clinicians, Masters educated child life specialists, Masters prepared nurse practitioners and Masters prepared social workers.

19.5.2 Caveats and Comments on the Cancer Parenting Programme

EC is a programme, not individual therapy. Therapy is uniquely responsive to the emerging issues, both manifest and latent, that a client brings into sessions with a therapist. Because it is fully manualised, the EC Programme requires that the counsellor deliver the programme regardless of each ill parent's unique history, prior parenting style and practices, culture or country of origin. The programme is behavioural medicine, much like penicillin is a medication whose efficacy has been tested for a specific type of organism. The EC Programme is not meant to replace individual therapy. It is a focused, targeted programme whose outcomes are to enhance parenting behaviour, skills and confidence and to diminish cancer-related distress in the child and diagnosed mother during the first year of diagnosis and treatment. It can be an adjunct to additional therapy or counselling; it is not a replacement for those services.

19.6 Current and Future Directions

Provider systems and individual professionals are exploring ways to offer this programme through third-party billing, through support from non-profit organisations, and as part of agency-sponsored psychological counselling services for parents with cancer. Third party billing using mental health codes has been successful in using the diagnostic categories of 'adjustment disorder' or 'anxiety disorder'.

Given the evidence for efficacy on mothers' and children's outcomes, the EC Programme has now been expanded and is being tested on parents of either gender with any type of non-metastatic cancer. This expanded programme is called, When Mommy or Daddy Get Cancer: A Cancer Parenting Programme and is being tested as a Phase II clinical trial funded by the Lance Armstrong Foundation.

A new version of the cancer parenting programme has also been developed for diagnosed parents with an adolescent. It is currently being tested in a Phase II clinical trial, funded by the Fred Hutchinson Cancer Research Center. The adolescent-focused programme is called The Connecting Programme. Because parents are sometimes too ill to travel to the clinic to receive the EC Programme, it is also being tested in a Phase II trial as a telephone-delivered intervention. Long-range, pending outcomes from the Phase II trial, a more rigorous clinical trial will be needed to test the efficacy of a telephone-delivered version of the EC Programme.

Ultimately, the goal of the EC Programme and its extensions to parental cancers of all types, its application to adolescents, and its delivery as a clinic-based or telephone-delivered intervention, is to prevent unnecessary distress and suffering in both the ill parent and dependent child. The EC Programme complements medical treatment for cancer with a programme that helps heal the parent–child dyad [57]. Families are enabled to thrive, not merely survive, the cancer.

References

1. Christ, G.H., Siegel, K. and Christ, A.E. (2002) Adolescent grief: "It never really hit me... until it actually happened". *The Journal of the American Medical Association*, **288**, 1269–1278.
2. Christ, G., Siegel, K. and Sperber, D. (1994) Impact of parental terminal cancer on adolescents. *American Journal of Orthopsychiatry*, **64**, 605–613.
3. Siegel, K., Mesagno, F.P., Karus, D. *et al.* (1992) Psychosocial adjustment of children with a terminally ill parent. *Journal of the American Academy of Child and Adolescent Psychiatry*, **31**, 327–333.
4. Lewis, F.M. (2009) Advancing family focused oncology nursing research, in *Advancing Oncology Nursing Science* (eds J.M. Phillips and C.R. King), Oncology Nursing Society Publishing Division, Pittsburgh, PA, pp. 409–434.
5. Lewis, F.M. (2010) The family's "stuck points" in adjusting to cancer, in *Psycho-Oncology*, 2nd edn (ed. J. Holland), Oxford University Press, Oxford, pp. 511–515.
6. Kennedy, V.L. and Lloyd-Williams, M. (2009) How children cope when a parent has advanced cancer. *Psycho-Oncology*, **18**, 886–892.
7. Zahlis, E.H. (2001) The child's worries about the mother's breast cancer: sources of distress in school-age children. *Oncology Nursing Forum*, **28**, 1019–1025.
8. Issel, L.M., Ersek, M. and Lewis, F.M. (1990) How children cope with mother's breast cancer. *Oncology Nursing Forum*, **17**, 5–13.
9. Fann, J.R., Thomas-Rich, A.M., Katon, W.J. *et al.* (2008) Major depression after breast cancer: a review of epidemiology and treatment. *General Hospital Psychiatry*, **30**, 112–126.
10. Fallowfield, L.J., Hall, A., Maguire, G.P. *et al.* (1990) Psychological outcomes of different treatment policies in women with early breast cancer outside a clinical trial. *British Medical Journal*, **301**, 575–580.
11. Goldberg, J.A., Scott, R.N., Davidson, P.M. *et al.* (1992) Psychological morbidity in the first year after breast surgery. *European Journal of Surgical Oncology*, **18**, 327–331.
12. Cummings, E.M. and Davies, P. (1994) Maternal depression and child development. *Journal of Child Psychology and Psychiatry*, **35**, 73–112.
13. Goodman, S.H. and Brumley, H.E. (1990) Schizophrenic and depressed mothers: relational deficits in parenting. *Developmental Psychology*, **26**, 31–39.
14. Orvaschel, H. (1983) Maternal depression and child dysfunction, in *Advances in Child Clinical Psychology*, vol. **6** (eds B.B. Lahey and A.E. Kazdin), Plenum Press, New York, pp. 169–197.
15. Hammen, C., Burge, D. and Stansbury, K. (1990) Relationship of mother and child variables to child outcomes in a high-risk sample: a causal modeling analysis. *Developmental Psychology*, **26**, 24–30.
16. Zahlis, E.H. and Lewis, F.M. (1998) Mothers' stories of the school-age child's experience with the mother's breast cancer. *Journal of Psychosocial Oncology*, **16**, 25–43.
17. Shands, M.E., Lewis, F.M. and Zahlis, E.H. (2000) Mother and child interactions about the mother's breast cancer: an interview study. *Oncology Nursing Forum*, **27**, 77–85.
18. Barnes, J., Kroll, L., Burke, O. *et al.* (2000) Qualitative interview study of communication between parents and children about maternal breast cancer. *British Medical Journal*, **321**, 479–482.
19. Lewis, F.M. and Darby, E.L. (2004) Adolescent adjustment and maternal breast cancer: a test of the "faucet hypothesis". *Journal of Psychosocial Oncology*, **21**, 83–106.
20. Vannatta, K., Ramsey, R.R., Noll, R.B. *et al.* (2010) Associations of child adjustment with parent and family functioning: comparison of families of women with and without breast cancer. *Journal of Developmental and Behavioral Pediatrics*, **31**, 9–16.
21. Maccoby, E.E. and Martin, J.A. (1983) Socialization in the context of the family: parent-child interaction, in *Handbook of Child Psychology*, Socialization, Personality, and Social Development, Vol. **IV** (ed. P.H. Mussen), John Wiley & Sons, Inc., New York, pp. 1–101.
22. Egeland, B., Carlson, E. and Sroufe, L.A. (1993) Resilience as a process. *Development and Psychopathology*, **5**, 517–528.
23. Lewis, F.M., Hammond, M.A. and Woods, N.F. (1993) The family's functioning with newly diagnosed breast cancer in the mother: the development of an explanatory model. *Journal of Behavioral Medicine*, **16**, 351–370.
24. Lewis, F.M. and Hammond, M.A. (1996) The father's, mother's and adolescent's functioning with breast cancer. *Family Relations*, **45**, 1–10.
25. Woods, N.F. and Lewis, F.M. (1995) Women with chronic illness: their views of their families' adaptation. *Health Care for Women International*, **16**, 135–148.
26. Lewis, F.M., Ellison, E.S. and Woods, N.F. (1985) The impact of breast cancer on the family. *Seminars in Oncology Nursing*, **1**, 206–213.
27. Armsden, G.C. and Lewis, F.M. (1993) The child's adaptation to parental medical illness: theory and clinical implications. *Patient Education and Counseling*, **22**, 153–165.
28. Armsden, G.C. and Lewis, F.M. (1994) Behavioral adjustment and self-esteem among school-age children of mothers with breast cancer. *Oncology Nursing Forum*, **21**, 39–45.

29. Wellisch, D.K. (1981) Family relationships of the mastectomy patient: interactions with the spouse and children. *Israel Journal of Medical Science*, **17**, 993–996.

30. Wellisch, D.K., Gritz, E.R., Schain, W. *et al.* (1991) Psychological functioning of daughters of breast cancer patients. Part I: daughters and comparison subjects. *Psychosomatics*, **32**, 324–335.

31. Wellisch, D.K., Gritz, E.R., Schain, W. *et al.* (1992) Psychological functioning of daughters of breast cancer patients. Part II: characterizing the daughter of the breast cancer patient. *Psychosomatics*, **33**, 171–179.

32. Compas, B.E., Worsham, N.L., Epping-Jordan, J.E. *et al.* (1994) When mom or dad has cancer: markers of psychological distress in cancer patients, spouses and children. *Health Psychology*, **13**, 507–515.

33. Compas, B.E., Worsham, N.L., Ey, S. *et al.* (1996) When mom or dad has cancer II: coping, cognitive appraisals, and psychological distress in children of cancer patients. *Health Psychology*, **15**, 167–175.

34. Grant, K.E. and Compas, B.E. (1995) Stress and anxious-depressed symptoms among adolescents: searching for mechanisms of risk. *Journal of Consulting and Clinical Psychology*, **63**, 1015–1021.

35. Welch, A.S., Wadsworth, M.E. and Compas, B.E. (1996) Adjustment of children and adolescents to parental cancer: parents and children's perspectives. *Cancer*, **77**, 1409–1418.

36. Achenbach, T.M. (1991) *Manual for the Youth Self-Report and 1991 Profile*, University of Vermont, Department of Psychiatry, Burlington, VT.

37. Achenbach, T.M. and Edelbrock, C.S. (1978) The classification of child psycho-pathology: a review and analysis of empirical efforts. *Psychological Bulletin*, **85**, 1275–1301.

38. Achenbach, T.M. and Edelbrock, C. (1983) *Manual for the Child Behavior Checklist and Revised Child Behavior Profile*, University of Vermont, Department of Psychology, Burlington, VT.

39. Brown, R.T., Fuemmeler, B., Anderson, D. *et al.* (2007) Adjustment of children and their mothers with breast cancer. *Journal of Pediatric Psychology*, **32**, 297–308.

40. Harris, C.A. and Zakowski, S.G. (2003) Comparisons of distress in adolescents of cancer patients and controls. *Psycho-Oncology*, **12**, 173–182.

41. Sigal, J.J., Perry, J.C., Robbins, J.M. *et al.* (2003) Maternal preoccupation and parenting as predictors of emotional and behavioral problems in children of women with breast cancer. *Journal of Clinical Oncology*, **21**, 1155–1160.

42. Visser, A., Huizinga, G.A. and Hoekstra, J.H. (2005) Emotional and behavioural functioning of children of a parent diagnosed with cancer: a cross-informant perspective. *Psycho-Oncology*, **14**, 746–758.

43. Clemmons, D. (2009) The significance of motherhood for adolescents whose mothers have breast cancer. *Oncology Nursing Forum*, **36** (5), 571–577.

44. Lewis, F.M., Casey, S.M., Brandt, P.A. *et al.* (2006) The Enhancing Connections programme: a pilot evaluation of a cognitive-behavioral intervention for mothers and children affected by breast cancer. *Psycho-Oncology*, **15**, 486–497.

45. Birenbaum, L.K., Yancy, D.Z., Phillips, D.S. *et al.* (1999) School-age children and adolescents' adjustment when a parent has cancer. *Oncology Nursing Forum*, **26**, 1639–1643.

46. Howes, M.J., Hoke, L., Winterbottom, M. *et al.* (1994) Psychosocial effects of breast cancer on the patient's children. *Journal of Psychosocial Oncology*, **12**, 1–21.

47. Lewis, F.M. and Hammond, M.A. (1992) Psychosocial adjustment of the family to breast cancer: a longitudinal analysis. *Journal of the American Medical Women's Association*, **47**, 194–200.

48. Lewis, F.M., Woods, N.F., Hough, E.E. *et al.* (1989) The family's functioning with chronic illness in the mother: the spouse's perspective. *Social Science and Medicine*, **29**, 1261–1269.

49. Watson, M., St. James-Roberts, I., Ashley, S. *et al.* (2006) Factors associated with emotional and behavioral problems among school age children of breast cancer patients. *British Journal of Cancer*, **94**, 43–50.

50. Osborn, T. (2007) The psychosocial impact of parental cancer on children and adolescents: a systematic review. *Psycho-Oncology*, **16**, 101–126.

51. Grabiak, B.R., Bender, C.M. and Puskar, K.R. (2007) The impact of parental cancer on the adolescent: an analysis of the literature. *Psychooncology*, **16**, 127–137.

52. Semple, C.J. and McCance, T. (2010) Parents' experience of cancer who have young children: a literature review. *Cancer Nursing*, **33**, 110–118.

53. Bandura, A. (1997) *Self-efficacy: The Exercise of Control*, W.H. Freeman and Company, New York.

54. Bandura, A. (2001) Social cognitive theory: an agentic perspective. *Annual Review of Psychology*, **52**, 1–26.

55. Bandura, A. (2004) Health promotion by social cognitive means. *Health Education and Health Behavior*, **31**, 143–164.

56. Lewis, F.M., Fletcher, K.A., Cochrane, B.B. *et al.* (2008) Predictors of depressed mood in spouses of women with breast cancer. *Journal of Clinical Oncology*, **26**, 1–7.

57. Lewis, F.M. (2004) Family-focused oncology nursing research: a healing paradigm for future studies. *Oncology Nursing Forum*, **31**, 288–292.

20 Psychosocial Interventions for Elderly Cancer Patients: How Old Would You Be If You Did Not Know How Old You Are?

Lea Baider[1] and Lodovico Balducci[2]

[1]Sharett Institute of Oncology, Hadassah University Hospital, Jerusalem, Israel
[2]H. Lee Moffitt Cancer Center and Research Institute, Tampa, Florida

20.1 Introduction

...If we do not honour our past, we lose our future. If we destroy our roots, we cannot grow old. (F. Hundertwasser, cited from mosaicart-source.wordpress.com)

How do we know old age? How do we know when other people are old? How do we know when we are old ourselves? As we move chronologically through our lives, old age becomes increasingly and inescapably apparent in the physical, functional and psychological changes that take place in our bodies and minds. It is conceived that images of old-age are embedded in the specific historical, social and cultural contexts of each person. As a cultural construct, images of an older person do not simply reflect the facts about how ideally we should look, but project social ideas and beliefs about aging and the place of older people within society.

Stereotypical thinking about aging means that many older people find their relationships with others conditioned by misconceptions as 'all older people get sick', 'all elderly people are isolated and lonely' or 'older people are tired and indifferent to the dynamics of the world'. The norms and values of society erode the perception of the older person as fully human, and the result leads the older person to become gradually isolated from social and intellectual interactions with those who are seen as normally competent [1].

20.2 Cancer in the Elderly: Clinical Evaluation

Cancer is mostly a disease of aging. In the US, 50% of all neoplasms already occur in 12% of the population, that is over 65. By the year 2030, individuals over 65 are expected to account for 20% of the population and 70% of all cancer patients. Cancer has also become the first cause of death for Americans up to the age of 85 [2]. Cancer in older people is rapidly becoming a global, multifaceted problem involving biological, social and economic issues.

The health and the support of the elderly patient have gained prominence due to a combination of three factors that include:

- Increased prevalence of cancer in older people due to the aging of the population, the increased incidence of cancer in the elderly and the more prolonged survival of cancer patients, including the oldest ones [2]. The malignancies that are most prevalent after age 70 include cancers of the breast, prostate, large bowel, lung and oesophagus, brain tumours, myelodysplasia, acute leukaemias and lymphomas.

- Disabling consequences of cancer and its treatment. Even in a highly selected series of cancer patients 70 and older, the prevalence of dependence in Instrumental Activities of Daily Living (IADL) was as high as 70% and the prevalence

Handbook of Psychotherapy in Cancer Care, First Edition. Edited by Maggie Watson and David W. Kissane.
© 2011 John Wiley & Sons, Inc. Published 2011 by John Wiley & Sons, Inc.

of potentially disabling comorbidity as high as 90% [3–5]. Common disabling manifestations of cancer include bone metastases that may cause severe pain, anaemia, that is associated with fatigue and in extreme cases congestive heart failure and coronary ischaemia, sarcopenia associated with decreased survival, functional dependence, frailty and increased risk of therapeutic complications. Disabling manifestations of cancer treatment include deconditioning following surgery and radiation therapy, neutropenia and neutropenic infections that may include prolonged hospitalisations and occasionally cause the patient's demise, anaemia and mucositis which may compromise the patient's nutrition and lead to sarcopenia [6].

- Reduction in the pool of potential caregivers, due to the disappearance of the extended family and entrance into the work force of women who used to be the traditional caregivers of the elderly [7].

This characteristic introduces the construct of frailty, that is extremely important for its clinical consequences and the delivery of any psychological intervention. The frail person is one whose disability may be precipitated even by minimal stress [8].

The Comprehensive Geriatric Assessment (CGA) focuses on the following parameters:

- function;
- comorbidity;
- geriatric syndromes;
- living conditions;
- polypharmacy;
- nutrition;
- emotional screening; and
- cognitive screening.

At present, the CGA represents the best validated and most clinically useful assessment of physiological age [9].

20.3 Quandaries and Reliability of Interventions

We move beyond the question of whether psychological intervention is possible with elderly cancer patients to a consideration of whether the intervention process needs to be adapted for the aged. Gerontologists have explored and substantiated the possible changes that need to be made for any psychological intervention to maximise success with the very vulnerable population of elderly cancer patients [10]. Adaptations due to illness and age would need to respond to change in the social, cultural and familial context of the elderly.

Interventions for elderly cancer patients have tended to become more oriented towards understanding the person as s/he is now, towards setting and achieving relatively short-term and specific goals and towards including an understanding of the social-cultural-familial context within which the individual is embedded.

Age is not specifically evaluated in most reviews of psycho-oncology interventions for adults. The fact that older patients report lower levels of distress is often interpreted as their having less need or urgency for learning new skills, communication and support. This may potentially mask the underlying problems that older patients experience during their long illness trajectory (for specific reviews, see [11–14]).

Studies that directly compare psychological interventions with psychotropic medications found psychological interventions to be equally effective or more effective based on client self-reported questionnaires [15, 16].

Pinquart and Sörenson [17] explored aspects of interventions that led to higher effect sizes in studies of psychological interventions with older adults. They found greater reduction of depression and greater improvement of life satisfaction in: (i) psychoeducational interventions, (ii) interventions that targeted people who were depressed before treatment rather than those that targeted a presumably 'at-risk' group, (iii) tailored therapy protocols (nine sessions) and (iv) therapies delivered by qualified therapists on geriatric care.

However, most research interventions on older people are still guided by the physical symptomatology (co-morbidity) and/or focus on depression. The scarce evidence-based, psychological intervention studies [18–21] for older cancer patients have shown conspicuously the psychological need, which challenges our field to provide this unmet need.

20.4 Psychosocial Theories on Ageing: Basis for Interventions

20.4.1 Life Strengths

Clinicians as well as researchers dealing with aging have turned to the handful of theoretical models of being old. In particular, the writings of Erikson [22] formulated a stage theory of development in terms of successive psychological tasks to be carried out through the life span culminating in old age.

Table 20.1	Targets to improve perceived self-efficacy in cancer patients: psychoeducational therapy	
	Impact of diagnosis, treatment and disease progression on many patients	**Improvements associated with increased self-efficacy**
Cognition	Helplessness, despair	Ability to exert some control, 'fight back'
Affect	Dysphoric mood: anxiety and depression	Improved mood: less anxiety and depression
Physical	Uncontrollable symptoms: pain, fatigue, nausea	Some control over physical symptoms
Behaviour	Withdrawal from activities: work, social	Improved interactions with others

Kivnick [23] developed a method for assessing what she described as 'life strengths' in elderly clients in long-term care, based on updated versions of Erikson's eight concepts. Kivnick argued that if care providers consider people's functional needs together with their abilities, they are less likely to exaggerate their disabilities and miss chances of enhancing the quality of their lives.

Based on Erikson's theoretical model of psychosocial developmental life stages, Holland and colleagues [21] developed an evidence-based psychoeducational intervention with elderly cancer patients. Two groups of elderly patients were given different instructions for the intervention. In the first group, readings from authors such as Erikson and Vaillant were included as a trigger for the exploration of the patients' personal stories of illness. The second group was more structured, with discussions of very specific subjects during seven sessions:

- coping with cancer and aging;
- facing the unknowns of cancer and aging;
- loneliness and the stigma of cancer and aging;
- making peace with one's life: who am I?
- wisdom and the keepers of meaning.

20.4.2 Self-Efficacy Theory

Bandura's [24] self-efficacy model demonstrated the importance of self-referent thought in psychosocial functioning, that is, the patient's appraisal of his/her ability to cope with a specific situation. Perceived self-efficacy, as a construct for elderly patients, may prove to be a powerful predictor of adjustment to specific stressful events such as the sequelae of cancer.

Based on Bandura's self-efficacy model, Cunningham and colleagues [25] developed and tested a psychoeducational programme comprising seven weekly, 2-hour sessions. This programme was specifically designed to enhance the cancer patients' sense of control over emotional states. It taught standard coping skills, relaxation, positive mental imagery, stress control, cognitive restructuring, goal setting and discussed general issues of life style change. A workbook and two audiotapes were issued to all participants, home practice being strongly advocated. The authors concluded that the intervention improved quality of life in most elderly cancer patients (Table 20.1).

20.4.3 Chronic Disease Self-Management Programme (CDSMP)

Farrell and colleagues [26] examined to see if participation in a chronic disease self-management programme (CDSMP) improved self-efficacy, health and self-management behaviours in an underserved, older population. The CDSMP teaching process was based on Bandura's self-efficacy theory (see also [27]) and includes strategies that encourage the development of a personal exercise programme and the enhancement of cognitive symptom management, problem solving and communication skills. Examples of activities in this programme include: inviting a 'significant' person (family or friend) to join the participant in listening to his/her favourite song, inviting a grandchild to join in searching for old family photos and visiting places with significant others that are connected to the past. Farrell and colleagues identified (i) meaning, (ii) health consequences associated with traditional dietary practices and (iii) communication with health care providers. These topics were incorporated into the weekly brainstorming and problem-solving activities for the older participants (Table 20.2).

20.4.4 Coping and Communication Support Intervention

Rose and colleagues [20] describe the development of a coping and communication support (CCS)

Table 20.2	Instruments, number of Items and types of scales to address variables [22]		
Research question	**Variables**	**Items**	**Type of scale**
1. What change in self-efficacy occurred?	Self-efficacy scale, scored as how confident they were to manage fatigue, discomfort/pain, emotional distress	6	Likert
	Self-efficacy health scale – degree participants believed that they could influence or change their health	1	Likert
2. What change in self-management behaviours occurred?	Physical activities scale – exercises, walking, bicycling, swimming	5	Single number
	Cognitive symptoms – progressive muscle relaxation, imagery, meaning	6	Likert
	Communication with health provider, asked questions, discussed problems	3	Likert

intervention for advanced cancer patients. The CCS intervention is implemented with newly diagnosed late-stage cancer patients who are middle-aged and older. It is tailored to patients' needs and preferences and designed to support them over the period of time when life goals and care goals are expected to shift. Based on a model of successful aging over the lifespan [28], the intervention offers patients coping skills, communication and support and recognises the importance of health information processing style in cancer communication.

20.4.4.1 Initial Care Conference
An initial care conference establishes a connection between the patient and family member/s and the Coping and Communication Support Programme (CCSP) to set the stage for telephone follow-up.

20.4.4.2 CCS Follow-Up Phone Contacts
The schedule for telephone contacts is flexible and tailored to patient preference. Telephone contacts offer opportunities to: (i) explore the physical, emotional, functional and social impact of advanced cancer and its treatment; (ii) prepare patients psychologically for future therapy or progression of disease; (iii) identify personal goals and goals of treatment; (iv) identify further needs for information/support; (v) enhance expression of affect; (vi) support hope and appropriate psychological defence; (vii) foster independence; (viii) facilitate coping; (ix) optimise social support; (x) address practical problems; and (xi) refer patients for symptom management, informational needs and support.

Preliminary data on middle-aged and older patients indicate that older patients voice similar preferences for engagement in the intervention.

20.5 Elderly Cancer Patient Interventions

20.5.1 Narratives – Reminiscence – Life Review

20.5.1.1 Reminiscence
Reminiscence – the processing of remembering prior life events – serves a specific function for elders' need to look back on their lives and derive a sense of accomplishment and meaning. 'Did my life make a difference? Did it mean anything?' Life review as a universal event in the lives of aging people is prompted by the awareness of illness and the proximity of death [29]. Elders may find their memories a source of great joy at a time when their social support networks are dwindling or they are confronted with cancer.

Reminiscence group intervention is designed to help elderly cancer patients retrieve positive events and feelings through the process of reminiscing. Although it does not focus on helping elders resolve lifelong conflicts, therapists cannot dismiss negative memories. Grief, loss and other painful experiences need to be acknowledged as part of the tapestry of the patient's subjective recounting of the past – 'I am now what my memory recalls me being.' This intervention is specifically geared to guiding elders to remember events that reinforce the belief that they are worthwhile and valued as persons. The group adds an important dimension to the use of reminiscence. What has been of significant subjective importance to any individual can be confirmed by a more collectively objective valuation.

Mosher-Ashley and Barrett [30] described this process as remembering 'victories over life challenges'. When elders are faced with stressful life events – such as learning about chronic health problems or painful isolation – they tend to focus on the past or future.

Zinn [31] approached reminiscence as a chronological process in which the therapist meets with the elderly patient for 10 sessions. Subjects are devoted to each of the major developmental stages to improve self-esteem, to help the elder identify the major accomplishments of those life stages and coping strengths. In that way, the elderly patients may recall how they handled difficult times during specific times in their lives. The goal is to generate and recount positive family memories from these times in their lives. The topics selected are determined by the goals of the reminiscence intervention for the specific elderly needs.

20.5.1.2 Narratives: Stories to Tell

What is a story? What do I mean when I use the concept of narrative or story? A story enables people to link together the events they experience, using the ways of viewing things, or their personal constructs, to do so. This linking occurs over time. Integration is therefore a defining characteristic of stories, or narratives, but it can vary from being tight and inflexible to loose and easily changed over time [32].

It is particularly important to the elderly to hear, and of course tell, stories about people like themselves. They have a special need to maintain their identities, despite their illness, in the face of less and less confirmation for them. Patient narratives maintain stability and connection, emphasise shared meanings and facilitate emotional communication in and outside families over fears of abandonment and death.

Illness narratives are life-review stories that families tell about their experiences with serious and persistent illness. These primarily oral narratives help promote continuity and mastery over the challenges of disease by facilitating coping, adaptation, meaning, attribution and coherence. The dominant themes of any narrative are largely determined by the temporal and relational contexts, and the social-cultural framework, within which stories are created and shared. Illness narratives have a significant impact on family members' responses, myths and worldviews about health, illness and medicine [33].

For most individuals, serious illness provokes what narrative sociologists term a biographical disruption or the interruption of a future-oriented trajectory, that is based implicitly on presumptions of health [34]. The illness may be perceived by older patients as a direct invasion into their sense of time and space, plans, decisions and commitments. With each new symptomatology, anger and disappointment become part of the daily uncertainties. Therapists should guide patients to accept the illness as a reality and to rediscover how to maintain a sense of emotional control through the use of humour, reframing, revising and reorganising priorities.

20.5.1.3 Life Review

'How did I become an old person?' The focus of life review is primarily on the creative development of self-concept, perceived here as our ideas about who we are, who we have been and who we will be [35]. Life review most commonly arises in therapy when working with grieving patients who must construct a new view of themselves that extends past the illness and when 'new' emotions must be integrated into the self. Some physical traumas that result in chronic illness and disability require a new view of the self as a person lacking abilities that had previously been taken for granted [36].

Domains of the patient's life experience:

- Family of origin, including patient's birthplace, immigration and acculturation experiences, narrative of parents' and significant others' lives.
- Patient's perception of social, work and professional identity.
- Children and other aspects of family life in adulthood.
- Work history and patient's evaluation of it.
- Patient's sense of ethnicity, gender and social class as influences on life.
- Body image and important changes in body since illness.
- Religious and spiritual history or life view – systems of belief.
- Experiences of past and present illnesses – loss and transition.
- Experiences of death as a trajectory of grief – adaptation.
- How much time is left? What things are left to accomplish?

The Life Review and Experience Form (LREF), developed by Burnside and Haight [37], offers a protocol covering areas such as death, grief, fear, religion, school, hardships, sex, work, and relationships over the life span, losses, achievements and intimacy.

Life review process:

- What kind of life they had?
- What would they leave the same?
- What are their satisfactions and disappointments?
- What are they most proud of?
- How have significant life events affected their lives?
- How can negative events be balanced against more positive events in their lives?

Life reviews are never completed, despite the fact that they can be objectively finished. In fact, when time is known to be limited by life-threatening illness, or when frailty is predictable in the near future due to progressive illness, planning for the remainder of life typically takes on greater urgency. Deciding what issues need to be completed and what unfinished business in life and relationships should be finished is of greater urgency when the time is known to be limited. In this sense, planning for the future requires more therapeutic energy for terminal cancer patients than for other elderly patients where denial becomes the search for hope and cure.

20.6 Forgiveness: Life – Illness – Death

Forgiveness is centred in a subjective sense of morality, which in its simplest form is concerned with the quest for the good. When people seek the good, they do so in relation to others [38].

20.6.1 Phase Model of Forgiveness

Enright and the Human Development Study Group on Forgiveness [39] developed a model of forgiveness that could be significantly integrated as an intervention model for the older cancer population. The phase model of forgiveness describes four phases (see Figure 20.1) that form a developmental progression:

1. Uncovering phase: The person's insight about whether the injustice and subsequent injury have compromised his/her life.

2. Decision phase: A decision to forgive is a cognitive process, not one in which forgiveness is completed.

3. Work phase: The one forgiving may begin to experience some self-compassion.

4. Deepening phase: Insights often stimulate other thoughts: Have I needed others' forgiveness in the past? What was it like for me when I was forgiven? Am I motivated to interact in new ways?

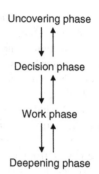

Figure 20.1 *Developmental nature of the phases.*

20.6.2 Forgiveness Tailored to Interventions (see Table 20.3)

Early clinical case studies and a growing body of more recent evidence-based research interventions suggest that, although the amelioration of psychological symptoms in elderly cancer patients is a complex and difficult challenge, the use of forgiveness therapy may be particularly helpful in promoting emotional health, enhancing a sense of self-awareness and addressing their deep emotional pain and compassion [40]. Forgiveness interventions are integral to emotion constructs, such as feelings of loss, loneliness, anger and fear.

20.6.3 Model of Forgiveness Applied to Cancer

In one of the most recent interventions with elderly terminally-ill cancer patients, Hansen *et al.* [41] describes the model of forgiveness applied to cancer. The authors tested the effectiveness of a four-week forgiveness therapy programme in improving the quality of life of elderly terminally-ill cancer patients.

Table 20.3	Intervention process of forgiveness

Session	Topics
1	Introduction to forgiveness; possible psychological defences
2	Exploration of issues leading to one's own anger, frustration
3	Acknowledging that one has been hurt
4	Commitment to forgive oneself, other
5	Reframing, empathy, compassion
6	Spirituality, meaning
7	Accepting pain, growth due to the event
8	Focusing on one's own changes caused by the event

Adapted from Ref. [34].

Referral was self-selective, with staff inviting older, physically-able patients to participate. Participants were randomly assigned to a forgiveness therapy group or to a wait-listed control group, which received forgiveness therapy in the second four-week period. They were asked to describe a perceived injustice, provide demographic information (age, gender, marital status and family members), indicate their medical diagnosis and identify one instance of being subjected to what they perceived to be a deep hurt and injustice. The intervention was created to recognise and respect the specific needs of older adults at the end of life. The group facilitator followed a structure for each of the four sessions: summarise the previous session, introduce new principles with unit material, discuss the principles of the unit, discuss the participants' reflections of their personal stories and responses to the principles, present handouts summarising the principal points of the unit, and provide topics to reflect upon between sessions.

Hansen and colleagues [41] reported that, as people forgive, their anger decreases, allowing for improved psychological well-being and improved relationships. One of the key therapist interventions is helping the patient confront anger and helplessness through a process of emotional forgiveness. The findings here are consonant with the goals of palliative care professionals, in that the intervention enhanced emotional health in the face of physical decline. Despite the paucity of formal data and evidence-based outcomes for this intervention, the authors strongly suggested that patients who forgive benefit from a concomitant decrease in anger, depression, anxiety and related symptoms.

Enright [38] and Hansen *et al.* [41] encourage patients to 'reinterpret' past and present events through emotional reframing. This allows therapists to reflect on the patients' ways of feeling and perceiving the significant people around them. This intervention includes some teaching and learning. Patients have a chance to reflect on the meaning of forgiveness, who or what hurt them, the depth of anger and how this alters with time, perceptions of change and other aspects of the forgiveness process (Table 20.3).

20.7 Cognitive-Behavioural Therapy

Through a process of relearning, people can change both their emotional responses to events and situations and the behaviour that follows. Elders need to first learn which situations in the process of illness trigger painful thoughts and emotions that are difficult to control.

Cognitive-behavioural therapy (CBT), which was adapted for use with elders by McInnis-Dittrich [42], is based on the assumption that both cognitive and behavioural responses to events are learned. CBT can be done individually or in groups. Groups should be limited to 8–12 participants particularly with older patients. The purpose should be clearly stated, and particular comorbidities not suitable for the group should be defined. Since candidates for group participation are not targets for research, selection can be through medical and social agency referrals or advertisements by oncology and geriatric departments.

The process of CBT involves the following distinct phases:

1. Preparation: Present clear ideas about the result of participating in the group process:

   a. How situations, thoughts, feelings and behaviour are connected.
   b. What we want to be different in our lives.

2. Collaboration-identification: This process is intended to empower the elderly patient to regain control over life as a part of enhancing quality of life:

   a. Explore situations in which the elder is aware of being depressed or anxious.
   b. See how certain situations and events are followed by particular feelings. What did the event mean to me?
   c. Connect situations or events, the cognitive response or thought, and the subsequent feelings.
   d. Help elders to identify those once pleasurable activities and to commit time to resuming them.

3. **Change phase**:

   a. Identify and correct cognitive distortions. What is dysfunctional about the way I am thinking (e.g. mind reading, self-blaming, unrealistic demands on others, unrealistic expectations of self and exaggerated self-importance)?
   b. What can I do to make myself feel better?' Take positive steps to empower myself to regain mastery over the environment (Figure 20.2).

Cognitive-behavioural intervention offers elderly people opportunities to examine the connections between what they think and how those thoughts affect subsequent feelings and behaviours [42]. The sense of self-awareness that develops as they

1. Please rate your mood using the 9-point scale shown below. If you felt good, put a higher number on the chart below. If you felt 'so-so,' mark a 5. And if you felt low or depressed, mark a lower number.

1	2	3	4	5	6	7	8	9
Very depressed				'So-so'				Very happy

2. Please briefly give reasons that have an influence on your feelings

Time of day	Mood score	Reasons why I felt this way

3. What do you think could help change your negative feelings?

4. Whom do you think could help you?

Figure 20.2 *Mood and feelings form.*

participate in CBT is intended to be carried over beyond the therapeutic relationship so that if troubling thoughts develop in future situations, they have learned how to identify the source of those thoughts and feelings and to develop corrective actions on their own.

Rather than attempt to orient elderly people with dementia to time and space, validation therapy respects and uses their confused reality, not the caregiver's, to understand what they are trying to communicate [43, 44].

Cognitive impairment (CI) in the general population is broadly classified as reversible or non-reversible. The major cause of reversible CI in hospitalised patients is delirium [45]. For cancer patients, an additional classification would include: CI directly attributable to the location or treatment of brain tumours or metastases, CI secondary to depression and fatigue independent of tumour location [46], premorbid characteristics of patients at risk for developing specific tumours (e.g. elevated rates of alcoholism (and consequent CI) among head and neck tumour patients [47], patients presenting with paraneoplastic syndrome (most frequently seen in lung

cancer) and finally, CI subsequent to chemotherapy [48] or whole-brain radiation.

When possible, underlying causes of CI are treated (e.g. malnutrition, fatigue, polymedication). Higher-functioning individuals frequently search for memory groups or computerised 'cognitive gyms' to improve their functioning, but little is known about the efficacy of these approaches in elderly cancer patients.

20.8 Life and Hope: Transforming Fear into Hope

A grounded theory to uncovering the processes by which older palliative care patients maintain their hope may lead to the development of strategies for fostering hope in this population. By increasing hope, we may be able to contribute to patients' quality of life, which is a goal of end-of-life care [49, 50]. In order to live with hope, the participants described the basic social process of transforming and creating new hope. Hope is dynamic: 'well, it changes, that's for sure'. The participants had made a conscious decision to change or transform their fears into hope: 'What you can do is you can make life in your mind or your behaviour that can make it easier in your life [49, p. 37].'

Duggleby and Wright [51] describe acceptance as an aspect of reconciliation of life and death. This acknowledgement does not preclude the use of denial as a protective mechanism. Denial as a coping response may act as a self-protection mechanism for palliative care patients, enabling them to defend themselves from threats and therefore enhancing their perception of control and self-efficacy. Hope is situational, so denial could be used as a coping mechanism by compartmentalising one aspect of the participants' lives and acknowledging 'life the way it is' in other aspects. The two concepts are not mutually exclusive.

20.9 Selected Therapies: Intervention Techniques with Groups of Elderly Cancer Patients

1. Card games – meaning of their choice (e.g. myths, habitat, relationships).

2. Music group – remembrance, meaning and hope, CD/type selected by each member.

3. Reminiscence and meaning – personal photos in developmental time, place, relationships.

4. Important people – meaning of relationship – when? – why? – mutuality.

Most of the exercises above work best with small groups and can be quite useful with the patients' families. Each intervention theme offers a supportive backdrop against which to practice adaptation and new coping styles, to learn to distinguish between function and dysfunction and to reflect on aspects of life as a challenge and hope (for complete therapy protocols, write to Lea Baider).

20.10 Case Examples

20.10.1 Card Game Intervention

Habitat: It is the last of the three card-game group sessions, with nine elderly participants with different cancer diagnoses and stages of the illness.

Ilana is 77 years old, mother of three, with terminal pancreatic cancer – liver and colon metastasis. She chose her card, which was totally blank. In a very low tone of voice, as if she were in an internal monologue instead of interacting with the group, Ilana said:

'I am going there...the numbness of life...no breath, no colours, no smells. It is the nothingness...

At home, at nights, I wander around looking at the white ceiling, wanting to penetrate into the nothingness of the walls. It is not fear...it is what I do not know...'

PARTICIPANT: *But you are now here, alive. Why don't you choose the colourful cards that are full with people and nature instead of deathly blank ones?...*
ILANA: *Because I know that I am dying, and I need to feel and see my death...*
PARTICIPANT: *What about feeling that you are alive and talk to us?...*
ILANA: *I am afraid of feeling alive...and this card reflects exactly how I really feel...totally blank...The card is me...a reflection of my mind and my body...*

The group interaction allowed Ilana to talk about her psychological pain and isolation and gave the therapist the opportunity to extrapolate to all the group members' subjective experiences of hopelessness and loss. Ilana's reflection on the card she chose may be perceived by the group as a threat to their own frail vulnerability. The therapist bridged the gap between Ilana's fears and anxieties of death and her capacity for joyful life events and meaningful encounters with family and friends. The dynamic process should be the acceptance of how to live simultaneously with dualities and contradictory emotions.

20.10.2 Music Group

The music group is a five-session therapy intervention comprising 10–14 patients with different cancer diagnoses and stages of the illness. Each participant brings a CD or tape with music that was very significant at a particular period in their life.

Daniel is an 82-year-old widower and first-generation Holocaust survivor of the Dachau concentration camp. He has metastasised colon cancer. He brought a tape of two old Yiddish wedding songs. During the music time, Daniel is in the centre of the room and swaying along with the music as most of the other participants sing along. Two others join him in the dance.

DANIEL: *This is the dance I danced at my wedding, on the boat coming to Israel as a refugee; and it is also the melody I danced to at my granddaughter's wedding – with the drain bag attached to my body. I was so happy and so grateful to God to be alive...I danced and danced, and all the memories of my life*

*were with me. When I become sad, I play this music
and I dance, and I cry, and I laugh...but I dance...*
PARTICIPANTS: *Daniel, the next time, you should
invite all of us, and we will dance with you.*

Several participants acknowledged that they had the
same kind of music at their wedding and also at their
children's and grandchildren's weddings, and that they
would like to learn from Daniel how to dance...

Participants shared their stories of the music and
moments in their lives...

(The dialogues from these two clinical vignettes
were translated from Hebrew. The first author was the
therapist.)

20.11 Overview of Evidence for Therapeutic Benefit

Meta-analyses on interventions for the elderly population were briefly cited above along with several
qualitative therapies for elderly cancer patients. A more
recent study quantifies the feasibility of a 'dignity'
therapy using a randomised and control design [52].
Unfortunately, the methodologies of most of the interventions cited above were poorly designed, not randomised and lacked any control group, making the
interpretation of the outcomes unreliable and hard to
generalise from. There is a need for well-designed
studies concerning elderly cancer patients, their informal elderly caregivers and families and the role of the
medical staff and mental health professionals. Herein
lies an opportunity for professional reflection, research
and pursuit of available resources syntonic to elderly
patients' physical and psychological needs in order to
enhance the quality of their life [53].

The first author's personal view is not to focus
rigidly on one particular screening instrument for
elderly patients and informal caregivers, but rather
to begin with a basic interpersonal interview in
order to interact freely and empathically with the
patient – listening, asking and responding. The goal
is to identify undetected distress symptoms and unmet
needs of elderly patients and to give voice to the
silent experience of their life, illness and pending
death [54–56].

20.12 Conclusion

> *...In the depth of winter, I finally learned that within
> me there lay an invincible summer...* Albert Camus,
> *Return to Tipasa* (1952), as translated in *Lyrical and
> Critical Essays* (1968), p. 169.

Cancer in the elderly has become a health priority
worldwide and health authorities are increasingly providing information to the aging population concerning
cancer epidemiology, medical treatment options and
psychosocial resources. The ability to successfully
negotiate cross-cultural issues in the clinical setting
and to develop improved therapeutic services for
elderly cancer patients plays an important role in
today's practice of oncology. Such ability is based
on the therapist's level of competence and sensitivity
to the role that culture plays in the patient-doctor
relationship as well as the acquisition of specific skills
and attitudes [57].

Any study of elderly people with cancer requires
an integrative evaluation of aging containing physiological, psychological and behavioural variables [58].
The literature already presents a variety of venues to
identify this particular population at risk [54]. Much
of the psychosocial risk reflects not only their physical
restrictions but issues such as loneliness, dependency,
loss, sense of unfulfillment, guilt and shame related to
their unspoken emotions and the vulnerability brought
on by illness and aging.

Our message clearly reflects the need for broader
evidence-based studies that embrace wide-scope
predictors, theoretical constructs, standardised-
control-randomised designs and objective outcomes.
Notwithstanding this unmet need, we are aware of
the limitations of the interventions described above,
particularly in the mostly unchartered areas of family
dynamics, loneliness of the elderly patient and informal caregiver interventions – given the pivotal role
of the caregiver in the management of cancer in the
older aged person [59].

Identifying interventions with reliable evidence and
empirical data may facilitate the delivery of more tailored interventions, ameliorating the unpredictability of
illness and guided by the enhancement of the patient's
sense of self-value, meaning from the past and hope
for their life in the present.

References

1. Vaillant, G. (2002) *Aging Well*, Little Brown, New York.
2. Jemal, A., Thun, M.J., Ries, L.A. *et al.* (2008) Annual report
   to the nation on the status of cancer, 1975–2005, featuring
   trends in lung cancer, tobacco use, and tobacco control. *Journal of the National Cancer Institute*, **100** (23), 1672–1694.
3. (a) Ingram, S.S., Seo, P.H., Martell, R.E. *et al.* (2002)
   Comprehensive assessment of elderly cancer patients: the
   feasibility of self-report methodology. *Journal of Clinical
   Oncology*, **c20**, 770–775 ; (b) Balducci, L. and Beghe, C.
   (2002) Management of cancer in the older person. *Clinical
   Geriatrics*, **10**, 54–60.

4. Baxter, N.N., Durham, S.B., Phillips, K.A. *et al.* (2009) Risk of dementia in older breast cancer survivors: a population-based cohort study of the association with adjuvant chemotherapy. *Journal of the American Geriatrics Society*, **57** (3), 403–401.

5. Said, M.W. and Lichtman, S.M. (2009) Chemotherapy options and outcomes in older patients with colorectal cancer. *Critical Reviews in Oncology/Hematology*, **72**, 155–169.

6. Balducci, L. (2009) Pharmacology of antineoplastic medications in older cancer patients. *Oncology*, **23**, 78–85.

7. Wolff, J.L. and Kasper, J.D. (2006) Caregiver of frail elderly. Updating a national profile. *Gerontologist*, **46** (3), 344–356.

8. Walston, J., Hadley, E.C. and Ferrucci, L. (2006) Research agenda for frailty in older adults. *Journal of the American Geriatrics Society*, **54**, 991–1001.

9. Extermann, M. and Hurria, A. (2007) Comprehensive geriatric assessment for older patients with cancer. *Journal of Clinical Oncology*, **25**, 1824–1831.

10. Balducci, L., Cohen, H.J., Engstrom, P.F. *et al.* (2005) Senior adult oncology clinical practice guidelines in oncology. *Journal of the National Comprehensive Cancer Network*, **3** (4), 572–590.

11. Spoletini, I., Gianni, W., Repetto, L. *et al.* (2008) Depression and cancer: an unexplored and unresolved emergent issue in elderly patients. *Critical Reviews in Oncology/Hematology*, **65**, 143–155.

12. Weinberger, M.I., Roth, A.J. and Nelson, C.J. (2009) Untangling the complexities of depression diagnosis in older cancer patients. *The Oncologist*, **14**, 60–66.

13. Nelson, C.J., Weinberger, M.I., Balk, E. *et al.* (2009) The chronology of distress, anxiety and depression in older prostate cancer patients. *The Oncologist*, **14**, 891–899.

14. Chustecka, Z. (2009) Depression in older cancer patients. *Journal of General Internal Medicine*, **24** (Supp. 2), 417–424.

15. Balducci, L. and Beghe, C. (2002) Management of cancer in the older person. *Clinical Geriatrics*, **10**, 54–60.

16. Osborn, R.L., Demoncada, A.C. and Feuerstein, M. (2006) Psychosocial interventions for depression, anxiety, and quality of life in cancer survivors: meta-analyses. *International Journal of Psychiatry in Medicine*, **36**, 13–34.

17. Pinquart, M. and Sörenson, S. (2001) How effective are psychotherapeutic interventions with older adults? A meta-analysis. *Journal of Mental Health and Aging*, **7**, 207–240.

18. Query, J.L. and Wright, K. (2003) Assessing communication competence in an online study: toward informing subsequent interventions among older adults with cancer. *Health Communication*, **15**, 203–218.

19. Lapid, M.I., Rummans, T.A., Brown, P.D. *et al.* (2007) Improving the quality of life of geriatric cancer patients with a structured multidisciplinary intervention: a randomized controlled trial. *Palliative and Supportive Care*, **5**, 107–114.

20. Rose, J.H., Radziewicz, R., Bowman, K.F. *et al.* (2008) A coping and communication support intervention tailored to older patients diagnosed with late-stage cancer. *Clinical Intervention in Aging*, **3**, 77–95.

21. Holland, J., Poppito, S., Nelson, C. *et al.* (2009) Reappraisal in the eighth cycle stage: a theoretical psychoeducational intervention in elderly patients with cancer. *Palliative and Supportive Care*, **7**, 271–279.

22. Erikson, E.H. (1982) *The Life Cycle Completed*, Norton, New York.

23. Kivnick, H.G. (1993) Everyday mental health: a guide to assessing life strengths. *Generations*, **17** (1), 13–20.

24. Bandura, A. (1977) Self-efficacy: toward a unifying theory of behavioral change. *Psychological Review*, **84**, 191–215.

25. Cunningham, A.J., Lockwood, G.A. and Cunningham, J.A. (1991) A relationship between perceived self-efficacy and quality of life in cancer patients. *Patient Education and Counseling*, **17**, 71–78.

26. Farrell, K., Wicks, M.N. and Martin, J.C. (2004) Chronic disease self-management improved with enhanced self-efficacy. *Clinical Nursing Research*, **13**, 289–308.

27. Loring, K.R., Sobel, D., Ritter, P. *et al.* (2001) Effects of a self-management program on patients with chronic disease. *Effective Clinical Practice*, **4**, 256–262.

28. Baltes, P.B. (1997) On the incomplete architecture of human ontogeny: selection, optimization and compensation as foundation of developmental theory. *American Psychology*, **52**, 366–380.

29. Butler, R.N., Lewis, M.I. and Sunderland, T. (1998) *Aging and Mental Health: Positive Psychological and Biomedical Approaches*, Allyn and Bacon, Boston.

30. Mosher-Ashley, P.M. and Barrett, P.W. (1997) *A Life Worth Living: Practical Strategies for Reducing Depression in Older Adults*, U.S. Health Professions Press, Baltimore.

31. Zinn, J.O. (2005) The biographical approach: a better way to understand behavior in health and illness. *Health, Risk and Society*, **71**, 1–9.

32. Pinnegar, S. and Daynes, G. (2007) Locating narrative inquiry historically: thematic in the turn to narrative, in *Handbook of Narrative Inquiry: Mapping A Methodology* (ed. D.J. Clandinin), Sage, Thousand Oaks, CA, pp. 3–34.

33. Lindenmeyer, A., Griffiths, F., Green, E. *et al.* (2008) Family health narratives: midlife women's concepts of vulnerability to illness. *Health*, **12**, 275–293.

34. Garro, L.C. (2003) Narrative troubling experiences. *Transcultural Psychiatry*, **40** (1), 5–43.

35. Coleman, P.G. (1996) Identity management in later life, in *Handbook of the Clinical Psychology of Aging* (ed. R.T. Woods), John Wiley & Sons, Ltd, Chichester, pp. 93–115.

36. Knight, B.G., Nordhus, I.H. and Satre, D.D. (2003) Psychotherapy with the older client: an integrative approach, in *Comprehensive Handbook of Psychology*, Clinical Psychology, Vol. **8** (eds I.B. Weiner, G. Stricker and T.A. Widiger), John Wiley & Sons, Inc., New York, pp. 453–468.

37. Burnside, I. and Haight, B. (1998) Reminiscence and life review: therapeutic interventions for older people. *Nurse Practitioner*, **29**, 55–61.

38. Enright, R.D. and Fitzgibbons, R.P. (2000) *Helping Clients Forgive: An Empirical Guide for Resolving Anger and Restoring Hope*, American Psychological Association, Washington, DC.

39. Enright, R.D., Human Development Study Group (1991) The moral development of forgiveness, in *The Handbook of Moral Behavior and Development*, vol. **1** (eds W. Kurtiner and J. Gewirtz), Erlbaum, pp. 123–151.

40. Baskin, T.W. and Enright, R.D. (2004) Intervention studies on forgiveness: a meta-analysis. *Journal of Counseling and Development*, **82**, 79–90.

41. Hansen, M.J., Enright, R.D., Baskin, T.W. *et al.* (2009) A palliative care intervention in forgiveness therapy for elderly terminally ill cancer patients. *Journal of Palliative Care*, **25**, 51–60.

42. McInnis-Dittrich, K. (2002) *Social Work with Elders: A Biopsychosocial Approach to Assessment and Intervention*, Allyn and Bacon, Boston.

43. Laidlaw, K., Thompson, L.W., Siskin, L.D. *et al.* (2003) *Cognitive Behavior Therapy with Older People*, John Wiley & Sons, Inc., New York.

44. Jansen, C.E., Miaskowski, C., Dodd, M. *et al.* (2005) A metaanalysis of studies of the effects of cancer chemotherapy on various domains of cognitive function. *Cancer*, **104**, 2222–2233.

45. Stagno, D., Gibson, C. and Breitbart, W. (2004) The delirium subtypes: a review of prevalence, phenomenology, pathophysiology, and treatment response. *Palliative Support Care*, **2**, 171–179.

46. Luciani, A., Jacobsen, P.B., Extermann, M. *et al.* (2008) Fatigue and functional dependence in older cancer patients. *American Journal of Clinical Oncology*, **31**, 424–430.

47. McCaffrey, J.C., Weitzner, M., Kamboukas, D. *et al.* (2007) Alcoholism, depression, and abnormal cognition in head and neck cancer: a pilot study. *Otolaryngology – Head and Neck Surgery*, **136**, 92–97.

48. Heck, J.E., Albert, S.M., Franco, R. *et al.* (2008) Patterns of dementia diagnosis in surveillance, epidemiology, and end results breast cancer survivors who use chemotherapy. *Journal of the American Geriatric Society*, **56**, 1687–1692.

49. Buckley, J. and Herth, K. (2004) Fostering hope in terminally ill patients. *Nursing Standard*, **19** (10), 33–41.

50. Duggleby, W. and Wright, K. (2004) Elderly palliative care cancer patients' descriptions of hope-fostering strategies. *International Journal of Palliative Nursing*, **10** (7), 352–359.

51. Duggleby, W. and Wright, K. (2005) Transforming hope: how elderly palliative patients live with hope. *Canadian Journal of Nursing Research*, **37**, 70–84.

52. Hall, S., Chochinov, H., Harding, R. *et al.* (2009) A phase II randomized controlled trial assessing the feasibility, acceptability and potential effectiveness of "Dignity Therapy" for older people in care homes. *BMC Geriatrics*, **9**, 1–8.

53. Kotkamp-Mothes, N., Slawinsky, D., Hindermann, S. *et al.* (2005) Coping and psychological well being in families of elderly cancer patients. *Critical Reviews in Oncology/Hematology*, **55**, 213–229.

54. Garssen, B. and de Kok, E. (2008) How useful is a screening instrument? *Psycho-Oncology*, **17**, 726–728.

55. Palmer, S.C. and Coyne, J.C. (2003) Screening for depression in medical care: pitfalls, alternatives and revised priorities. *Journal of Psychosomatic Research*, **54**, 279–287.

56. Vodernaier, A., Linden, W. and Siu, C. (2009) Screening for emotional distress in cancer patients: a systematic review of assessment instruments. *Journal of the National Cancer Institute*, **101**, 1–25.

57. Surbone, A., Kagawa-Singer, M., Terret, C. *et al.* (2007) The illness trajectory of elderly cancer patients across cultures: SIOG position paper. *Annals of Oncology*, **18**, 633–638.

58. Balducci, L. (2009) Pharmacology of antineoplastic medications in older cancer patients. *Oncology*, **23** (1), 78–85.

59. Goldzweig, G., Andritsch, E., Hubert, A. *et al.* (2009) Psychological distress among male patients and male spouses: what do oncologists need to know? *Annals of Oncology* (published online: 11 October 2009), doi: 10.1093/annonc/mdp398

21 Reconstructing Meaning in Bereavement

Robert A. Neimeyer

Department of Psychology, University of Memphis, Memphis, TN, USA

21.1 The Clinical Context

Nearly three years after an aggressive metastatic bone cancer ended her husband John's life within three weeks of its diagnosis, Mary recalled:

I was a basket case.... It was not a peaceful death, it was agony. I just remember after everyone left, after John died I got in bed with him and held him for over an hour until the nurses told me I had to leave. I couldn't, I really couldn't grasp it because we had been so close for 18 years, and I just was so unprepared to let him go. The first night in the hospital that I spent with him, I said, 'Well, John, you can't go anywhere. You know you mean everything to me.' I said, 'You are my north, my south, my east and west. I can't make it without you. You are everything to me.' And he said to me, 'Honey, you are to me, too. And I'll always be here for you. I'll always be with you.'

[After his death] it was completely, completely disorienting, to be without him physically... and mentally and emotionally and psychologically and spiritually. It was the whole enchilada.... I lost a great deal of weight. I couldn't sleep. I found myself being up at night till three or four in the morning and then some days not even getting dressed until four in the afternoon. I found myself kissing his pictures. I found myself having my housekeeper wash his clothes as if he were on a trip and would be coming back. I found myself not being able to accept the fact that he was really gone. I mean I was just overwhelmed with the grief. I got through the funeral and... then I collapsed.... And it went on and on and on. I went to his graveyard over an hour away twice a day, even when the roads were closed for winter weather.

My grown children got very concerned about me, and convinced me I needed some help. When I saw you [in therapy] it had been seven or eight months and I was a basket case.

What do cases like Mary's teach us about the complexities of loss, both as clinical challenges and normative human experiences? What do they suggest about what is entailed in adapting to a life in which we confront the painfully real absence of the loved one as a physical being? And how do survivors find new orientation to a world made suddenly strange by the loss, in a way that calls for practical, psychological, social and perhaps even spiritual transitions as they move towards an unknown future? My goal in this chapter is to address such questions from the standpoint of contemporary theory and research on bereavement, with the goal of mining their implications for clinical intervention. In so doing I will tack between discussion of emerging models and their research evidence on the one hand, and brief description of therapeutic techniques and their application on the other.

21.2 Theoretical Perspectives: the Changing Landscape of Loss

As research demonstrates, until quite recently the dominant – and typically the only – model of adaptation to loss incorporated in medical and social work curricula was based on popularisations of stage theory [1], derived loosely from clinical observations of psychological adjustment to the end-of-life in combination with work on phases of adaptation to bereavement in the work of Bowlby [2]. Among the tacit assumptions of such models were that responses to loss could be

Handbook of Psychotherapy in Cancer Care, First Edition. Edited by Maggie Watson and David W. Kissane.
© 2011 John Wiley & Sons, Inc. Published 2011 by John Wiley & Sons, Inc.

adequately described in terms of a sequential patterning of emotional reactions that began in disbelief or denial of the difficult reality, and passed through some form of separation distress (e.g. yearning, pining, angry protest against the reality of the loss) and mourning before moving towards acceptance, recovery, or the like. Accordingly, in keeping with a psychoanalytic model of *trauerarbeit*, the work of mourning [3], therapy was construed chiefly as a process of encouraging *catharsis*, the free expression of grief-related emotions, and *decathexis*, the gradual process of reviewing and breaking the bonds to the deceased so as to permit the mourner to invest psychic energy in new relationships. Recent scholarship has documented how this conception of grieving was rapidly assimilated by popular discourses of grief, holding sway in the self-help as well as professional literature until the final years of the twentieth century [4].

Much, however, has changed in recent years, as over 5000 scholarly and scientific articles on grief have appeared since the publication of the landmark Institute of Medicine report on bereavement research in 1984 [5]. As a result of the bootstrapping of new models and findings, nearly every aspect of the traditional twentieth century model of bereavement has been called into question, making room for novel conceptualisations of adaptation to loss, and with them, new clinical practices. For example, recent empirical attempts to document the phasic progression of natural death bereavement (e.g. through cancer or heart failure) have failed to detect crests in various indicators of grief-related disbelief, anger, yearning, depression and acceptance that accord with the series of dominant reactions posited by stage theory [6, 7], although limited evidence supports the possibility that each of the indicators reaches its own relative maximum value in a sequence compatible with the model. In general, for natural death bereavement, acceptance seems to be the dominant response throughout the first two years of adjustment, from the earliest weeks, and separation distress in the form of yearning and sadness are the most salient of the 'negative' indicators throughout, whereas anger and disbelief occur consistently at low levels. Importantly, however, in cases of violent death (through suicide, homicide or fatal accident), the course of adaptation is much more turbulent, with disbelief eclipsing other responses for mourners in the earliest weeks of loss, and normative indicators of separation distress such as yearning for the loved one being subordinated and perhaps obscured by high levels of anger, disbelief and depression [6]. Similarly, empirically informed evaluations of the 'grief

work' hypothesis call into question the assumptions that expression of negative affect plays a curative role in adaptation to loss [8, 9], or that 'resolution' of grief typically involves breaking, rather than continuing the bond to the loved one [10, 11].

With the decline in authority of these once-dominant models has come a great variety of new theoretical approaches to understanding the experience of bereavement in both its adaptive and maladaptive aspects, building on contemporary cognitive, coping, systemic and even neurological perspectives [12, 13]. Among these are the *dual process model*, which posits an oscillation in attention between a 'loss orientation' to grief work and reorganising the image of the deceased and a 'restoration orientation' to changed roles and goals [14], and the *two-track model*, which examines not only the mourner's biopsychosocial symptomatology, but also his or her changing and ongoing relationship to the loved one, as revealed in attachment-related emotions, thoughts and practices in the course of everyday life [15]. Importantly, these and other contemporary theories have recently seen the development of validated assessment tools to support more informed research and practice relevant to their application [15, 16]. In addition to such new models, traditional perspectives such as attachment theory, which carries significant implications for how securely and insecurely attached mourners negotiate the stress of separation, are receiving overdue empirical scrutiny and support, not only in relation to the loss of human attachment figures [17], but also in relation to the loss of pets, where strong but anxious patterns of attachment are associated with less favourable psychological outcomes [18].

One particularly relevant development in grief theory and research concerns the refinement of diagnostic criteria for *complicated grief* (CG) [19, 20], also termed prolonged grief disorder because of its considerable chronicity and debilitating consequences [21]. In contrast to older and looser formulations of 'pathological' or 'abnormal' grief, the diagnosis of CG has been carefully vetted by 15 years of empirical research, resulting in clinically useful and evidence-based criteria for its identification (see Table 21.1). As a pattern of maladaptive response to the separation distress associated with the loss of a significant attachment through death, the core of the syndrome consists of a preoccupation with the deceased commonly experienced as intense and unremitting yearning, compounded by additional symptoms of loneliness, bitterness, difficulty accepting the death, a diminished sense of self, perceived

Table 21.1	Proposed diagnostic criteria for complicated grief (prolonged grief disorder)[a]
Category	**Definition**
A	*Event*: Bereavement (loss of a significant other)
B	*Separation distress*: The bereaved person experiences yearning (e.g. craving, pining or longing for the deceased; physical or emotional suffering as a result of the desired, but unfulfilled, reunion with the deceased) daily or to a disabling degree
C	*Cognitive, emotional and behavioural symptoms*: The bereaved person must have five (or more) of the following symptoms experienced daily or to a disabling degree
1	Confusion about one's role in life or diminished sense of self (i.e. feeling that a part of oneself has died)
2	Difficulty accepting the loss
3	Avoidance of reminders of the reality of the loss
4	Inability to trust others since the loss
5	Bitterness or anger related to the loss
6	Difficulty moving on with life (e.g. making new friends, pursuing interests)
7	Numbness (absence of emotion) since the loss
8	Feeling that life is unfulfilling, empty or meaningless since the loss
9	Feeling stunned, dazed or shocked by the loss
D	*Timing*: Diagnosis should not be made until at least six months have elapsed since the death
E	*Impairment*: The disturbance causes clinically significant impairment in social, occupational or other important areas of functioning (e.g. domestic responsibilities)
F	*Relation to other mental disorders*: The disturbance is not better accounted for by co-morbid major depressive disorder, generalised anxiety disorder or posttraumatic stress disorder

[a] Adapted from Prigerson *et al.* [21].

purposelessness about a future without the loved one and a persistent feeling of emotional numbness, in the presence of significant impairment in one's social, occupational or family roles. Importantly, such symptoms only become diagnostic of CG when they persist for a minimum of six months, at which point they reliably forecast a variety of troubling medical and psychological sequelae, including cardiac events, immune system dysfunction, hypertension, anxiety, substance abuse and suicide, even after depressive and posttraumatic stress symptomatology are controlled [21]. However, it is important to bear in mind that CG is best conceived of as the extreme end of a continuum that includes more normative grief responses, underscoring the value of assessing the intensity of associated symptoms, rather than simply their presence or absence [22].

A close consideration of Mary's report in our first session of therapy gave ample evidence of complicated and prolonged grieving, to an extent that was life-vitiating and even life-threatening. Perhaps significantly in light of the form of cancer that ended her husband's life, she described his death as 'bone-shattering' for her, leaving her 'completely unable to accept the fact that he was gone'. She spoke plaintively of 'wanting him back, well', and reported calling his voice mail repeatedly just to hear his voice, 'unable to grasp that he couldn't call back'. In these and other respects, her yearning for him was an aching constant in her life, and she noted that with his death, she had lost her

'rock' and her 'anchor'. She also felt as if she had lost herself, as she described how she 'felt encased in so much grief that I don't even know who I am anymore'. Once an outgoing, social person, she confessed that with her intractable grief over the eight months since John's death, she had felt 'abandoned' by many people, including – she noted in a moment of candour – by John himself. Facing a future that felt bleak and lonely, she found herself entertaining vague suicidal thoughts, though the devastating suicide of a relative a few years before dissuaded her from acting on them. In summary, she clearly met the criteria for a CG diagnosis presented in Table 21.1. Just as clearly, she seemed 'stuck' in the loss orientation of the dual process model, unable to find her way towards anything but the most temporary restoration, and preoccupied not only with serious biopsychosocial symptomatology of depression and despair in terms of the two-track model, but also with overpowering needs to reestablish some form of relationship with John in a way that suggested an insecure and dependent form of attachment.

21.3 Grief and the Quest for Meaning

To be maximally useful, a clinical perspective on bereavement should go beyond a clear description of adverse outcomes; it should also posit scientifically assessable processes implicated in such outcomes and generate useful practical procedures for redressing them. Research associated with what has come to be called a *meaning reconstruction* perspective [23, 24] has moved consistently in this direction, with a considerable yield of supportive evidence deriving from the work of multiple investigators. Importantly, it also has dovetailed with other contemporary models mentioned above to contribute to a more comprehensive conceptualisation of grief in its adaptive and maladaptive aspects.

In both a classical [25] and contemporary [26] constructivist perspective, human beings are viewed as self-organising makers of meaning, punctuating the ceaseless flow of experience into significant episodes and organising them into patterns so as to anticipate, interpret and negotiate life's complexity in some viable fashion. This need to impart a modicum of predictability and intelligibility to experience is nowhere clearer than in the social world, where we construct intricate and often intimate connections with others, effectively braiding our efforts at meaning-making with theirs in passionately intersubjective relationships that are mutually self-defining [27]. Ultimately, these processes of personal and social construction give rise to a self-narrative [28], defined as 'an overarching cognitive-affective-behavioural structure that organises the 'micro-narratives' of everyday life into a 'macro-narrative' that consolidates our self-understanding, establishes our characteristic range of emotions and goals and guides our performance on the stage of the social world" (p. 53–54).

Viewed in this perspective, the death of a significant attachment figure can threaten to invalidate, sometimes profoundly, the survivor's secure grounding in a life that once 'made sense', but no longer does. Grieving therefore entails *reaffirming or reconstructing a world of meaning that has been challenged by loss* [29]. Stated more colloquially, adapting to the death of a loved one commonly requires 'relearning the self' and 'relearning the world', as both are frequently changed significantly by the very present absence of the other [30]. At its most devastating, such losses are seismic events that shake the foundations of our personal realities [31], sometimes shattering core assumptions that the universe is predictable, benign and intelligible [32]. When this happens – when our self-narrative appears unable to assimilate the hard reality of the loved one's death and its sweeping implications for our ongoing lives – we are commonly launched into a search for meaning in the 'event story' of the death itself, as well as in the 'back story' of our relationship to the deceased [33]. In the ideal case, reaffirming the loving history of a connection, that is reorganised, but not relinquished, can restore the attachment security

necessary to integrate the event story of the loss into our evolving self-narrative, in a way that averts a chronic crisis of meaning.

Evidence from numerous studies documents the relationship between challenges to survivors' worlds of meaning and their trajectories through bereavement. For example, in one prospective, longitudinal study of older widows and widowers, the great majority of whom lost their spouses to cancer, those who struggled with a 'search for meaning' about their partner's death at 6 and 18 months post-loss continued to wrestle with more intense and persistent grief and depression as much as four years later, even controlling for prior symptomatology [34]. Similarly, in a large cohort of bereaved young adults, survivors who failed to 'make sense' of the loss or find any 'silver lining' in it in the form of personal benefits (e.g. revised life priorities or personal growth) suffered the highest levels of CG symptoms across the first two years of bereavement, whereas the passage of time alone was unrelated to levels of distress [35]. Moreover, breakdown in sense-making has proven to be such a significant mediator of bereavement outcome that it appears to account for nearly all of the difference observed between natural death losses (e.g. cancer, heart failure) on the one hand and typically more traumatising forms of violent death losses (suicide, homicide, fatal accident) on the other [36].

A two-part study of parents who lost children to both violent and natural death sheds further light on the relationship between meaning making following this particularly tragic form of loss and CG an average of six years later. In the first part of the study, a quantitative assessment of parents' self-reported ability to make sense of the death was found to be much the strongest predictor of their adaptation, accounting for five times more of the intensity of their normal grief symptoms (e.g. crying, missing the child) and 15 times more of the intensity of CG symptoms (e.g. withdrawal from other relationships, bitterness) than was accounted for by such factors as the mode of death (natural or violent), gender of the parent, or number of months since the loss [37]. In the second part of this investigation, a mixed methods design was used to identify the *kind* of sense-making or benefit-finding in which parents engaged, and how these specific clusters of meaning making related to bereavement outcome. Content coding the narrative themes reported in the parents' own words, the investigators found that the most common sense made of the loss was that it was God's will, or that they would reunite with the child in the afterlife. Other common meanings centred on the imperfection of the world and the frailty of life. Common unsought benefits in the loss were a deepened commitment to helping others, enhanced compassion in the face of suffering and a keener appreciation of life. Underscoring the importance of meaning-making in predicting bereavement outcomes, those parents who reported finding no sense or no benefit in the experience were four times more likely to meet criteria for CG than those who found at least some meaning in the loss. Attributing the death to God's will and focusing on how the child was no longer suffering were the sense making themes most strongly associated with reduced CG, just as enhanced spirituality and revised life priorities were the benefits that best predicted fewer complications.

Finally, it is worth underscoring that meaning-making in the context of bereavement may predict not only less posttraumatic stress and grief, but also more posttraumatic *growth* [31]. For example, a prospective study of adaptation to later life loss of a spouse demonstrated that sense making at 6 and 18 months post-loss forecast subsequent positive emotion states such as excitement and accomplishment as much as four years later [34]. Such findings underscore the importance of monitoring positive psychological states and resilience in the wake of bereavement, as these do not simply seem to be merely the inverse of adverse symptomatology [38], and could be properly considered targets of clinical intervention in their own right [39].

Considering the case of Mary in light of the meaning reconstruction model, it was easy to hear echoes of the decimation of her framework of sustaining meaning in her allusion to having lost 'her north, her south, her east and her west' with John's passing, as well as in her incredulity about the aggressive cancer that ended his life with so little forewarning. In view of the spiritual themes commonly invoked by survivors searching for some sense in their loss, it was notable that Mary frequently spoke of feeling betrayed or abandoned by God, especially in our early sessions, feeling that 'He took everything of value from my life, and all that is left is just garbage.' Still, she confessed, there were 'small signs that God cares ... tiny things like helping me drive 3 hours in an ice storm to spend 15 minutes at John's grave, or letting me have Christmas with him before taking him away'. It was such germinal signs of renewal that we sought to cultivate as we shifted from assessing the impact of Mary's loss on her functioning to helping her find a 'through line' that integrated the loss into a larger and evolving self-narrative that gave it meaning, and conserved the significance of her life as well as John's.

21.4 Techniques for Reconstructing Meaning in Loss

With the advent of the meaning reconstruction model and related cognitive [40] and integrative [41] approaches to CG have come efforts to construct interventions to help bereaved individuals make sense of their unwelcome transition, using both experientially intense in-therapy procedures [33, 42–44] and out-of-therapy reflective exercises [28, 29, 45, 46]. Given the role of narration as an organising principle for meaning-making [47, 48], its action can be observed in the neurological activation of centres of autobiographical memory in f-MRI studies of grieving subjects [49]. Narrative processes entail the 'restorative retelling' of the loss under conditions that promote its integration [50, 51], as well as a variety of other techniques for reorganising the relationship to the deceased in meaningful terms [29]. Table 21.2 presents a sampling of these procedures.

Table 21.2	Representative meaning-oriented interventions in grief therapy
Method	**Definition**
Retelling the event story of the death	After shoring up client resources for revisiting the story of the loss, replaying it in slow motion detail to promote narrative mastery and coherence.
Accessing various narrative voices	Braiding together strands of narration of the loss focusing on the objective-external story, the emotion-focused internal story and the reflexive, meaning-making story to foster a more comprehensive integration of the experience.
Imaginal dialogues	Engaging the bereaved in symbolic conversations with or about the deceased using visualisation or empty chair methods to facilitate completion of unfinished business and ongoing access to the continuing bond.
Journaling and letter writing	Writing personally and reflectively about the loss to oneself, to the deceased or to real or imagined others to promote articulation, symbolisation and renegotiation of meaning.
Biographical methods	Recording the back story of the deceased person's life and its connection to the bereaved individual's own to honour the loved one and to assist in the integration of the loss into the bereaved person's self-narrative.
Life imprint	Reflecting on the role of the deceased in shaping the bereaved individual's enduring characteristics at levels ranging from concrete gestures and mannerisms to abstract principles and life purposes.

21.4.1 Retelling the 'Event Story' of the Death

Perhaps the most fundamental method for assisting the bereaved in coming to terms with the loss is to facilitate its retelling, that is, to invite the story of the loss in a 'holding environment' that permits its safe articulation, exploration and integration. Procedurally, this entails first establishing a relationship of trust between client and therapist, or in the case of group therapy, between the individual and other members, predicated on a shared understanding of treatment goals, the cultivation of an atmosphere of acceptance, and agreement on strategies for soothing the client if he or she experiences a level of arousal that exceeds a manageable 'window of tolerance'. In addition, therapist and client may work together to identify resources in the client's spiritual beliefs and secular philosophy, social world and relationship to the deceased that can help frame the loss and sustain the survivor in the hard work of reengaging a potentially traumatic account of the loss [51]. In the case of loss of the loved one through progressive disease, retelling commonly involves eliciting the story of the illness, the death itself and its immediate aftermath, extending through the funeral or memorial service. Akin to prolonged exposure treatments for trauma, retelling or 'revisiting' protocols entail encouraging the client to 'stay with' the emotionally arousing account of the loss for 15–30 minutes, during which the therapist provides prompting to attend to the painful details that are often 'edited out' of a conventional description. For example, 'hot spots' or points of vivid grief or other anguish may be revisited multiple times in succession until they are processed fully, with lessened arousal. In the case of particularly traumatising deaths, I find the slow-motion 'replay' of the relevant scenes to consume a full session or more, potentially reinforced by the digital recording of the client's story for him or her to listen to between sessions, making notes of any passages that triggered additional insights or emotions, or that invite further processing in therapy. The overall goal of retelling is to foster narrative mastery of the event, thus helping the client to integrate the hard reality of the death into an ongoing self-narrative that includes, but is not defined by the separation.

21.4.2 Accessing Various Narrative Voices

A useful companion to the retelling procedure is fostering engagement with the material in alternate narrative voices, namely, the external, internal and reflexive

styles [52, 53]. In its most basic form, retelling focuses on the *external* narrative, that is the scene-by-scene reconstruction of significant episodes (e.g. the point of detection of initial worrying symptoms, initial diagnosis, death), at quite specific levels (e.g. the expression on the face of the attending physician, the scene of the death), as the client gradually assimilates the event and its implications. However, this process can be facilitated by prompting for the *internal* narrative of the same episodes, focusing on the client's emotional and bodily reactions during the scenes (e.g. 'What feelings came to you when you first heard the doctor say that your son's cancer was 'not a curable disease?' or 'I noticed that your hand seemed to go instinctively to your stomach when you said that. What was happening in your body, just then?'). At other points, especially when the client has finished relating a specific episode, the therapist can also prompt for the *reflexive*, meaning-making narrative voice (e.g. 'What sense did you make of what was happening at that time? What sense do you make of it now?'). In this elaboration of retelling, the goal is to foster a fuller integration of not only the significant event memories surrounding the loss, but also of those personal reactions to it that can deepen understanding over time.

21.4.3 Imaginal Dialogues

In life as in art, of course, stories are often *performed* as well as related. As vividly evocative as retelling can be, the visualisation and enactment of narratives concerning the loss are typically more so, contributing to the powerful experiential learning that generates new meaning and possibility in action [26]. This is particularly appropriate when the therapist is making use of psychodramatic procedures to seek new solutions to old problems related to the event story of the loss [54], as well as when the client is seeking to reaffirm, revisit, revise or reconstruct some aspect of the 'back story' of the attachment relationship to the deceased. Most commonly, this takes the form of a facilitated 'conversation' with the deceased, held either in visualisation or placed symbolically in an empty chair, to whom the client expresses his or her preoccupations, feelings and the needs implicit in them [55]. It is frequently helpful to encourage the client to then take the position of the loved one and respond, alternating seats until some form of resolution of the emotional problem occurs in dialogue [56], often entailing forgiveness of one or both parties for sensed failures in the relationship, or affirmation of mutual love. Importantly, the goal of such work is less to 'say goodbye' than it is to renegotiate the terms of the ongoing relationship, in keeping with contemporary continuing bonds [10] or two-track [15] models of bereavement.

Imaginal dialogues are not limited to encounters between the client and the deceased, however. For example, it can be useful to ask the client to take the role of the lost loved one, and allow the therapist to interview him or her about the client's strengths, special qualities and coping resources that will help with adaptation in a time of transition [57]. Offering notes on the interview can be surprisingly affirming to the client, who may draw on them as a narrative resource to help secure a sense of connection to the other, who remains accessible in memory and conversation.

21.4.4 *Journaling and Letter Writing*

As research on the expressive writing paradigm has demonstrated, sifting through one's responses to a traumatic event on paper can be quite therapeutic, even in the absence of therapist feedback, often achieving moderate effect sizes that increase in the months that follow the intervention [58, 59]. Although some studies of this form of intervention have yielded less impressive effects in the case of bereavement than in the case of other difficult life experiences, this may be attributed to their recruitment of bereaved people who did not require intervention, perhaps in combination with reliance on generic instructions as opposed to relevant prompts for the writing [46]. For this reason, clinical applications of the method could usefully focus on the challenges in processing the meaning of a problematic loss that commonly arise in the context of CG.

Among these applications would be *written versions of the retelling procedures* described above, inviting an expanded account of the most difficult aspects of the loss, along with associated emotions and meanings. Framing the writing as a *letter to the deceased* can also be a healing practice, using the correspondence as an opportunity to express the significance of the relationship and its loss for the author, perhaps followed by a 'response' written to the self on behalf of the deceased loved one. Variations on this method can include *opening an email account in the name of the deceased*, inviting an ongoing 'dialogue' that has the advantages of verisimilitude (by actually sending the message and having a response arrive in one's inbox) and consistency (leaving a coherent thread of accessible 'exchanges' that can be reviewed periodically for evidence of one's growth through grief). Such practices seem less esoteric from the standpoint of a dialogical model of the self, which views

'individuals' as comprised of the incorporated voices of others, with whom we remain in conversation and relationship [60]. From this perspective, corresponding with the other in this symbolic fashion promotes greater correspondence within the self, in the sense of promoting coherence rather than segregation of affectively charged sub-systems of resonant meaning.

Other forms of therapeutic letter writing can include *past-future self letters*, in which the bereaved person might be invited to pen a letter back to the client as if from the vantage point of a hypothetical future self, who has integrated the loss in a healthy fashion and has moved forward with life, or *notes to hypothetical others* who have suffered a similar loss, offering perspective or advice regarding what steps in healing might be possible now [61]. Such techniques make use of the client's imagination to address very real life challenges, but from a standpoint that encourages compassion and creativity instead of criticism. More realistic alternatives include *letters of gratitude*, in which the client writes to actual people (perhaps in the form of a joint letter to all those who attended the loved one's memorial service) expressing appreciation for their role in the life of the deceased as well as the survivor, expressing hopeful intentions to move forward and petitioning their support in doing so.

21.4.5 *Biographical Methods*

It might be said that grief is a biographical emotion, in the sense that it represents the affective motivation to orient to and extend the life of the deceased [62]. Accordingly, methods that help the bereaved honour that life or explore its implications for their own can be relevant to their post-loss adaptation. Examples would include traditional memorial media such as *biographies*, *scrapbooks*, *photo albums* and *memory boxes* containing significant memorabilia, as well as more recent electronic media such as *virtual memorials* and *blogs* that capture images and vignettes of the deceased loved one's life, often inviting the contributions of others.

A second form of biographical method entails reflecting on one's own life as a survivor, and drafting a 'table of contents' for one's self-narrative that conveys the role of significant losses that punctuate the flow of experience into meaningful episodes or life phases. This *chapters of our lives* exercise can be augmented as a therapeutic tool by any of a number of reflective prompts that foster engagement with the basic themes that underpin the narrative and that consider how life and loss might take on different meanings from the vantage points of various observers, ages or narrative genres (tragedy, history, heroic saga, etc.) [29, 63]. Similarly, more visual depictions of one's life course and the role of loss in it can be explored through the use of *life line* procedures, in which the important events of life and their emotional significance can be depicted over time in a chart, where the horizontal axis represents years and the vertical represents positive to negative developments. Integrating simple symbols of important transitions and inviting verbal sharing with the therapist or group can provide validation for the client and understanding for those working with him or her in reorienting to life after loss.

21.4.6 Life Imprint

Whether viewed in terms of psychodynamic introjection, behavioural modelling or a postmodern blurring of the personal and social world, most contemporary psychological theories recognise that our sense of identity is comprised substantially of the importation of aspects of others into the self. Accordingly, it can be fruitful to reflect systematically on those features of oneself derived from another – in this case the deceased – in a way that extends or continues that person's 'presence' in the world beyond the boundaries of his or her literal life [64, 65]. These life imprints can be felt at levels that range from our mannerisms, characteristic facial expressions or gestures, through our basic personality and patterns of social interactions, to our core values and life purposes. Noting these in a reflective journal entry, and then considering which of these imprints one wants to affirm, and how, or alternatively relinquish, can be an engaging self awareness assignment, or a prompt to further processing in therapy. A variation on the life imprint involves soliciting the imprints that our loved one left in the lives of others, which tends to honour and affirm the deceased, build bonds of community in shared grief and demonstrate vividly how he or she continues to have a place in the world in the lives of many others.

21.5 Clinical Illustration of Therapy as Meaning Reconstruction

Therapy with Mary drew usefully on several of these narrative procedures. Alerted to the possible benefit of honouring her husband's legacy by a memorial card Mary proudly shared near the end of our first session, I suggested she set aside some time to journal about

the development of her love relationship with John, capturing some of the endearing memories of their lives together in a way that might be shared with their adult children. Mary did so eagerly for the next couple of weeks, crying and laughing as she recalled and recorded memorable moments in their courtship and long marriage. As she noted, she 'did not want to allow John's memory to erase', and began to think of writing a book to 'capture what was special about him and all the hysterical things we did'. This seemed both to legitimate the pain of her loss and provide an affirmation of who he was, in a way that let her move gradually into her lack of resolution about the way he died. Specifically, we drew on retelling procedures to help her process the story of the death, allowing her to give voice to how she was 'flooded with images of his final days', especially his poorly controlled end-stage pain and her anger at physicians who seemed to proffer false hope of his recovery. As she began to make sense of the traumatic suddenness of his death in a few short weeks of hospitalisation, she became able to speak of his dying with less overwhelming emotion, and to identify features of her relationship with John that required further attention. Inquiring about whether she continued to speak with him, and if so, how the 'conversation' evolved, opened the door to facilitated empty chair conversations with him, in which she forgave him for leaving her, and received reassurances of his undying love. Gradually, she reengaged her religious beliefs and community, working towards a deepened spirituality that accommodated the reality of suffering and death without implying abandonment by God. As six months of therapy drew towards an end, Mary summarised the pivotal moment in our work that tipped her away from a prolonged, complicated response to John's death and towards a restoration that opened her to new career prospects and renewed interest in the social world:

> You've been so helpful, like a godsend, really. No one had told me about writing about our relationship, about John. That was the most incredibly helpful thing to me, like a release. One widow suggested journaling about my feelings, but the timing was wrong, and it just made me feel worse . . . .

> I had no idea that this journey could be so profound, and so fraught with pain. And I know I'm not there yet, but I have taken steps in the right direction.

A follow up with Mary two years after therapy concluded led to some brief work on a new relationship she was pursuing, but confirmed her ability to find sustainable meaning in her loss, as well as in her ongoing life.

21.6 Overview of Efficacy of Meaning-Making Interventions

Although a meaning reconstruction approach to grief therapy is a relatively recent development, increasing research supports the efficacy of its central procedures. As with all bereavement interventions, existing evidence suggests that to be effective, professional therapy should be offered to clients who show clinically significant signs of distress or complication, insofar as those persons experiencing minimal or normative grief will typically adapt to their loss with the support of their families and communities [66]. When professional intervention is indicated, however, a growing number of cognitive behavioural, narrative and integrative treatments have begun to demonstrate their relevance in randomised controlled trials. For example, tailored 'complicated grief therapy' or CGT features restorative retelling procedures that prompt explicit and detailed processing of the event story of the death and reconnecting in imaginal conversations with the deceased, as well as the projection of new goals in a changed world. Significantly, such procedures are found to substantially outperform interpersonal therapy for depression when offered to clients meeting criteria for CG, across the course of 16 sessions of therapy [55]. Similarly, hybrid exposure-based treatment combined with cognitive restructuring has been found to be effective in treating complicated, prolonged bereavement, with some evidence that the exposure component (consisting of sustained contact with the story of the loss and associated emotions) may be especially efficacious [67]. Other controlled studies have investigated the outcome of writing interventions that provide carefully targeted prompts to assist clients in taking perspective on their loss, with impressive effects. For example, one study recruited bereaved college students, and instructed them to write across a total of three sessions with a focus on (i) emotional expression and exploration about the loss, (ii) attempting to 'make sense' of the experience, (iii) seeking some form of benefit or life lesson in the unwelcome transition, or (iv) simply writing about the room in which they sat as a control for nonspecific factors (such as distraction) associated with writing itself. Results demonstrated the efficacy of all three active interventions relative to the control condition, with the further implication that the benefit-finding condition was especially helpful.

Moreover, gains continued to accrue over the three months that followed the intervention [68], a finding commonly observed in studies of writing interventions [46]. This finding is further reinforced by research administering narrative assignments (e.g. to describe the loss in detail, discuss the sense made of it, reopen 'correspondence' with the deceased, and formulate a coping plan and project a meaningful future) wholly via the Internet to community members suffering CG [69]. Common features of these demonstrably efficacious interventions include (i) establishment of clinically significant need, and particularly CG, as a criterion of treatment, (ii) sustained processing of the event story of the death, with an emphasis on its most difficult aspects, (iii) evocative engagement with the symbolic presence of the loved one in spoken or written dialogue, (iv) facilitation of sense-making or benefit-finding regarding the loss experience and (v) reorganisation of life goals in light of the loss. Especially in light of the equivocal efficacy of traditional grief therapy [70], these results are encouraging, and argue for the value of further research to establish the mechanisms of effective meaning-oriented therapy. The recent validation of a measure for tracking the integration of successful life experiences [71], a key component of the meaning reconstruction model [72], makes such process-outcome research feasible.

21.7 Service Development to Build a Programme

The techniques described in this chapter are applicable by psychologists, social workers, pastoral care staff and psychiatrists. Hospice and palliative care services aim to integrate bereavement care into the totality of their programmes, and continuity of service provision is a key feature of family-centred models from the time of first entry of a patient into an oncology programme. A focus on the meaning of illness, suffering, loss and resilience would seem to be compatible with this emphasis.

21.8 Conclusion

The foregoing strategies represent some of the available experiential and narrative procedures for fostering client meaning-making and reconstruction of a continuing bond in the wake of loss [29, 46]. When invoked at appropriate junctures of therapy and when tailored to the needs and strengths of each client, such methods can make a useful contribution to bereavement adaptation, as recent studies of narrative procedures using facilitated retelling, various forms of letter writing and journaling about the sense and benefits to be found in the loss are beginning to document. It is my hope that the clinical refinement of the meaning-making processes that people of all cultures naturally bring to bear on the experience of bereavement will continue to enrich the practice of grief therapy when the intrinsic healing efforts of bereaved individuals and communities are insufficient to deal with grievous loss.

References

1. Kubler-Ross, E. (1969) *On Death and Dying*, Macmillan, New York.
2. Bowlby, J. (1980) *Attachment and Loss: Loss, Sadness and Depression*, Basic, New York.
3. Freud, S. and Strachey, J. (1917/1957) Mourning and melancholia, *The Complete Psychological Works of Sigmund Freud*. Hogarth Press, London, pp. 152–170.
4. Dennis, M.R. (2011) Popular culture and the paradigm shifts in grief theory and therapy. *Death Studies*, in press.
5. Osterweis, M., Solomon, F. and Green, M. (eds) (1984) *Bereavement*, National Academy Press, Washington, DC.
6. Holland, J. and Neimeyer, R.A. (2010) An examination of stage theory of grief among individuals bereaved by natural and violent causes: a meaning-oriented contribution. *Omega*, **61**, 105–122.
7. Maciejewski, P.K., Zhang, B., Block, S.D. and Prigerson, H.G. (2007) An empirical examination of the stage theory of grief. *Journal of the American Medical Association*, **297**, 716–723.
8. Stroebe, M. (1992) Coping with bereavement: a review of the grief work hypothesis. *Omega*, **26**, 19–42.
9. Wortman, C.B. and Silver, R. (2001) The myths of coping with loss revisited, in *Handbook of Bereavement Research* (eds M. Stroebe, R. Hansson, W. Stroebe and H. Schut), American Psychological Association, Washington, DC, pp. 405–430.
10. Klass, D., Silverman, P.R. and Nickman, S. (1996) *Continuing Bonds: New Understandings of Grief*, Taylor & Francis, Washington, DC.
11. Stroebe, M., Gergen, M., Gergen, K. and Stroebe, W. (1992) Broken hearts or broken bonds: love and death in historical perspective. *American Psychologist*, **47**, 1205–1212.
12. Neimeyer, R.A., Winokuer, H., Harris D. and Thornton, G. (eds) (2011) *Grief and Bereavement in Contemporary Society: Bridging Research and Practice*, Routledge, New York.
13. Stroebe, M., Hansson, R., Schut, H. and Stroebe W. (eds) (2008) *Handbook of Bereavement Research and Practice*, American Psychological Association, Washington, DC.
14. Stroebe, M. and Schut, H. (1999) The dual process model of coping with bereavement: rationale and description. *Death Studies*, **23**, 197–224.
15. Rubin, S. (1999) The two-track model of bereavement: overview, retrospect and prospect. *Death Studies*, **23**, 681–714.
16. Caserta, M.S. and Lund, D.A. (2007) Toward the development of an Inventory of Daily Widowed Life (IDWL): guided by the dual process model of coping with bereavement. *Death Studies*, **31**, 505–535.
17. Parkes, C.M. and Prigerson H. (2009) *Bereavement*, 4th edn, Routledge, London & New York.
18. Field, N.P., Orsini, L., Gavish, R. and Packman, W. (2009) Pet loss. *Death Studies*, **33**, 334–355.
19. Prigerson, H.G., Bierhals, A.J., Kasl, S.V. *et al.* (1996) Complicated grief as a distinct disorder from bereavement-related depression and anxiety. *American Journal of Psychiatry*, **153**, 1484–1486.
20. Prigerson, H.G. and Maciejewski, P.K. (2006) A call for sound empirical testing and evaluation of criteria for complicated grief proposed by the DSM V. *Omega*, **52**, 9–19.
21. Prigerson, H.G., Horowitz, M.J., Jacobs, S.C. *et al.* (2009) Prolonged grief disorder: psychometric validation of criteria proposed for DSM-V and ICD-11. *PLoS Medicine*, **6** (8), 1–12.
22. Holland, J.M., Neimeyer, R.A., Boelen, P.A. and Prigerson, H.G. (2009) The underlying structure of grief: a taxometric investigation of prolonged and normal reactions to loss. *Journal of Psychopathology and Behavioral Assessment*, **31**, 190–201.
23. Neimeyer, R.A. (ed.) (2001) *Meaning Reconstruction and the Experience of Loss*, American Psychological Association, Washington, DC.
24. Neimeyer, R.A. (2006) Widowhood, grief and the quest for meaning: a narrative perspective on resilience, in *Spousal Bereavement in Late Life* (eds D. Carr, R.M. Nesse and C.B. Wortman), Springer, New York, pp. 227–252.
25. Kelly, G.A. (1955) *The Psychology of Personal Constructs*, Norton, New York.
26. Neimeyer, R.A. (2009) *Constructivist Psychotherapy*, Routledge, London and New York.
27. Leitner, L.M. and Faidley, A.J. (2002) Disorder, diagnosis, and the struggles of humanness, in *Studies in Meaning* (eds J.D. Raskin and S.K. Bridges), Pace University Press, New York, pp. 99–121.
28. Neimeyer, R.A. (2004) Fostering posttraumatic growth: a narrative contribution. *Psychological Inquiry*, **15**, 53–59.
29. Neimeyer, R.A. (2002) *Lessons of Loss: A guide to Coping*, Center for the Study of Loss and Transition, Memphis, TN.
30. Attig, T. (1996) *How We Grieve: Relearning the World*, Oxford University Press, New York.
31. Calhoun, L. and Tedeschi, R.G. (eds) (2006) *Handbook of Posttraumatic Growth*, Lawrence Erlbaum, Mahwah, NJ.
32. Janoff-Bulman, R. and Berger, A.R. (2000) The other side of trauma, in *Loss and Trauma* (eds J.H. Harvey and E.D. Miller), Brunner Mazel, Philadelphia.
33. Neimeyer, R.A. and Sands, D.C. (2011) Meaning reconstruction in bereavement: From principles to practice, in *Grief and Bereavement in Contemporary Society: Bridging Research and Practice* (eds R.A. Neimeyer, H. Winokuer, D. Harris and G. Thornton), Routledge, New York.
34. Coleman, R.A. and Neimeyer, R.A. (2010) Measuring meaning: Searching for and making sense of spousal loss in later life. *Death Studies*, **34**, 804–834.
35. Holland, J., Currier, J. and Neimeyer, R.A. (2006) Meaning reconstruction in the first two years of bereavement: the role of sense-making and benefit-finding. *Omega*, **53**, 173–191.
36. Currier, J.M., Holland, J. and Neimeyer, R.A. (2006) Sense making, grief and the experience of violent loss: toward a mediational model. *Death Studies*, **30**, 403–428.

37. Keesee, N.J., Currier, J.M. and Neimeyer, R.A. (2008) Predictors of grief following the death of one's child: the contribution of finding meaning. *Journal of Clinical Psychology*, **64**, 1145–1163.

38. Bonanno, G.A. (2004) Loss, trauma and human resilience. *American Psychologist*, **59**, 20–28.

39. Neimeyer, R.A., Hogan, N. and Laurie, A. (2008) The measurement of grief: psychometric considerations in the assessment of reactions to bereavement, in *Handbook of Bereavement Research: 21st Century Perspectives* (eds M. Stroebe, R.O. Hansson, H. Schut and W. Stroebe), American Psychological Association, Washington, DC, pp. 133–186.

40. Boelen, P., van den Hout, M. and van den Bout, J. (2006) A cognitive-behavioral conceptualization of complicated grief. *Clinical Psychology: Science and Practice*, **1** (13), 109–128.

41. Horowitz, M.J., Siegel, B., Holen, A. *et al.* (1997) Diagnostic criteria for complicated grief disorder. *American Journal of Psychiatry*, **154**, 904–910.

42. Neimeyer, R.A. (2004) *Constructivist Psychotherapy [VHS video/DVD]*, American Psychological Association, Washington, DC.

43. Neimeyer, R.A. (2008) *Constructivist Psychotherapy Over Time [DVD]*, American Psychological Association, Washington, DC.

44. Neimeyer, R.A., Burke, L., Mackay, M. and Stringer, J. (2010) Grief therapy and the reconstruction of meaning: from principles to practice. *Journal of Contemporary Psychotherapy*, **40**, 73–83.

45. Neimeyer, R.A. (2010) *Strategies of Grief Therapy [Online Continuing Education Program]*, American Psychological Association.

46. Neimeyer, R.A., van Dyke, J.G. and Pennebaker, J.W. (2009) Narrative medicine: writing through bereavement, in *Handbook of Psychiatry in Palliative Medicine* (eds H. Chochinov and W. Breitbart), Oxford University Press, New York, pp. 454–469.

47. Bruner, J. (1990) *Acts of Meaning*, Harvard University Press, Cambridge, MA.

48. Rubin, D.C. and Greenberg, D.L. (2003) The role of narrative in recollection: a view from cognitive psychology and neuropsychology, in *Narrative and Consciousness* (eds G.D. Fireman, T.E. McVay and O.J. Flanagan), Oxford University Press, New York, pp. 53–85.

49. Gundel, H., O'Conner, M., Littrell, L. *et al.* (2003) Functional neuroanatomy of grief: an f-MRI study. *American Journal of Psychiatry*, **160**, 1946–1953.

50. Rynearson, E.K. (1999) *Retelling Violent Death*, Brunner Routledge, New York.

51. Rynearson, E.K. (ed.) (2006) *Violent Death*, Routledge, New York.

52. Angus, L. and Hardke, K. (1994) Narrative processes in psychotherapy. *Canadian Psychology*, **35**, 190–203.

53. Neimeyer, R.A. and Levitt, H. (2001) Coping and coherence: a narrative perspective, in *Stress and Coping* (ed. C.R. Snyder), Oxford University Press, New York, pp. 47–67.

54. Neimeyer, R.A. and Arvay, M.J. (2004) Performing the self: Therapeutic enactment and the narrative integration of loss, in *The Dialogical Self in Psychotherapy* (eds H.J.M. Hermans and G. Dimaggio), Brunner Routledge, New York.

55. Shear, K., Frank, E., Houch, P.R. and Reynolds, C.F. (2005) Treatment of complicated grief: a randomized controlled trial. *Journal of the American Medical Association*, **293**, 2601–2608.

56. Greenberg, L., Elliott, R. and Rice, L. (1993) *Facilitating Emotional Change*, Guilford, New York.

57. Neimeyer, R.A., Burke, L., Mackay, M. and Stringer, J. (2010) Grief therapy and the reconstruction of meaning: from principles to practice. *Journal of Contemporary Psychotherapy*, **40**, 73–83.

58. Esterling, B.A., L'Abate, L., Murray, E.J. and Pennebaker, J.W. (1999) Empirical foundations for writing in prevention and psychotherapy. *Clinical Psychology Review*, **19**, 79–96.

59. Pennebaker, J. (1996) *Opening Up*, Guilford, New York.

60. Hermans, H. and Dimaggio, G. (eds) (2004) *The Dialogical Self in Psychotherapy*, Routledge, New York.

61. Neimeyer, R.A. (2001) *Lessons of Loss: A Guide to Coping*, Brunner Routledge, Philadelphia.

62. Walter, T. (1996) A new model of grief: bereavement and biography. *Mortality*, **1**, 7–25.

63. Neimeyer, R.A. (2006) Narrating the dialogical self: toward an expanded toolbox for the counselling psychologist. *Counselling Psychology Quarterly*, **19**, 105–120.

64. Neimeyer, R.A. (2010) The life imprint, in *Favorite Counseling and Therapy Techniques* (ed. H. Rosenthal), Routledge, New York.

65. Vickio, C. (1999) Together in spirit: keeping our relationships alive when loved ones die. *Death Studies*, **23**, 161–175.

66. Currier, J.M., Neimeyer, R.A. and Berman, J.S. (2008) The effectiveness of psychotherapeutic interventions for the bereaved: a comprehensive quantitative review. *Psychological Bulletin*, **134**, 648–661.

67. Boelen, P.A., de Keijser, J., van den Hout, M. and van den Bout, J. (2007) Treatment of complicated grief: a comparison between cognitive-behavioral therapy and supportive counseling. *Journal of Clinical and Consulting Psychology*, **75**, 277–284.

68. Lichtenthal, W.G. and Cruess, D.G. (2010) Effects of directed written disclosure on grief and distress symptoms among bereaved individuals. *Death Studies*, **34**, 475–499.

69. Wagner, B., Knaevelsrud, C. and Maercker, A. (2006) Internet-based cognitive-behavioral therapy for complicated grief: a randomized controlled trial. *Death Studies*, **30**, 429–453.

70. Neimeyer, R.A. and Currier, J.M. (2009) Grief therapy: evidence of efficacy and emerging directions. *Current Directions in Psychological Science*, **18**, 252–256.

71. Holland, J.M., Currier, J.M., Coleman, R.A. and Neimeyer, R.A. (2011) The Integration of Stressful Life Experiences Scale (ISLES): development and initial validation of a new measure. *International Journal of Stress Management*, **17**, 325–352.

72. Gillies, J. and Neimeyer, R.A. (2006) Loss, grief and the search for significance: toward a model of meaning reconstruction in bereavement. *Journal of Constructivist Psychology*, **19**, 31–65.

References

Index